Management of Hazardous Material Emergencies

Editors

STEPHEN W. BORRON
ZIAD KAZZI

EMERGENCY MEDICINE
CLINICS OF NORTH AMERICA

www.emed.theclinics.com

Consulting Editor
AMAL MATTU

February 2015 • Volume 33 • Number 1

ELSEVIER

1600 John F. Kennedy Boulevard • Suite 1800 • Philadelphia, Pennsylvania, 19103-2899

http://www.theclinics.com

EMERGENCY MEDICINE CLINICS OF NORTH AMERICA Volume 33, Number 1
February 2015 ISSN 0733-8627, ISBN-13: 978-0-323-35437-0

Editor: Patrick Manley
Developmental Editor: Casey Jackson

Emergency Medicine Clinics of North America (ISSN 0733-8627) is published quarterly by Elsevier Inc., 360 Park Avenue South, New York, NY, 10010-1710. Months of issue are February, May, August, and November. Business and Editorial Offices: 1600 John F. Kennedy Boulevard, Suite 1800, Philadelphia, PA 19103-2899. Customer Service Office: 6277 Sea Harbor Drive, Orlando, FL 32887-4800. Periodicals postage paid at New York, NY, and additional mailing offices. Subscription prices are $155.00 per year (US students), $315.00 per year (US individuals), $523.00 per year (US institutions), $220.00 per year (international students), $450.00 per year (international individuals), $642.00 per year (international institutions), $220.00 per year (Canadian students), $385.00 per year (Canadian individuals), and $642.00 per year (Canadian institutions). International air speed delivery is included in all Clinics' subscription prices. All prices are subject to change without notice. **POSTMASTER:** Send address changes to Emergency Medicine Clinics of North America, Elsevier Periodicals Customer Service, 11830 Westline Industrial Drive, St. Louis, MO 63146. Customer Service (orders, claims, online, change of address): Elsevier Periodicals Customer Service, 11830 Westline Industrial Drive, St. Louis, MO 63146. Tel: 1-800-654-2452 (U.S. and Canada); 314-453-7041 (outside U.S. and Canada). Fax: 314-453-5170. E-mail: journalscustomerservice-usa@elsevier.com (for print support); journalsonline support-usa@elsevier.com (for online support).

Reprints. For copies of 100 or more of articles in this publication, please contact the Commercial Reprints Department, Elsevier Inc., 360 Park Avenue South, New York, NY 10010-1710. Tel.: 212-633-3874; Fax: 212-633-3820; E-mail: reprints@elsevier.com.

Emergency Medicine Clinics of North America is covered in MEDLINE/PubMed (Index Medicus), Current Contents/Clinical Medicine, EMBASE/Excerpta Medica, BIOSIS, SciSearch, CINAHL, ISI/BIOMED, and Research Alert.

Contributors

CONSULTING EDITOR

AMAL MATTU, MD, FAAEM, FACEP
Professor and Vice Chair, Department of Emergency Medicine, University of Maryland
School of Medicine, Baltimore, Maryland

EDITORS

STEPHEN W. BORRON, MD, MS
Professor of Emergency Medicine and Medical Toxicology, Paul L. Foster School of
Medicine, Medical Director, West Texas Regional Poison Center, Texas Tech University
Health Sciences Center at El Paso, El Paso, Texas

ZIAD KAZZI, MD
Assistant Professor, Department of Emergency Medicine, Emory University; Medical
Toxicologist, National Center for Environmental Health, Centers for Disease Control and
Prevention, Atlanta, Georgia

AUTHORS

CYNTHIA K. AARON, MD
Professor, Wayne State University School of Medicine, Children's Hospital of Michigan
Regional Poison Control Center, Detroit Medical Center, Detroit, Michigan

VIKHYAT S. BEBARTA, MD, Lt Col, USAF, MC
Medical Toxicology, Department of Emergency Medicine, San Antonio Military Medical
Center, San Antonio, Texas

LUIZ BERTELLI, PhD
Los Alamos National Laboratory, Albuquerque, New Mexico

STEPHEN W. BORRON, MD, MS
Professor of Emergency Medicine and Medical Toxicology, Paul L. Foster School of
Medicine, Medical Director, West Texas Regional Poison Center, Texas Tech University
Health Sciences Center at El Paso, El Paso, Texas

JENNIFER BUZZELL, MS
National Center for Environmental Health, Centers for Disease Control and Prevention,
Atlanta, Georgia

DAVID CAWTHON, PhD
Project Toxicologist, Center for Toxicology and Environmental Health, North Little Rock,
Arkansas

DORAN CHRISTENSEN, DO
Associate Medical Director, Radiation Emergency Assistance Center/Training Site, Oak
Ridge, Tennessee

CHARLOTTE CLARK, CEMHP
Hospital Emergency Management, Grady Health System, Atlanta, Georgia

ROBERT N.E. FRENCH, MD, MPH
Assistant Professor, Department of Emergency Medicine, Yale School of Medicine, and Medical Director, Yale New Haven Center for Emergency Preparedness and Disaster Response, Yale New Haven Health System, New Haven, Connecticut

ROBERT J. GELLER, MD
Department of Pediatrics, Emory University School of Medicine, Atlanta, Georgia

MICHAEL G. HOLLAND, MD, FACMT, FAACT, FACOEM, FACEP
Associate Professor, Department of Emergency Medicine; Medical Toxicologist, Upstate New York Poison Center, SUNY Upstate Medical University, Syracuse, New York; Occupational Physician, Center for Occupational Health, Glens Falls Hospital, Glens Falls, New York; Senior Medical Toxicologist, Center for Toxicology and Environmental Health, North Little Rock, Arkansas

CAROL J. IDDINS, MD
U.S. Department of Energy; Associate Director, Radiation Emergency Assistance Center/ Training Site; Oak Ridge Institute for Science and Education; Oak Ridge Associated Universities, Oak Ridge, Tennessee

ZIAD KAZZI, MD
Assistant Professor, Department of Emergency Medicine, Emory University; Medical Toxicologist, National Center for Environmental Health, Centers for Disease Control and Prevention, Atlanta, Georgia

ANDREW M. KING, MD
Assistant Professor, Wayne State University School of Medicine, Children's Hospital of Michigan Regional Poison Control Center, Detroit Medical Center, Detroit, Michigan

MARK KIRK, MD
Chemical Defense Program, Health Threats Resilience Division, Office of Health Affairs, US Department of Homeland Security, Washington, DC

JOSHUA KLAPOW, PhD
Professor, Department of Health Care Organization and Policy, University of Alabama at Birmingham School of Public Health; Chip Rewards, Inc, Birmingham, Alabama

JERROLD B. LEIKIN, MD, FACP, FACEP, FAACT, FACMT, FACOEM
Director of Medical Toxicology, NorthShore University HealthSystems-OMEGA, Clinical Professor, University of Chicago Pritzker School of Medicine, Glenview, Illinois

LISA C. McCORMICK, DrPH
Assistant Professor, Department of Health Care Organization and Policy, University of Alabama at Birmingham School of Public Health, Birmingham, Alabama

CHARLES McKAY, MD, FACMT, FACEP
Associate Medical Director, Connecticut Poison Control Center; Vice President, American College of Medical Toxicology; Division of Medical Toxicology, Department of Emergency Medicine, Hartford Hospital, Hartford, Connecticut; University of Connecticut School of Medicine, Farmington, Connecticut

BROOKS L. MOORE, MD
Department of Emergency Medicine, Emory University School of Medicine, Atlanta, Georgia

ELIZABETH J. SCHARMAN, PharmD, DABAT, BCPS, FAACT
Department Clinical Pharmacy, Professor, WVU School of Pharmacy; Director, WV Poison Center, West Virginia

GABRIEL S. TAJEU, MPH
Doctoral Candidate and Graduate Fellow, Department of Health Care Organization and Policy, University of Alabama at Birmingham School of Public Health, Birmingham, Alabama

ANTHONY J. TOMASSONI, MD, MS, FACEP, FACMT
Assistant Professor, Department of Emergency Medicine, Medical Director, Yale New Haven Center for Emergency Preparedness and Disaster Response, Yale New Haven Health System, Yale University School of Medicine, New Haven, Connecticut

RICHARD TOVAR, MD, FACEP, FACMT
Medical Toxicology, Clinical Forensic Medicine, TacticalTox, Delafield, Wisconsin

FRANK G. WALTER, MD, FACEP, FACMT, FAACT
Professor of Emergency Medicine, College of Medicine; Professor of Pharmacy Practice and Science, College of Pharmacy, The University of Arizona, Tucson, Arizona

Contents

> Toxidromes aid emergency care providers in the context of the patient presenting with suspected poisoning, unexplained altered mental status, unknown hazardous materials or chemical weapons exposure, or the unknown overdose. The ability to capture an adequate chemical exposure history and to recognize toxidromes may reduce dependence on laboratory tests, speed time to delivery of specific antidote therapy, and improve selection of supportive care practices tailored to the etiologic agent. This article highlights elements of the exposure history and presents selected toxidromes that may be caused by toxic industrial chemicals and chemical weapons. Specific antidotes for toxidromes and points regarding their use, and special supportive measures, are presented.

> Hospital planning for chemical or radiological events is essential but all too often treated as a low priority. Although some other types of disasters like hurricanes and tornadoes may be more frequent, chemical and radiological emergencies have the potential for major disruptions to clinical care. Thorough planning can mitigate the impact of a chemical or radiological event. Planning needs to include all 4 phases of an event: mitigation (preplanning), preparation, response, and recovery. Mitigation activities should include the performance of a hazards vulnerability analysis and identification of local subject-matter experts and team leaders.

> Accurate identification of the hazardous material is essential for proper care. Efficient hospital security and triage must prevent contaminated

victims from entering the emergency department (ED) and causing secondary contamination. The decontamination area should be located outside the ambulance entrance. Decontamination priorities are protection of the health care worker, utilization of Level C personal protective equipment, and proper decontamination of the exposed patient. Decontamination proceeds in a head-to-toe sequence. Run-off water is a hazardous waste. Hospital and Community Management Planning for these emergencies is essential for proper preparation and effective response to the hazardous materials incident.

Mark Kirk and Carol J. Iddins

Most approaches toward chemical and radiological/nuclear (CRN) incidents focus on the clinical skills of the first receiver. These skills are certainly important and are addressed throughout this article. Information management skills are often overlooked. Emergency physicians must competently amass information elements most critical to know during a crisis, choosing an appropriate resource to rapidly find reliable information. During large-scale CRN incidents, the emergency physician needs to use information for: planning, incident management, toxicant management, disposition/definitive care, and recovery management. Information management and synthesis are crucial throughout the phases of the disaster cycle: planning, response, mitigation, and recovery.

Stephen W. Borron and Vikhyat S. Bebarta

Asphyxiants deprive the body of oxygen. Simple asphyxiants displace oxygen from the lungs, whereas systemic asphyxiants interfere with transport of oxygen by hemoglobin or with mitochondrial oxidative phosphorylation. Asphyxiants may be gases, liquids, or solids, or their metabolites. The typical clinical picture of asphyxiant poisoning is one of progressive mental status changes, alteration of breathing, progressively abnormal vital signs, coma, seizures, and eventually cardiovascular collapse and death. Treatment of asphyxiant poisoning is aggressive supportive care, with control of the airway and ventilation and maintenance of cardiac output. Supportive care is often enhanced by the administration of specific antidotes.

Richard Tovar and Jerrold B. Leikin

This article reviews toxic chemicals that cause irritation and damage to single and multiple organ systems (corrosion) in an acute fashion. An irritant toxic chemical causes reversible damage to skin or other organ system, whereas a corrosive agent produces irreversible damage, namely, visible necrosis into integumentary layers, following application of a substance for up to 4 hours. Corrosive reactions can cause coagulation or liquefaction necrosis. Damaged areas are typified by ulcers, bleeding, bloody scabs, and eventual discoloration caused by blanching of the skin, complete areas of alopecia, and scars. Histopathology should be considered to evaluate questionable lesions.

Organophosphates (OPs) and carbamates have a wide variety of applications, most commonly as pesticides used to eradicate agricultural pests or control populations of disease-carrying vectors. Some OP and carbamates have therapeutic indications such as physostigmine. Certain organophosphorus compounds, known as nerve agents, have been employed in chemical warfare and terrorism incidents. Both classes inhibit acetylcholinesterase (AChE) enzymes, leading to excess acetylcholine accumulation at nerve terminals. In the setting of toxicity from either agent class, clinical syndromes result from excessive nicotinic and muscarinic neurostimulation. The toxic effects from OPs and carbamates differ with respect to reversibility, subacute, and chronic effects. Decontamination, meticulous supportive care, aggressive antimuscarinic therapy, seizure control, and administration of oximes are cornerstones of management.

Numerous examples of chemical contamination of food, water, or medication have led to steps by regulatory agencies to maintain the safety of this critical social infrastructure and supply chain. Identification of contaminant site is important. Environmental testing and biomonitoring can define the nature and extent of the event and are useful for providing objective information, but may be unavailable in time for clinical care. Clinical diagnosis should be based on toxidrome recognition and assessment of public health implications. There are several resources available to assist and these can be accessed through regional poison control centers or local/state public health departments.

After a radiation emergency that involves the dispersal of radioactive material, patients can become externally and internally contaminated with 1 or more radionuclides. Internal contamination can lead to the delivery of harmful ionizing radiation doses to various organs and tissues or the whole body. The clinical consequences can range from acute radiation syndrome to the long-term development of cancer. Estimating the amount of radioactive material absorbed into the body can guide the management of patients. Treatment includes, in addition to supportive care and long term monitoring, certain medical countermeasures like Prussian blue, calcium diethylenetriamine pentaacetic acid (DTPA) and zinc DTPA.

This article reviews the literature pertaining to psychological impacts in the aftermath of technological disasters, focusing on the immediate psychological and mental health consequences emergency department physicians and first responders may encounter in the aftermath of such disasters. First receivers see a wide spectrum of psychological distress, including acute onset of psychiatric disorders, the exacerbation of existing psychological and psychiatric conditions, and widespread symptomatology even in the absence of a diagnosable disorder. The informal community support systems that exist after a natural disaster may not be available to communities affected by a technological disaster leading to a need for more formal mental health supportive services.

Preparation for, and response to, hazardous materials emergencies requires both preplanning and just-in-time information management. The development of an emergency operations plan and a hazardous materials incident response plan involves many steps and implicates numerous resources: institutional, governmental, and private. This article provides checklists for development of plans and guidelines, with numerous references to information and material resources. An important component of readiness is revision. The availability of resources, human and informatics, as well as the means for accessing them, inevitably changes over time. The reader is advised to update all links and telephone numbers on a regularly scheduled basis.

EMERGENCY MEDICINE
CLINICS OF NORTH AMERICA

RELATED INTEREST

Emergency Medicine Clinics, February 2014 (Vol. 32, No. 1)
Clinical Toxicology
Silas W. Smith, and Daniel M. Lugassy, *Editors*

DOWNLOAD
Free App!

Review Articles
THE CLINICS

NOW AVAILABLE FOR YOUR iPhone and iPad

PROGRAM OBJECTIVE

The goal of *Emergency Medicine Clinics of North America* is to keep practicing emergency medicine physicians and emergency medicine residents up to date with current clinical practice in emergency medicine by providing timely articles reviewing the state of the art in patient care.

LEARNING OBJECTIVES

Upon completion of this activity, participants will be able to:

1. Review hospital preparedness for hazardous material emergencies including chemical and radiological emergencies.
2. Recognize resources for toxicological information and assistance.
3. Discuss psychological aspects of chemical and radiological disasters.

ACCREDITATION

The Elsevier Office of Continuing Medical Education (EOCME) is accredited by the Accreditation Council for Continuing Medical Education (ACCME) to provide continuing medical education for physicians.

The EOCME designates this enduring material for a maximum of 15 *AMA PRA Category 1 Credit*(s) ™. Physicians should claim only the credit commensurate with the extent of their participation in the activity.

All other health care professionals requesting continuing education credit for this enduring material will be issued a certificate of participation.

DISCLOSURE OF CONFLICTS OF INTEREST

The EOCME assesses conflict of interest with its instructors, faculty, planners, and other individuals who are in a position to control the content of CME activities. All relevant conflicts of interest that are identified are thoroughly vetted by EOCME for fair balance, scientific objectivity, and patient care recommendations. EOCME is committed to providing its learners with CME activities that promote improvements or quality in healthcare and not a specific proprietary business or a commercial interest.

The planning committee, staff, authors and editors listed below have identified no financial relationships or relationships to products or devices they or their spouse/life partner have with commercial interest related to the content of this CME activity:
Cynthia K. Aaron, MD; Vikhyat S. Bebarta, MD; Luiz Bertelli, PhD; Stephen W. Borron, MD; Jennifer Buzzell, CHP; David R. Cawthon, PhD, DABT; Doran Christensen, DO; Charlotte Clark, EMHP; Robert N. E. French, MD, MPH; Robert J. Geller, MD; Kristen Helm; Michael G. Holland, MD, FACMT, FAACT, FACOEM, FACEP; Brynne Hunter; Carol J. Iddins, MD; Ziad N. Kazzi, MD; Andrew M. King, MD; Mark Kirk, MD; Joshua C. Klapow, PhD; Indu Kumari; Sandy Lavery; Jerrold B. Leikin, MD; Patrick Manley; Amal Mattu, MD; Lisa C. McCormick, DrPH; Charles A. McKay, Jr, MD, FACMT, FACEP, ABIM; Jill McNair; Brooks L. Moore, MD; Elizabeth J. Scharman, PharmD, DABAT, BCPS, FAACT; Gabriel S. Tajeu, MPH; Anthony J. Tomassoni, MD, MS, FACEP, FACMT; Richard Tovar, MD, FACEP, FACMT.

The planning committee, staff, authors and editors listed below have identified financial relationships or relationships to products or devices they or their spouse/life partner have with commercial interest related to the content of this CME activity:
Frank G. Walter, MD, FACEP, FACMT, FAACT is a consultant/advisor for Heyltex Corporation, DxTerity Diagnostics and IB Consultancy.

UNAPPROVED/OFF-LABEL USE DISCLOSURE

The EOCME requires CME faculty to disclose to the participants:

1. When products or procedures being discussed are off-label, unlabelled, experimental, and/or investigational (not US Food and Drug Administration [FDA] approved); and
2. Any limitations on the information presented, such as data that are preliminary or that represent ongoing research, interim analyses, and/or unsupported opinions. Faculty may discuss information about pharmaceutical agents that is outside of FDA-approved labelling. This information is intended solely for CME and is not intended to promote off-label use of these medications. If you have any questions, contact the medical affairs department of the manufacturer for the most recent prescribing information.

TO ENROLL

To enroll in the *Emergency Medicine Clinics* Continuing Medical Education program, call customer service at 1-800-654-2452 or sign up online at http://www.theclinics.com/home/cme. The CME program is available to subscribers for an additional annual fee of $235 USD.

METHOD OF PARTICIPATION

In order to claim credit, participants must complete the following:

1. Complete enrolment as indicated above.
2. Read the activity.
3. Complete the CME Test and Evaluation. Participants must achieve a score of 70% on the test. All CME Tests and Evaluations must be completed online.

CME INQUIRIES/SPECIAL NEEDS

For all CME inquiries or special needs, please contact elsevierCME@elsevier.com.

Foreword

Management of Hazardous Materials Emergencies

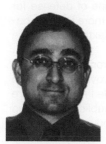

Amal Mattu, MD
Consulting Editor

As I pondered how to write the foreword for this issue of *Emergency Medicine Clinics of North America*, I came to a simple realization—I really don't know much about hazardous materials (HAZMAT) at all. I don't even think I could clearly define what they are, though I think I could eventually recognize them if I saw them. The problem is that by the time I recognized what I was dealing with, it might very well be too late for the patient...and for me!

In emergency medicine, we spend most of our time dwelling on the management of common complaints, such as chest pain, abdominal pain, and back pain, among many other complaints. We read about and teach our trainees about high-risk entities, such as myocardial infarction, stroke, aortic dissection, and pulmonary embolism. We spend a great deal of our time managing lower-risk but high-frequency complaints, such as viral syndromes, bumps, bruises, and lacerations. But where do HAZMAT exposures fall into this mix? The complications of these exposures span the gamut of low risk all the way up to high risk and deadly. Fortunately for all of us, they are very uncommon, but when they do occur, they may pose significant public health risks and dangers to entire families or towns. Given that the first site of arrival for these patients would be the emergency department, it certainly seems sensible, even mandatory, for all of us to be well-educated in recognizing and managing HAZMAT exposures. With this bit of newfound respect for HAZMAT emergencies, I went to the textbooks to see what I could quickly learn before writing this foreword.

First, I reviewed three popular texts that focus on core curriculum review for those that are studying for the Written Certification Examination in emergency medicine. I found in each of the texts a page or two regarding hydrocarbons, organophosphates, and an occasional mention of phosgene. Perhaps there was enough content there to answer a couple of questions on the exam, but the texts were severely lacking in terms of providing real recommendations about how to manage patients. When I reviewed our own residency's curriculum, I found at best only an occasional mention of

Emerg Med Clin N Am 33 (2015) xv–xvi
http://dx.doi.org/10.1016/j.emc.2014.10.003
0733-8627/15/$ – see front matter © 2015 Elsevier Inc. All rights reserved.

exposures to some of the relevant agents in assorted toxicology lectures, but nothing truly of any substance over the past several years. Next, I reviewed three of the "classic," comprehensive textbooks in emergency medicine. Surely, I thought, these would provide a practical approach to managing minor and major HAZMAT exposures. I was pleased to find that each did provide some information regarding site control and decontamination, but nevertheless, they were still somewhat lacking in depth. Given that we in the emergency department are the first line of defense for major public health emergencies, it seems that we need to know far more than the basics that are provided in the current popular emergency medicine textbooks that are available to us.

Fortunately for our sake and for the public's sake, Dr Stephen Borron, Dr Ziad Kazzi, and an outstanding group of authors have stepped forward to provide us a much needed resource that discusses in necessary depth how to provide immediate care to the victims of HAZMAT exposures and also how to protect the public from spread of these exposures. In the following pages, all of us that are poorly educated and (therefore) poorly prepared for HAZMAT emergencies will learn exactly what we *should have* been learning in our training programs and when studying for the Certification Exams. After an excellent introductory article, which really hammers home the importance for all of us to be experts in HAZMAT emergencies, the contributors continue to discuss a potpourri of key topics. They discuss some individual toxins, such as industrial agents, irritants, corrosives, asphyxiants, and cholinergic agents. They also discuss some key issues pertaining to personal and public health, including how to use protective equipment, hospital preparedness, food/water/medication contamination, and mental health consequences of chemical and radioactive agents. Finally, they provide a critically important checklist for HAZMAT preparedness in the Appendix.

This issue of *Emergency Medicine Clinics of North America* represents an important addition to the emergency medicine literature. Experienced emergency physicians, emergency medicine trainees, and the public will benefit tremendously from the expertise provided in the pages that follow. The guest editors and authors are commended for providing a single resource that covers a broad spectrum of HAZMAT exposures in a succinct, clinically relevant, and cutting-edge manner.

Amal Mattu, MD
Department of Emergency Medicine
University of Maryland School of Medicine
Baltimore, MD 21201, USA

E-mail address:
amattu@smail.umaryland.edu

Preface

Management of Hazardous Material Emergencies

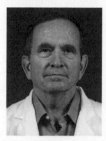 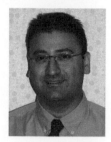

Stephen W. Borron, MD, MS   Ziad Kazzi, MD

Editors

As this issue of *Emergency Medicine Clinics of North America* goes to press, the United States is extraordinarily preoccupied with a number of health concerns indirectly related to the topic of this tome, hazardous materials preparedness. The nation has recently suffered its first death due to Ebola and observed the first case of transmission of the disease in this country. Pediatric intensive care units throughout the country are struggling with respiratory illness caused by Enterovirus D 68. Unrest in the Middle East has raised the specter of a domestic terrorist attack by sympathizers of the so-called Islamic State. Each of these events potentially involves hazardous materials, biological, chemical, or radiologic in nature. Each, likewise, underscores the necessity of a resilient public health infrastructure, for training and education of health care workers and first responders, and for updated all-hazards planning for disasters and their management. We hope that this issue of the *Emergency Medicine Clinics of North America* will further prepare its readers to safely and effectively respond to unfamiliar emergencies threatening the public health.

Stephen W. Borron, MD, MS
3800 North Mesa Street
Suite A2-507
El Paso, TX 79902, USA

Ziad Kazzi, MD
Emergency Medicine
Emory University
531 Asbury Cir-Annex, Suite N340
Atlanta, GA 30322, USA

E-mail addresses:
stephen.borron@ttuhsc.edu (S.W. Borron)
zkazzi@emory.edu (Z. Kazzi)

Emerg Med Clin N Am 33 (2015) xvii
http://dx.doi.org/10.1016/j.emc.2014.10.001
0733-8627/15/$ – see front matter © 2015 Elsevier Inc. All rights reserved.

Introduction: Hazardous Materials and Radiologic/ Nuclear Incidents: Lessons Learned?

Stephen W. Borron, MD, MS

On the night of December 3, 1984, the world was made acutely aware of the potential for devastation and death that can accompany the production of chemicals, when some 40 tons of methyl isocyanate were released into the air surrounding the Union Carbide India Limited facility in Bhopal, India. This event has been adeptly chronicled by Broughton.[1] The sequence of technical failures that led to this tragedy would seem almost comedic, were it not for the 3800 immediate deaths and thousands of lives forever changed. There remains some controversy about whether this was an accident aggravated by the combination of poor maintenance, and mechanical and human failures, or an act of sabotage. Whatever the case, some of the lessons we supposedly learned were that:

1. Regulation is only as good as its enforcement. Local government was said to be aware of safety problems at the Union Carbide plant but failed to act on them owing to fear of economic effects of plant closure. At the time of the Bhopal incident, the vent gas scrubber (a safety device) had been shut down for 3 weeks; a safety valve failed, permitting the mixing of 1 ton of water with 40 tons of methyl isocyanate, leading to an exothermic reaction; the refrigeration unit, which normally would have cooled the methyl isocyanate, had been shut down. The gas flare safety system had likewise been shut down. And so, the methyl isocyanate was released.[1]
2. Zoning laws should prohibit the placement of facilities that manufacture, store, or use large quantities of extremely hazardous materials alongside public facilities and housing units. According to Broughton,[1] the site of Union Carbide India Limited was zoned for light industrial and commercial use, not for hazardous industry. A slum colony sprang up in the area adjacent to the plant.
3. The public has a right to know when such materials are being used or stored in their community. This information should be easily accessible from public officials. This was the crux of the Emergency Planning and Community Right-to-Know Act of 1986, passed by the US Congress in response to this event. According to Patel,[2] the people living around Union Carbide India Limited were warned of potential hazards associated with the plant, but ignored them because they did not know how to react to them and because the dangers had been downplayed by local officials.

Department of Emergency Medicine, Paul L Foster School of Medicine, Texas Tech University Health Sciences Center, 4801 Alberta Avenue, Suite B3200, El Paso, TX 79905, USA
E-mail address: stephen.borron@ttuhsc.edu

Emerg Med Clin N Am 33 (2015) 1–11
http://dx.doi.org/10.1016/j.emc.2014.09.003
0733-8627/15/$ – see front matter © 2015 Elsevier Inc. All rights reserved.

4. The response to hazardous materials release requires education, training, equipment, and supplies. There was no mass casualty emergency action plan in Bhopal. The problem was compounded by a shortage of hospital beds and physicians; local hospitals were overwhelmed without specific knowledge of the gas involved.[1]
5. Inadequate response to such releases may result in extraordinary loss of life, health, and economic well-being, which may last for years. An estimated 3800 people immediately lost their lives. Thousands of others have suffered chronic ocular, respiratory, reproductive, genetic, and neurobehavioral problems. Forty years later, the residents of Bhopal continue to suffer.

Flash forward to April 17, 2013, when a farm supply wholesaler, Adair Grain, Inc (also known as West Fertilizer), storing 270 tons of ammonium nitrate, erupted in an explosion and conflagration in the Central Texas town of West. Fifteen people lost their lives and another 160 or more were injured. This incident, like many that came before it, did not have to happen. But for the immediate response of emergency physicians, nurses, and emergency medical services personnel, the outcomes would undoubtedly have been worse. So what did we learn again?

1. Regulation is only as good as its enforcement. Under the Chemical Facility Anti-Terrorism Standards Act, fertilizer plants and depots are required to report holdings of more than 400 pounds of ammonium nitrate to the Department of Homeland Security (DHS).[3] Despite holding 270 tons of ammonium nitrate, Adair Grain never filed any "top-screen reports," which would have triggered oversight by DHS of safety plans. Neither the Environmental Protection Agency nor the Occupational Safety and Health Administration regulate the handling or storage of ammonium nitrate.[3]
2. Zoning laws should prohibit the placement of facilities that manufacture, store, or use large quantities of extremely hazardous materials alongside public facilities and housing units. West Fertilizer was located immediately across the railroad tracks from West Intermediate School and fewer than 500 feet from West High School. It was fewer than 1000 feet from a nursing home and an assisted living facility, near an apartment complex and numerous private residences. When the West fertilizer plant was built in 1962, it was surrounded by farms and ranches. Recent construction of the schools apparently did not take into account in their risk analysis, if there was one, the West Fertilizer facility's ammonium nitrate storage. Fortunately, the explosion occurred at 7:20 PM, after school was out. The intermediate school was flattened. Without a doubt, had the explosion occurred during the school day, the death and injury toll would have been much greater.
3. The public has a right to know when such materials are being used or stored in their community. This information should be easily accessible from public officials. Incredibly, in this case the Attorney General of Texas disagrees. Shortly after the event at West, the Attorney General ruled that neither the Department of State Health Services nor local fire departments are at liberty henceforth to disclose locations of hazardous materials to the public, suggesting rather that regarding chemical companies and the public: "You know where they are if you drive around. You can ask every facility whether or not they have chemicals or not. You can ask them if they do, and they can tell you, well, we do have chemicals or we don't have chemicals, and if they do, they tell which ones they have."[4]
4. Response to hazardous materials release requires education, training, equipment and supplies. This time, the emergency medical response was much better. Since 9/11, training and provision of equipment for emergency response have increased dramatically owing to availability of federal funding. The medical response to this incident speaks to better preparedness on the part of providers.[5] It should be

noted, however, that this explosion occurred in a rural area. Had it occurred in an area of higher population density, the death and devastation could have been far greater.

5. Inadequate response to such releases may result in extraordinary loss of life, health, and economic well-being, which may last for years. Although the medical response was well adapted in the case of the West Fertilizer explosion, chemical safety and emergency planning on the part of the company and the city clearly were not. The loss of life in West was, fortunately, limited compared with Bhopal. However, the impact that these deaths and many injuries and the physical destruction that occurred will be felt for many years to come.

SO, JUST WHAT HAVE WE LEARNED?

This issue of *Emergency Medicine Clinics of North America* is timely; despite numerous hazardous materials and radiologic/nuclear incidents from which we have presumably learned lessons, these unfortunate incidents continue to occur and wreak havoc in the United States and throughout the world. Despite the increased emphasis on hazardous materials preparedness in the wake of 9/11, it seems we still have much to learn and new hazmat responses for which to prepare. It is our hope that these articles will help to cement the underpinnings of disaster preparedness among our readers. A look back at some of the historical hazardous materials exposures and the lessons thought to have been learned from them seems warranted.

We start with the early 20th century, because events that began in the 1920s and 1930s ultimately led to important legislation regarding occupational illnesses owing to chemicals and to a greater role for public health in the domain of industrial and occupational medicine.

GAULEY BRIDGE, WEST VIRGINIA

In the 1930s, Union Carbide employed contractors to drill and blast a 16,250-foot-long tunnel through a core of greater than 90% pure silica in the area of Gauley Bridge, West Virginia. Some 300 to 500 workers are estimated to have died of acute silicosis, sometimes in less than 2 weeks. This incident led to congressional hearings, popular movies, and, ultimately, strengthening of worker compensation laws. At the same time, erroneous conclusions were advanced by one of the most imminent radiologists of the time regarding the role of tuberculosis in death by acute silicosis.[6]

MANVILLE, NEW JERSEY

During the same decade, asbestosis was beginning to be described with increasing frequency in industry. An internal 1932 study performed at the Johns Manville plant in Manville, New Jersey, revealed an incidence of asbestosis of approximately 29% of the workforce. The study was not published until nearly 50 years later when information regarding its existence came to light in asbestos litigation.[7] Although asbestosis is a chronic disease, industry's reluctance to address it ultimately resulted in lawsuits and important occupational and environmental health and safety legislation that have impacted on acute hazardous materials exposures as well. Industry failed to follow the precautionary principle. Although the principle was not known by that name in the 1920s and 1930s, occupational physicians who monitored these workers were held to the higher precautionary principle of Hippocrates, "first do no harm," and might have done more to convince industry to do the same. It would take another 40 to

50 years, the discovery of asbestos-induced mesothelioma, and an avalanche of lawsuits, ending in bankruptcy of the asbestos industry, to drive this point home.

Surely, the collective historical acumen gained from the study of silicosis and asbestosis left no doubt that fibrogenic dust exposures must be controlled if workers are to be protected from debilitating lung diseases. And yet...new evidence exists for increases in the prevalence and severity of coal mine dust lung disease. Petsonk and colleagues[8] describe the recognition of a rapidly progressive pneumoconiosis in younger coal miners that continues to progress even after removal from exposure. Although dust diseases generally fall outside the purview of the emergency physician, the lessons with regard to hazardous exposures apply more broadly.

TEXAS CITY, TEXAS

West Fertilizer was not our first brush with ammonium nitrate's devastating danger. On April 16, 1947, a French-owned steamship, the SS Grandcamp, was docked at Texas City, Texas, near the Monsanto Chemical Company. The ammonium nitrate in the ship's hull caught fire early in the morning, then exploded at 9:12 AM. The first explosion killed the entire Texas City Fire Department, leaving it without defense when a second explosion occurred later that day on the SS High Flyer, also docked in Texas City and also carrying ammonium nitrate. A monument to the conflagration documents 576 persons dead; however, the exact number of dead will never likely be known. The injured numbered in the thousands with property losses in the millions. The resulting lawsuits were settled by the United States Supreme Court in 1962. The event led to changes in chemical manufacturing and new regulations for bagging handling and shipping of chemicals.[9]

OKLAHOMA CITY, OKLAHOMA

The explosive potential of ammonium nitrate was to rear its ugly head again on April 19, 1995, when Timothy McVeigh bombed the Alfred P. Murrah federal building, killing 168 people and injuring hundreds more.

TOKYO, JAPAN

One of the most dramatic acts of chemical terrorism occurred in Japan on March 30, 1995, carried out by operatives of Aum Shinrikyo, who released the organophosphate chemical warfare agent sarin in Tokyo subway cars. This was one of many attacks on the public by the cult, but undoubtedly the most disruptive.[10] In all, 640 victims were treated at St. Luke's International Hospital. No on-site (prehospital) decontamination was performed, resulting in numerous cases of secondary exposure. Owing to lack of personal protective equipment, approximately 23% of the hospital staff experienced secondary exposure to sarin.[11] Among the lessons learned, Okumura and colleagues[11] insist that hospitals must have adequate decontamination facilities, personal protective equipment, and that, in the case of sarin, atropine should be given before other treatments. Citing Sidell (relative to nerve agents), "the ABCs become the AABCs, with antidotes first."

GRANITEVILLE, SOUTH CAROLINA

On January 6, 2005, a freight train released approximately 11,500 gallons of chlorine, causing 9 deaths and sending more than 529 persons seeking medical treatment for chlorine exposure.[12] At least 6 hospitals in 2 states received patients. Those exposed to the release were told to report to decontamination units at University of South

Carolina at Aiken or at a high school. According to Mitchell and colleagues,[13] in one tent people exposed to the chemicals removed their clothes and were washed down, they then moved to a second tent where they were given medical attention. Wenck and colleagues[14] reported that victims fleeing the chlorine were intercepted and decontaminated, using wet decontamination. Emergency responders, in an abundance of caution, apparently determined that decontamination was necessary, perhaps owing to the irritant nature of chlorine. Exposure solely to gases usually requires no skin or mucous membrane decontamination to prevent secondary contamination of others.[15] Decontamination is time consuming, intrusive of personal privacy, and may put rescuers at risk owing to the requirement to wear personal protective equipment. The need for decontamination should be carefully considered in each event, using the best information available at the time and should be reviewed in after-action reports.

OTHER TRAIN DERAILMENTS

Transportation accidents of all kinds pose a risk of hazardous materials incidents. The dangers of seagoing cargo have already been illustrated, as has the train derailment in Graniteville. Train derailments are not infrequent, with 1280 reported to the Federal Railroad Administration in 2013. Total train accidents came to 1997, including 15 fires/violent ruptures.[16] Because trains carry an enormous amount of cargo, the potential impact of a train accident is much greater than other transportation accidents. The Hazardous Substances Emergency Events Surveillance System undertaken by the Agency for Toxic Substances and Disease Registry reported releases of hazardous materials from rail events occurring between 1999 and 2004 by 16 states participating in the system. Corrosive substances and irritant gases make up the largest number of releases (**Table 1**).

The Agency for Toxic Substances and Disease Registry made recommendations with regard to reducing mortality and morbidity from hazardous substance releases in transit. Of particular note to emergency physicians are the recommendations to develop emergency response plans before these events occur and to improve their ability to respond to incidents that involve human exposures to hazardous materials (**Box 1**).

DAMASCUS, SYRIA

On August 21, 2013, sarin was used in attacks on citizens in the Ghouta area of Damascus. Although the Syrian government denied involvement in the attacks, it subsequently agreed to give up its chemical weapon stores. The total number of dead and injured remains uncertain, but social media turned the event into an international outcry. At least 36 patients were evaluated by United Nations medical personnel 5 to 7 days after the exposure. Thirty-nine percent had persistent confusion and 5 of 36 had pinpoint pupils.[17]

HYDRAULIC FRACTURING

Petroleum exploration has long been among the most dangerous industries, with a death rate 7 times that of general industry. Thirty percent of these are due to highway crashes, and only about 3% are owing to harmful substance exposures.[18] The petroleum extraction industry is often cited by the Occupational Safety and Health Administration for confined space entry violations and failure to provide adequate personal protective equipment and, particularly, respiratory protection. The virtual

Table 1
Most common hazardous substances released during rail events: Hazardous Substances Emergency Events Surveillance system (16 states[a]; 1999–2004[b])

Substance	No. of releases[c]	%
Sulfuric acid	73	5.6
Sodium hydroxide	60	4.6
Hydrochloric acid	53	4.1
Ammonia	51	3.9
Methanol	36	2.8
Phosphoric acid	30	2.3
Mixture[d]	27	2.1
Argon	22	1.7
Ethylene glycol	22	1.7
Diesel fuel	19	1.5
Ethanol	17	1.3
Hydrogen peroxide	16	1.2
Potassium hydroxide	15	1.1
Alcohol NOS	11	0.8
Ammonium nitrate	11	0.8
Chlorine	11	0.8
Sodium chlorate	11	0.8

Abbreviation: NOS, not otherwise specified.
[a] Alabama, Colorado, Iowa, Louisiana. Minnesota, Mississippi. Missouri, New Jersey, New York, North Carolina Oregon, Rhode Island, Texas, Utah, Washington, and Wisconsin.
[b] Data from 2004 are preliminary.
[c] A total of 1299 substances were released during the 1165 rail events.
[d] Substances mixed before release (eg, benzene/toluene).
From Centers for Disease Control and Prevention. Public health consequences from hazardous substances acutely released during rail transit–South Carolina, 2005; selected States, 1999–2004. MMWR Morb Mortal Wkly Rep 2005;54(3):66; with permission.

explosion of hydraulic fracturing activity ("fracking") theoretically increases the risk of significant hazardous materials incidents, if only by sheer volume. Among the many chemicals known to be used in fracking fluids (many are trade secrets) and those that return to the surface after fracking, are hydrocarbons, such as benzene, toluene, ethyl benzene, and xylene. In addition to their toxicity, these compounds are extremely flammable. Hydrogen sulfide, a deadly asphyxiant and component of "sour gas" has been responsible for numerous injuries and deaths in the oil field. Corrosives and irritants such as glutaraldehyde, hydrochloric acid, acetic acid, potassium hydroxide, and ammonium chloride are used in fracking materials, as are alcohols, glycols, and glycol ethers. The dramatically increased vehicular traffic portends an increase in hazardous materials transportation incidents. Finally, there are numerous concerns surrounding technologically enhanced naturally occurring radioactive material (TENORM), which comes out of the ground as "produced water" or in pipe and tank scale. The predominant radionuclides vary by location, including uranium, radium and others. The US Environmental Protection Agency reports that the radiation levels in pipe and tank scale, whereas on average less than 200 pCi/g, can exceed 100,000 pCi/g.[19] To put this in perspective, the Government Accounting Office reports that the lifetime risk of cancer from exposure to uranium tailings containing radium at 5 pCi/g is 1 in 50. This is based on exposure to an

Box 1
Measures that government, employers, and first responders can implement to reduce morbidity and mortality from transit-associated hazardous substance releases

- Route hazardous materials away from densely populated areas, where feasible.
- Use Hazardous Substances Emergency Events Surveillance data or other federal, state, and local databases to determine where most releases occur.
- Develop emergency response plans before hazardous substance events occur, including a community-based public education campaign detailing proper evacuation (http://www.bt.cdc.gov/planning/evacuationfacts.asp), shelter-in-place plans (http://www.bt.cdc.gov/planning/shelteringfacts.asp), and decontamination procedures (http://www.bt.cdc.gov/planning/personalcleaning facts, asp).
- Deploy public warning systems (eg, sirens), practice drills, and public shelters.
- Ensure that employees who work with or around hazardous substances undergo continuous job safety training (eg, hazardous materials training) and have access to appropriate personal protective equipment.
- Ensure that emergency medical service and hospital emergency department staffs have the necessary guidance to plan for, and improve their ability to respond to, incidents that involve human exposure to hazardous materials (http://www.atsdr.cdc.gov/mhmi.html).
- Emphasize the importance of preventive maintenance of equipment and vehicles used in transport.[3,9]

From Centers for Disease Control and Prevention. Public health consequences from hazardous substances acutely released during rail transit–South Carolina, 2005; selected States, 1999–2004. MMWR Morb Mortal Wkly Rep, 2005;54(3):67.

individual residing on site after cleanup.[20] Illegal dumping of these materials has been reported in the news.[21] The long-term risks for hazardous materials incidents related to fracking are speculative, but communities heavily involved in oil and gas exploration are already feeling its impact in many ways.

RADIOLOGIC AND NUCLEAR INCIDENTS

Hazardous materials incidents can also be radiologic or nuclear in nature. The most common events seen are usually radiologic and are usually limited. They involve a small number of people and are seen in industrial, commercial, or medical settings where radioactive materials are utilized or mishandled.

GOIÂNIA, BRAZIL

Perhaps, the most significant incident involved the theft of a cesium-137 radiotherapy source in Goiania, Brazil, in 1987. This incident led to the death of 5 and the contamination of around 250 people. More than one hundred thousand people were monitored for contamination with cesium-137 and the incident had deep and long lasting psychological and economic consequences on the affected communities.[22] Steinhäusler[23] reports just a few of the economic costs: 42 houses required decontamination. Travelers spread the contamination up to 100 km; contaminated paper and lead were recovered as far away as 830 km from Goiânia.

MAYAPURI, DELHI, INDIA

More recently, a cobalt-60 radioactive source found its way into a crowded scrap metal market in Mayapuri, Delhi, India, in 2010[24] and led to the death of the scrap metal shop keeper and 7 injuries. In 2014, a truck carrying a cobalt-60 source was stolen in Mexico. The incident caused significant concerns, although it did not cause any known injuries.[25]

NUCLEAR POWER PLANT INCIDENTS

Fortunately, more severe incidents that occur at nuclear power plants are rare. Over the past several decades, there have been a handful of incidents with serious consequences to the environment or the public as classified by the International Nuclear and Radiological Event Scale[26]:

- Windscale Pile, Cumbria, The United Kingdom (1957)
- Three Mile Island, Harrisburg, Pennsylvania, USA (1979)
- Chernobyl, Former Soviet Union (1986)
- Fukushima, Japan (2011)

Although it is too early to assess the long-term adverse health effects from the Fukushima incident, review of the other events reveals that the primary adverse consequences, apart from the increase in thyroid cancer from the Chernobyl accident, are psychological and devastated a large number of individuals. The world dependence on energy and the number of nuclear power plants are both projected to increase in future years. Although the number of major incidents associated with this industry has been limited, the consequences can be dramatic and can be caused by either human error or natural disasters, like the Great Japan Earthquake and the resulting tsunami.

NUCLEAR WEAPONS

Certainly, the most dreaded scenario involving radiation is the detonation of a nuclear weapon or an improvised nuclear device. Although the world has seen more than 100 detonations, the only 2 that were not part of testing killed more than a 100,000 people and devastated Hiroshima and Nagasaki in Japan in 1945.

Current contingency planning in the United States assumes that the detonation of a 10-kiloton improvised nuclear device in an urban area would lead to more than one hundred thousand fatalities and to a greater number of injuries and displaced individuals who would seek medical evaluation.[27]

A large number of these individuals might be contaminated with radioactive material. The widespread consequences of such a dreadful incident reinforces the need for physicians and other health care providers to acquire a basic understanding of radiation injuries and the decontamination of patients who are contaminated with radioactive material that was dispersed in the environment after the detonation.

LONDON, UK

Last, physicians may encounter a single patient with exposure to radiation or contamination with radioactive material. A basic knowledge of the medical consequences of these possible scenarios is necessary to recognize these rare, yet potentially lethal events. The murder of Mr. Alexander Litvinenko in London in 2006 serves as a grim example of this type of situation.[28]

This issue of *Emergency Medicine Clinics of North America* is intended to facilitate the basic approach to a complex issue: Preparation for hazardous chemical and radiologic materials events impacting on the emergency department. It is not intended to be comprehensive, but rather an introduction for the practicing EM physician and a starting block for the EM physician involved in disaster management.

Tomassoni, French, and Walter provide an overview of frequently encountered toxic industrial chemicals. Because the number of chemicals used in commerce is enormous and are often unknown at the time of the initial chemical incident, they correctly point out the initial evaluation should focus on recognizable toxic syndromes or "toxidromes," which allow treatment to precede definitive identification of the substance or substances.

Moore, Geller, and Clark address the nuts and bolts of emergency department and hospital disaster preparedness, with specific attention to chemical and radiologic hazards. Regulations applicable to hospitals are addressed. An associated checklist (also found in the article by Borron) provides resources for development of a hospital emergency management plan.

Holland and Cawthon take on the important issues of personal protective equipment and decontamination, providing regulatory guidance and practical recommendations for both chemical and radiologic exposures.

Kirk and Iddins pull together the informational resources likely to be needed by the emergency physician in the first few hours after a hazardous materials incident, citing useful publications, telephone contacts, and web resources.

Borron and Bebarta discuss asphyxiants. This group of compounds is most likely to result in respiratory difficulties and/or loss of consciousness, posing a critical diagnostic and management challenge to practitioners.

Tovar and Leikin discuss an important group of compounds capable of causing skin, eye, respiratory, and gastrointestinal irritation or corrosive injury, depending on route of exposure and other physical parameters.

King and Aaron address a significant toxicologic issue, that of the organophosphate and carbamate compounds, which continue to pose threats both as agricultural chemicals, and in the case organophosphates, chemical weapons. Although these agrichemicals are gradually diminishing in use in developed countries, the risk of a chemical attack using organophosphate chemical warfare agents will likely remain with us for a long time.

McKay and Scharman tackle the issue of inadvertent and intentional contamination of food, medication, and water, all of which have resulted in death and serious injury. The recent contamination of the Elk River in West Virginia is described, along with the challenges in this type of investigation.

Kazzi, Buzzell, Bertelli, and Christensen discuss an enormous challenge for most emergency physicians, namely, assessing and managing patient with internal contamination by radionuclides. The discussion of decorporating agents ("antidotes") to radionuclides provides useful clinical information about these rarely encountered pharmaceuticals.

McCormick, Tajeu, and Klapow address the problem of dealing with mental health concerns that inevitably follow technological disasters, such as hazardous materials and radiologic incidents. They provide a cogent approach to addressing the concerns of the "worried well," those with preexisting mental conditions, and those at risk of developing more significant psychological problems, such as posttraumatic stress disorder.

Finally, Borron, aided by the generosity of his co-authors in this issue, amasses various resources and checklists that may be of use to emergency physician in a pinch, as well as recommendations for developing emergency management plans, stocking of antidotes, and obtaining appropriate personal protective equipment.

This collection of articles provides a useful review for some and an initiation for others into the complex domain of hazardous materials emergency response. The reader is encouraged to seek out additional education through continuing medical education courses, such as those provided by Advanced Hazmat Life Support, REAC/TS, the Federal Emergency Management Agency, the Centers for Disease Control and Prevention, and other agencies and institutions.

Although the hazardous materials emergencies of the last century or so have taught us valuable lessons, we have much to learn. To paraphrase the saying that you can never have too much money or good looks, for chemical disasters you can never have too much preparedness or practice. Or, as a former lieutenant governor, in a very different context, put it, "Drill baby, drill!"[29]

ACKNOWLEDGMENTS

The author sincerely thanks Dr Ziad Kazzi for his contributions to this Introduction and to this entire issue of *Emergency Medicine Clinics of North America*. His keen eye for detail and thoughtful comments have greatly facilitated this endeavor.

REFERENCES

1. Broughton E. The Bhopal disaster and its aftermath: a review. Environ Health 2005;4(1):6.
2. Patel T. Bhopal disaster. The Mandala Projects: Trade Environment Database. Available at: http://www1.american.edu/ted/bhopal.htm. Accessed October 23, 2014.
3. Reuters. Texas fertilizer plant had 1,350 times the amount of ammonium nitrate that would normally raise red flags. 2013. Available at: http://www.nydailynews.com/news/national/texas-fertilizer-plant-massive-amounts-unreported-ammonium-nitrate-article-1.1322766. Accessed August 28, 2014.
4. Root J. Abbott: ask chemical plants what's inside. July 1, 2014. Available from: http://www.texastribune.org/2014/07/01/abbott-ask-chemical-plants-whats-inside. Accessed August 19, 2014.
5. Zuzek C. The night West blew up. Tex Med 2013;109(7):41–5.
6. Cherniack MG. Historical perspectives in occupational medicine. Pancoast and the image of silicosis. Am J Ind Med 1990;18(5):599–612.
7. Borron SW, Forman SA, Lockey JE, et al. An early study of pulmonary asbestosis among manufacturing workers: original data and reconstruction of the 1932 cohort. Am J Ind Med 1997;31(3):324–34.
8. Petsonk EL, Rose C, Cohen R. Coal mine dust lung disease. New lessons from old exposure. Am J Respir Crit Care Med 2013;187(11):1178–85.
9. Texas City Disaster. 2010. Available at: http://www.tshaonline.org/handbook/online/articles/lyt01. Accessed August 19, 2014.
10. Chronology of Aum Shinrikyo's CBW activities. 2001. Available at: cns.miis.edu/reports/pdfs/aum_chrn.pdf. Accessed July 21, 2014.
11. Okumura T, Hisaoka T, Yamada A, et al. The Tokyo subway sarin attack–lessons learned. Toxicol Appl Pharmacol 2005;207(Suppl 2):471–6.
12. US Centers for Disease Control and Prevention. Public health consequences from hazardous substances acutely released during rail transit–South Carolina, 2005; selected States, 1999-2004. MMWR Morb Mortal Wkly Rep 2005;54(3):64–7.
13. Mitchell JT, Edmonds AS, Cutter SL, et al. Evacuation behavior in response to the Graniteville, South Carolina, chlorine spill. Boulder (CO): University of Colorado Natural Hazard Center; 2005.

14. Wenck MA, Van Sickle D, Drociuk D, et al. Rapid assessment of exposure to chlorine released from a train derailment and resulting health impact. Public Health Rep 2007;122(6):784–92.

15. Tauber DM. Personal protective equipment and decontamination. In: Walter FG, Schauben JL, Klein R, et al, editors. Advanced hazmat life support provider manual. Tucson (AZ): University of Arizona; 2014. p. 65–90.

16. Train accidents by type in major cause: source – FRA F 6180.54. 2014. Available at: http://safetydata.fra.dot.gov/OfficeofSafety/publicsite/Query/TrainAccident Damage.aspx. Accessed August 30, 2014.

17. Hurley WT. Chemoterrorism: nerve agents. In: Walter FG, Schauben JL, Klein R, et al, editors. Advanced hazmat life support provider manual. Tucson (AZ): University of Arizona; 2014. p. 367–86.

18. Witter RZ, Tenney L, Clark S, et al. Occupational exposures in the oil and gas extraction industry: State of the science and research recommendations. Am J Ind Med 2014;57(7):847–56.

19. Radiation Protection: TENORM sources. 2014. Available at: http://www.epa.gov/radiation/tenorm/sources.html. Accessed August 30, 2014.

20. Nuclear health and safety: Consensus on acceptable radiation risk to the public is lacking. Report number RCED-94-190. 1994. Available at: http://www.gpo.gov/fdsys/pkg/GAOREPORTS-RCED-94-190/html/GAOREPORTS-RCED-94-190.htm. Accessed August 30, 2014.

21. Dawson C. Fracking's new problem: radioactive waste. April 16, 2014. Available at: http://money.msn.com/investing/post–frackings-new-problem-radioactive-waste. Accessed August 30, 2014.

22. International Atomic Energy Agency (IAEA). The radiological incident in Goiania.1988. Available at: http://www-pub.iaea.org/mtcd/publications/pdf/pub815_web.pdf. Accessed August 5, 2014.

23. Steinhäusler F. Social and psychological effects of radiological terrorism. In: Khripunov I, Bolshov L, Nikonov D, editors. NATO science for peace and security series: human and societal dynamics. Brussels (Belgium): NATO; 2007. p. 176.

24. Dixit A. Protecting people and the environment: IAEA Code of Conduct on Safety and Security of Radioactive Sources. November 5, 2013. Available at: http://www.iaea.org/newscenter/news/2013/protectpeople.html. Accessed August 30, 2014.

25. International Atomic Energy Agency (IAEA). Mexico informs IAEA of theft of dangerous radioactive source. 2013. Available at: http://www.iaea.org/newscenter/news/2013/mexicoradsource.html. Accessed August 30, 2014.

26. International Atomic Energy Agency (IAEA). INES: The international nuclear and radiological event scale. 2008. Available at: https://www.iaea.org/Publications/Factsheets/English/ines.pdf. Accessed August 30, 2014.

27. Planning guidance for response to a nuclear detonation. 2010. 2nd edition. Available at: http://www.remm.nlm.gov/PlanningGuidanceNuclearDetonation.pdf. Accessed August 30, 2014.

28. Miller CW, Whitcomb RC, Ansari A, et al. Murder by radiation poisoning: implications for public health. J Environ Health 2012;74(10):8–13.

29. Drill, baby, drill. 2014. Available at: http://en.wikipedia.org/wiki/Drill,_baby,_drill. Accessed August 31, 2014.

Toxic Industrial Chemicals and Chemical Weapons

Exposure, Identification, and Management by Syndrome

Anthony J. Tomassoni, MD, MS[a],*, Robert N.E. French, MD, MPH[b], Frank G. Walter, MD[b]

KEYWORDS

- Toxidrome • Toxic industrial chemicals • Exposure history • Antidotes

KEY POINTS

- Causes of medical conditions resulting from chemical exposures may be elusive unless an exposure history is taken during the medical interview.
- Clinicians should address elements of the exposure history, using a systematic approach to improve the diagnostic accuracy of that history.
- Recognition of common toxidromes may facilitate diagnosis and treatment of patients exposed to unknown toxic chemicals.
- Understanding basic principles of toxicology and the significance of exposure limits can aid in the evaluation of exposed patients.
- Use of specific antidotes may rescue patients with specific exposures; therefore, clinicians should advocate for the availability of these agents.
- Clinicians should become familiar with the available resources for chemical exposures.

INTRODUCTION

With approximately 100,000 chemicals used each day in US industry, the range of hazardous materials situations that may challenge emergency care providers is daunting. Moreover, many of these chemicals have never been tested for safety with respect to environmental effects or human exposure.[1] Despite and because of technological advances, chemical spills and disasters will continue to occur, and these exposures

Disclosures: None.
[a] Department of Emergency Medicine, Yale New Haven Center for Emergency Preparedness and Disaster Response, Yale New Haven Health System, Yale University School of Medicine, 464 Congress Avenue, Suite 260, New Haven, CT 06519, USA; [b] College of Medicine, College of Pharmacy, The University of Arizona, 1501 North Campbell Avenue, Tucson, AZ 85724, USA
* Corresponding author.
E-mail address: anthony.tomassoni@yale.edu

Emerg Med Clin N Am 33 (2015) 13–36
http://dx.doi.org/10.1016/j.emc.2014.09.004
0733-8627/15/$ – see front matter © 2015 Elsevier Inc. All rights reserved.

emed.theclinics.com

may impact individuals or large populations. Although progress has been made in the use of "green chemistry," safer manufacturing processes, increasing use of personal protective equipment (PPE), and engineering controls, many of the chemicals in common use are potentially injurious. Increasing population density, settlement of high-risk areas, increasing dependence on industrial chemicals, human errors, and terrorism are among the many factors that cause disasters.[2] The expansion of terrorism coupled with the potential deployment of expedient chemical weapons makes it clear that emergency care providers must be prepared to handle exposures resulting from toxic industrial materials.

Although chemical exposures resulting from spills, terrorist attacks, and other dramatic events may result in immediate recognition, other less obvious or intentionally covert exposures may go unrecognized. This is especially true given the pace of today's emergency departments and medical offices.[3] It is important for emergency and primary care providers to document exposures and work-related conditions and to recognize opportunities for preventive care. Best practices may be facilitated by charting prompts and use of an exposure history form.[4]

The impact that even a brief exposure history may have on a patient's quality of life is illustrated by the following case. An exposure history taken by one of the authors (AJT) for a young adult construction worker without history of asthma who presented for care of bronchospasm revealed that he had recently begun using isocyanate-containing insulating materials. This use resulted in isocyanate sensitization, presumed isocyanate antibody production, and resultant asthma. The case was referred to occupational medicine and the presence of antibodies to isocyanate was confirmed. Identification of the cause of the patient's bronchospasm resulted in termination of isocyanate exposure with resultant improvement in his bronchospasm.[5] Chemical awareness, a high index of suspicion, an exposure history, and good follow through are essential for quality care of the patient with a possible chemical exposure.

It is useful for providers to think of exposures in terms of the acuity and urgency of the medical sequelae. Some exposures (eg, exposure to a high concentration of chlorine gas) may result in immediate effects (respiratory irritation and dyspnea secondary to lung injury and adult respiratory distress syndrome), whereas other exposures may result in short-term, delayed effects (exposure to a lesser concentration of chlorine may produce delayed pulmonary edema up to a day after exposure). Still other exposures may not be apparent for years, such as chemical carcinogenesis caused by benzene resulting in acute myelogenous leukemia. An understanding of the toxicologic principles of dose, route of exposure, and mechanism of toxicity combined with individual patient factors can aid in the establishment of a diagnosis and help with decision-making.

LESSONS LEARNED FROM PREVIOUS CHEMICAL DISASTERS

In addition to the immediate health, environmental, and economic effects of chemical releases, exposures may have severe long-term consequences. For example, on December 2–3, 1984, methyl isocyanate and other chemicals were released from a storage tank at a Union Carbide India plant that manufactured the carbamate insecticide carbaryl in Bhopal, India. This may qualify as the world's worst toxicologic disaster. More than 500,000 individuals were exposed in the impoverished towns surrounding the plant, and 3787 deaths were reported by the regional government.[6–9] Adult respiratory distress syndrome was the likely cause of death in most acute cases, with many deaths likely resulting from secondary respiratory infections. An increased number of stillbirths and spontaneous abortions were noted among the survivors.[10] The cause of this release remains unclear. Health data were restricted from publication until 1994.[9]

Lessons learned from this and other chemical disasters remind us that industrialization must not be dictated by market dynamics alone. Environmental public safety and public health regulations must be developed and put into place. Health care facilities must exist that have the capability to manage the consequences of an industrial accident. This may involve prepositioning of antidote, antidote stockpiling, and targeted education of health care providers and emergency responders. Unfortunately, many examples of hazardous industrial sites surrounded by dense populations exist.

BASIC CLINICAL PRINCIPLES OF HAZARDOUS MATERIALS TOXICOLOGY
Evaluating and Responding to Exposures

Timely recognition of the nature and scope of effects that may result from exposure to industrial chemicals is the sine qua non of quality care for those exposed. Keys to timely response include a thorough understanding of potential exposure routes and knowledge of the physical and chemical properties of the agents in question, and the ability to recognize clinical toxic syndromes (toxidromes). Obtaining an exposure history, providing supportive care, and obtaining and using antidotes may be lifesaving.

Diagnosis and treatment of a patient exposed to a hazardous industrial chemical may be relatively straightforward when the causative agent is a known workplace hazard and the patient is brought to a facility where expertise in the management of chemical exposures is available.

During emergencies, however, there may be multiple casualties, casualties may arrive before information about the hazard can be relayed to the treatment facility, and casualties may have coexisting traumatic injury. Real-time chemical monitoring to identify and quantify chemicals and characterize exposures is rarely available. Estimations of the magnitude of an exposure and the potential severity and consequences of that exposure may be based on limited information. Rapid intervention, albeit based on limited information, may influence patient outcomes.

- Staff and other patients must be protected from secondary exposure.
- Those with significant exposures must be differentiated from those who were either not exposed or had trivial exposures.
- In the absence of reliable identification of the toxic industrial chemical involved, casualties should be evaluated for presence of a toxidrome and treatment initiated accordingly.
- Decontamination should be initiated, if indicated, and when practical, the method of decontamination should be based on the agent involved and the route of exposure.
- Surge capacity and surge capability plans may need to be executed.
- Appropriate public health and public safety agencies and the regional poison control center should be notified.

Taking an Exposure History

Occupational and environmental exposures may present with nonspecific symptoms, or may mimic a common medical problem. The ability to elicit an exposure history empowers the clinician to detect, prevent, and treat diseases that may result from chemical exposure.

Cues and clues to facilitate accurate diagnosis

Identification of a toxic syndrome may facilitate formation of a differential diagnosis and aid in the recognition of an exposure to a toxic industrial chemical. Clues to the identity of the offending agent may lie in the occupation of the exposed individual or in the occupation of close contacts. For example, individuals who work as firefighters, wood and metal finishers, internal combustion engine mechanics, or in heavy traffic are more likely to be exposed to carbon monoxide and may present with headache. High-yield examples of symptoms that may result from environmental exposure are given in **Table 1**.[11] Other exposures may result in long-term effects. Some examples and their associated consequences are detailed in **Table 2**.[11]

Toxicity, exposure, and risk

Risk related to an exposure is typically directly proportional to the toxicity of the agent and the duration of exposure. The toxicity of an agent is of little importance if there is no potential for exposure. Although exposures are often a cost of doing business, risk is often mitigated through engineering controls aimed at preventing exposure and the use of PPE. Many attempts are made to determine acceptable risk, and much anxiety regarding actual and potential exposures results from poor understanding of environmental contamination and the long-term effects of

Table 1
Examples of environmental causes of medical problems

Symptoms and Diseases	Agent	Potential Exposures
Immediate or Short-Term Effects		
Dermatoses (allergic or irritant)	Metals (chromium, nickel), fibrous glass, solvents, caustic alkali, soaps	Electroplating, metal cleaning, plastics, machining, leather tanning, housekeeping
Headache	Carbon monoxide, solvents	Firefighting, automobile exhaust, wood finishing, dry cleaning
Acute psychoses	Lead, mercury, carbon disulfide	Removing paint from old houses, fungicide, wood preserving, viscose rayon industry
Asthma or dry cough	Formaldehyde, toluene diisocyanate, animal dander	Textiles, plastics, polyurethane kits, lacquer, animal handler
Pulmonary edema, pneumonitis	Nitrogen oxides, phosgene, halogen gases, cadmium	Welding, farming, chemical operations, smelting
Cardiac arrhythmias	Solvents, fluorocarbons	Metal cleaning, solvents use, refrigerator maintenance
Angina	Carbon monoxide, methylene chloride	Car repair, traffic exhaust, foundry, wood finishing
Abdominal pain	Lead	Battery making, enameling, smelting, painting, welding, ceramics, plumbing
Hepatitis (may become a long-term effect)	Halogenated hydrocarbons (eg, carbon tetrachloride)	Solvents use, lacquer use, hospital workers

From Goldman RH, Peters JM. The occupational and environmental health history. JAMA 1981;246(24):2833; with permission.

Table 2
Selected long-term effects and toxicants

Effects	Toxicant
Lung cancer	Arsenic, asbestos, nickel, uranium
Bladder cancer	Benzidine dyes and β-naphthylamine
Aplastic anemia/leukemia	Benzene, ionizing radiation
Neurologic effects	Carbon disulfide: extrapyramidal effects; Manganese: parkinsonian syndrome; Arsenic, lead, mercury, n-hexane and methyl butyl ketone: behavioral changes and/or neuropathies
COPD, pulmonary fibrosis, pleural plaques and mesothelioma	Asbestos
COPD (silicosis) and tuberculosis	Silica
COPD and chronic bronchitis (byssinosis/"brown lung disease")	Cotton fibers
Black lung disease	Coal dust
Pulmonary fibrosis	Beryllium

Abbreviation: COPD, chronic obstructive pulmonary disease.

exposure.[12] Risk assessment may be complicated by lack of exposure data, exposure to mixtures of chemicals, limited knowledge of the effects of the chemicals in question, and the limitations inherent in toxicology studies themselves. Chemical mixtures may result in additive effects, antagonistic effects, potentiating effects, or synergistic effects. Variables may include short- versus long-term exposure, concerns about teratology, reproductive toxicity, neurotoxicity, genotoxicity, irritating effects of chemicals, immune-mediated hypersensitivity, bioactivation, kinetics, products of combustion, antidote properties, and more.[13] Clinicians faced with questions from patients should draw on resources, such as poison centers, toxicologists, and occupational medicine physicians, for assistance in risk evaluation and to place patients' concerns in the proper context.

Routes of exposure

The common routes of exposure include inhalation, dermal (including mucous membrane and ocular) exposure, and ingestion. On occasion, injection (eg, spray gun) may play a role. The toxic syndrome that results from an exposure may be influenced by the route of exposure and is discussed later in this article.

Exposure, dose, and response

Comparison of the results of exposure within and across species is challenging. Genetic factors even within a single species result in variable responses to similar exposures. The dose response principle suggests that as the dose of a toxicant increases more individuals within a population are affected, and the magnitude of response by any individual increases. This relationship has many applications in toxicology, including the use of the "LD50," the dose of an agent lethal to 50% of a test population. Although a concept such as the LD50 is difficult to apply to an individual after a potentially toxic exposure, this and similar concepts are useful when establishing regulatory measures.[14] Further complicating the prediction of effects of exposure, some agents may induce repair mechanisms that actually reduce the effects of exposure at low doses.[15]

Bioactivation

Some toxicants, such as methylene chloride and paraquat, require metabolic transformation to maximize their injurious potential.[16] Sites of bioactivation may coincide with the target organs affected.[17] Unsurprisingly, these targets include the liver, kidney, and lung where substantial P-450 activity exists. Mechanisms of detoxification also exist and may limit toxic effects when they are in good repair.

Potential target organs and organ systems

Any organ or tissue may be the target of a toxicant. Some common examples of organs, toxicants, and effects are shown in **Table 3**.[18]

Sources of Exposure Information and Definitions

Clinicians are often faced with the need to make decisions regarding the selection of appropriate PPE and the decontamination, evaluation, stabilization, and potential transportation of a patient exposed to unfamiliar materials. They may also be called on to explain potential consequences of exposure to patients, families, employers,

Table 3
Selected target organs, toxicants, and some of their effects

Organ	Toxicants	Effects
Lung	1. Isocyanates, smoke (including tobacco smoke), particulates (silica, asbestos) 2. Paraquat 3. Asbestos	1. Asthma; chronic obstructive pulmonary disease 2. Pulmonary fibrosis (process accelerated by the administration of oxygen) 3. Mesothelioma
Liver	1. Carbon tetrachloride 2. Ethanol 3. Polychlorinated biphenyls 4. Arsenic 5. Vinyl chloride 6. Yellow phosphorous	1. Centrilobular necrosis 2. Hepatitis 3. Steatosis, necrosis 4. Neoplasm 5. Periportal necrosis 6. Acute hepatic failure
Kidney	1. Heavy metals, solvents 2. Toluene	1. Renal failure 2. Renal tubular acidosis
Blood	1. Benzene 2. Nitrates 3. Carbon monoxide	1. Aplastic anemia, acute leukemia, chronic myelogenous leukemia 2. Methemoglobinemia 3. Impaired oxygen transport
Cardiovascular	1. Carbon monoxide 2. Tobacco smoke	1. Angina (via loss of O_2-carrying capacity) 2. Accelerated cardiovascular disease
Nervous system, central	1. Hydrogen sulfide 2. Organic solvents	1. Central apnea 2. Encephalopathy
Nervous system, peripheral	n-hexane	Peripheral neuropathy
Skin	Halogenated aromatic hydrocarbons	Chloracne, dermatitis
Reproductive	Lead (female); carbon disulfide (male); consider also toxicants that may impair or be transmitted through lactation	Impaired fertility
Ocular	Alkali/acid	Corneal injury

and even unexposed concerned individuals. It is helpful for clinicians to arrange access to some basic references in advance of need. Because large disasters may disrupt network communications and/or the Internet, it is advisable to keep some references readily available in print format. Additionally, many public safety organizations employ professional hazardous materials technicians who are familiar with a variety of emergency response tools and services (lists of human and material resources are provided elsewhere in this issue).

Personal Protective Equipment

Clinicians who may be expected to handle victims of chemical exposure and decontamination personnel must be trained in appropriate selection and use of PPE. The Occupational Safety and Health Administration sets standards and provides information on the selection of PPE and employee training. Hazardous Waste Operations and Emergency Response rules (29 CFR 1910.120 Appendix B) delineate four levels of PPE required to protect workers under various site conditions. In most circumstances, emergency department personnel decontaminating or treating victims of chemical exposure previously decontaminated in the field may be adequately protected by the use of Level C or D PPE.[19] Detailed information on PPE and decontamination of adults and children is discussed elsewhere in this issue.

CLINICAL MANIFESTATIONS AND MANAGEMENT
Syndromic Recognition of Hazardous Materials

Given the myriad hazardous chemicals and the vast array of effects that may result from exposure, the clinician may benefit from placing these chemicals and their effects into groups with similar properties. Despite improved placarding of materials in transit and the widespread use of materials safety data sheets, circumstances arise where individuals sustain exposure to unknown chemicals in unknown concentration and for undefined periods of time. The severity and potential consequences of such an exposure must be rapidly and accurately assessed. Under such circumstances syndromic identification of agents is a powerful tool. The concept of the toxidrome, a constellation of clinical clues that point to the identity of a poison, is most useful.[20] Although each poison produces a toxidrome, some toxidromes are more common or more dramatic than others, and many members of a chemical class may produce that toxidrome. Timely and accurate toxidrome recognition may aid in identification of an unknown poison and lead to optimal patient treatment and salvage. Notable toxidromes of dangerous industrial chemicals, examples, symptoms, and cues to treatment are listed in **Table 4**.

Antidotes

Treatment for most dangerous industrial toxicants is limited to decontamination and supportive care. However, specific antidotes exist for a few industrial chemicals. It is imperative that clinicians recognize the opportunity to administer an antidote when one exists, because nearly all of these antidotes are most likely to be successful when used in a timely manner.

Toxicologists, emergency physicians, occupational medicine physicians, and others have a role along with poison centers and public health and emergency management agencies in stockpiling antidotes against hazardous toxicants that exist within and their catchment areas. These stockpiles should be based on hazard vulnerability analysis.[21,22] Selected antidotes to dangerous industrial chemicals are discussed in **Table 5**.

Table 4
Toxidromes associated with some dangerous industrial chemicals and chemical weapons

Toxidrome	Typical Toxicants	Predominant Route of Exposure	Typical Symptoms	Treatment
Irritant gas: highly water-soluble	Ammonia, formaldehyde, hydrogen chloride, sulfur dioxide	Inhalation	May cause mucous membrane and upper airway inflammation, edema, and corrosion. Symptoms include irritation, burning, coughing, airway swelling, stridor, laryngospasm, aphonia, shortness of breath, and respiratory arrest. Abnormal breath sounds, eye irritation, and runny nose may also be present.	Remove clothing if contaminated/malodorous; decontaminate those reporting skin/mucous membrane/eye irritation. Oxygen and supportive care as needed, early intubation for airway edema, positive pressure ventilation for pulmonary edema. Consult a toxicologist regarding potential role for nebulized sodium bicarbonate in the context of inhalation of agents that form acids in aqueous solution.
Irritant gas: moderately water-soluble	Chlorine	Inhalation	May cause inflammation, edema, and corrosion of the upper airway and the lungs. Symptoms include irritation, burning, coughing, wheezing, shortness of breath, noncardiogenic pulmonary edema and respiratory arrest. Airway swelling, stridor, laryngospasm, and aphonia are less likely than with highly water-soluble agents. Abnormal breath sounds, eye irritation, and runny nose may also be present.	Remove clothing if contaminated; decontaminate those reporting skin/mucous membrane/eye irritation. Administer oxygen. Supportive care. Endotracheal intubation may be required. Administer albuterol for bronchospasm. Admit those with significant exposure for 24-h observation because delayed effects may occur. Consider nebulized sodium bicarbonate: 3 mL of 4.2% for symptomatic chlorine exposure.

| Irritant gas: slightly water-soluble | Phosgene, nitrogen dioxide | Inhalation | Local irritant and corrosive effects. Symptoms include mild airway irritation. Coughing, wheezing, and shortness of breath caused by noncardiogenic pulmonary edema may lead to respiratory arrest. Abnormal breath sounds, eye irritation, and runny nose may also be present. | Remove clothing, and decontaminate those reporting skin/mucous membrane/eye irritation. Administer oxygen. Supportive care. Endotracheal intubation may be required. Administer albuterol for bronchospasm. Admit those with significant exposure for 24-h observation because delayed pulmonary edema may occur. |
| Asphyxiant: simple asphyxiant | Carbon dioxide, methane, nitrogen, propane | Inhalation | Displacement of oxygen from the ambient atmosphere, thereby decreasing the oxygen available to the lungs. Symptoms include shortness of breath, air hunger, rapid heart rate, chest pain, dysrhythmias, nausea/vomiting, confusion/ combativeness, syncope, coma, and respiratory arrest. | Administer oxygen. Remove clothing to eliminate odors. Supportive care. Endotracheal intubation may be required. |

(continued on next page)

Table 4
(continued)

Toxidrome	Typical Toxicants	Predominant Route of Exposure	Typical Symptoms	Treatment
Asphyxiant: systemic (chemical) asphyxiant	Isobutyl nitrite, carbon monoxide, hydrogen cyanide, hydrogen sulfide, hydrogen azide	Inhalation	Interference with oxygen transport and/or use. Symptoms may include shortness of breath, rapid heart rate, chest pain, dysrhythmias, pallor, diaphoresis, nausea/vomiting, confusion/combativeness, syncope, coma, respiratory arrest, vasodilation, hypotension or headache. Agents causing methemoglobinemia may result in bluish skin or chocolate-colored blood. Conjunctivitis and the odor of rotten eggs may indicate hydrogen sulfide poisoning. Carbon monoxide may present with flulike symptoms; cherry-red skin is a postmortem finding. Pulse oximetry may be falsely normal under some circumstances.	Administer oxygen. Remove clothing to minimize odor, and decontaminate if off-gassing solid/liquid agents persists. Eye decontamination as indicated. Supportive care. Endotracheal intubation may be required. Antidotes may be required. Patients exposed to structure fire may suffer from combined carbon monoxide and cyanide poisoning. Ingested cyanide or sulfide salts may react with gastric acid to form toxic gas. Special treatments: Carbon monoxide • Hyperbaric oxygen Methemoglobinemia • Methylene blue Cyanide • Sodium nitrite and/or sodium thio-sulfate, alternatively hydroxocobalamin Hydrogen sulfide • Possible roles for nitrites and/or hyperbaric oxygen No antidote to azides is known.

| Cholinergic | Organophosphate insecticides (dichlorvos, chlorpyrifos, guthion, diazinon, parathion) Carbamate insecticides, such as carbaryl Organophosphate nerve agents ("G" agents, soman, sarin, tabun, VX, and so forth) | Skin and mucous membranes; inhalation and ingestion possible; route of exposure may influence presenting symptoms (ie, inhalation, respiratory symptoms; ingestion, gastrointestinal symptoms; dermal, local fasciculations). | Causes inhibition of acetylcholinesterase resulting in acetylcholine excess. Symptoms include: Peripheral nervous system Muscarinic: Diarrhea, urination, miosis, bradycardia, bronchorrhea, bronchospasm, emesis, lacrimation, salivation, sweating Nicotinic: Mydriasis, tachycardia, weakness, hypertension, hyperglycemia, fasciculations Central nervous system: Confusion, convulsions and coma | Remove clothing. Decontaminate those exposed to mists, liquids, and so forth. Administer oxygen, supportive care. Early administration of antidotes may be required. Endotracheal intubation may be required. Albuterol for bronchospasm *after* antidotal therapy. Administration of adequate atropine blocks the effects of excess acetylcholine on its receptors and may be indicated for organophosphate and carbamate exposures. Administration of 2-PAM. 2-PAM is generally not indicated for carbaryl poisoning. Diazepam may prevent or terminate seizures. |

(continued on next page)

Table 4
(continued)

Toxidrome	Typical Toxicants	Predominant Route of Exposure	Typical Symptoms	Treatment
Corrosive	Acids (hydrochloric acid, nitric acid, sulfuric acid, and so forth) Bases (ammonium hydroxide, potassium hydroxide, sodium hydroxide, and so forth) Hydrofluoric acid, see below.	Skin and mucous membranes.	Irritant and corrosive local effects that cause burns of exposed tissues. Symptoms include: Respiratory: irritation, burns, edema of the airway and lungs, laryngospasm, dysphonia/aphonia Cardiovascular: tachycardia, hypovolemia, hypotension, dysrhythmia Nervous system: confusion, coma, methemoglobinemia (some oxidizers) or hypocalcemia (phosphorous, hydrofluoric acid) Skin, gastrointestinal system, eyes and mucous membranes: local corrosive effects, perforation Acids: coagulation necrosis Bases: liquefaction necrosis Hydrofluoric acid: reacts with calcium and magnesium	Remove clothing, and decontaminate with large amounts of water (or, for eyes, use sterile saline and Morgan lenses with topical anesthesia if available). In general, chemical burn blisters should be broken to release any entrapped chemical. Administer oxygen for respiratory contamination. Supportive care. Early endotracheal intubation may be required. Administer albuterol for bronchospasm.

| Corrosive | Hydrogen fluoride (hydrofluoric acid) | Inhalation, skin/eye contact or ingestion. Contact a toxicologist for assistance in management. | Irritating to skin, eyes, and mucous membranes. Inhalation may cause respiratory irritation or hemorrhage. Systemic effects include nausea, vomiting, gastric pain, cardiac arrhythmia. Dermal effects include pain, redness, and deep, slow healing burns with pain out of proportion to physical appearance. Exposure to dilute solution (10%) may result in delayed onset of symptoms (~6 h postexposure). Hypocalcemia may result from dermal exposure and may cause tetany, decreased myocardial contractility and cardiovascular collapse. Systemic hypocalcemia and even cardiac arrest may result when exposure is ingestion or topical exposure to 20% hydrofluoric acid over 20% or more body surface area. | Remove clothing because secondary contamination or off-gassing may occur. Supportive care and/or endotracheal intubation may be required. Treat arrhythmias with calcium and per advanced cardiovascular life support protocol. Irrigate irritated eyes with water or saline for at least 20 min. DO NOT induce emesis. DO NOT administer activated charcoal. Treat ingestions with 4–8 oz milk or water. Treat hypocalcemia with calcium gluconate or calcium chloride solution intravenously. Treat skin exposures with topical calcium gluconate gel. If pain persists >30 min. intra-arterial treatment with calcium gluconate may be indicated. Inhalation burns may require treatment with nebulized calcium gluconate 2.5%. |

(continued on next page)

Table 4
(continued)

Toxidrome	Typical Toxicants	Predominant Route of Exposure	Typical Symptoms	Treatment
Hydrocarbons and halogenated hydrocarbons	Chloroform, gasoline, propane, toluene, trichloroethylene	Inhalation of gases or vapors.	Inhalation can cause sleepiness to the point of narcosis (stupor and/or coma) and cardiac irritability. Hypoxia, narcosis, coma, sudden cardiac death caused by myocardial sensitization to endogenous catecholamines ("sudden sniffing death"). Aspiration or chemical pneumonitis. Cough, hypoxemia; nausea and vomiting if ingested. Defatting dermatitis.	Remove clothing, and decontaminate with water and mild liquid detergent (or, for eyes, use sterile saline and Morgan lenses with topical anesthesia if available). Administer oxygen as indicated. Supportive care. Avoid epinephrine where possible because of myocardial sensitization. Endotracheal intubation may be required. β-Blocker may be indicated for significant, persistent ventricular irritability induced by hydrocarbons. Consult a toxicologist and keep patients calm.
Seizures	Hydrazines (jet or rocket fuel)	Corrosive or irritating to the eyes, skin, nose, mucous membranes, throat and respiratory system. Seizures may present after ingestion.	Seizures	Supportive care. Benzodiazepines, barbiturates and/or propofol. Pyridoxine (vitamin B_6) in gram amounts for hydrazine ingestion. Hydrazine-induced seizures may be resistant to usual anticonvulsants and respond only to pyridoxine therapy.

Acidosis	Methanol (solvent or fuel)	Toxic exposure may occur by ingestion, inhalation or dermal routes.	Intoxication, acidosis, visual symptoms	Fomepizole or ethanol block metabolism to toxic metabolites. Supportive care. Dialysis may be indicated. Folate should be supplemented.
	Ethylene glycol (antifreeze, other)	Most exposures occur from the ingestion of antifreeze.	Intoxication, acidosis, crystaluria, renal failure	Fomepizole or ethanol blocks metabolism to toxic metabolites. Supportive care. Dialysis may be indicated. Pyridoxine and thiamine should be supplemented.
Hemolysis	Arsine (semiconductor manufacture, other)	Inhalation; Arsine is a highly toxic gas at extremely low concentrations.	Hemolysis	Supportive care. Exchange transfusion for plasma free hemoglobin level above 1.5 g/dL. No specific antidote.
Blister agents (vesicants)	Sulfur mustard (mustard gas, "H" agents)	Skin, eyes, inhalation. Damages DNA.	Delayed symptoms within 2–48 h. Red, itching skin leading to blisters. Irritated eyes, runny nose, hoarseness, cough, diarrhea, fever, nausea, vomiting. Bone marrow suppression may occur days later (radiomimetic effect).	Remove clothes that may be contaminated. Immediately wash area thoroughly, and flush eyes. Treatment is supportive. No antidote. Granulocyte colony–stimulating factor for bone marrow suppression.
Blister agents (vesicants)	Nitrogen mustard	Skin, eyes, inhalation. Damages DNA.	Delayed symptoms within several hours after exposure. Similar symptoms to sulfur mustard.	Remove clothes that may be contaminated. Immediately wash area thoroughly, and flush eyes. Treatment is supportive. No antidote. Granulocyte colony–stimulating factor for bone marrow suppression.

(continued on next page)

Table 4
(continued)

Toxidrome	Typical Toxicants	Predominant Route of Exposure	Typical Symptoms	Treatment
Blister agents (vesicants)	Lewisite	Exposure through skin, eyes, inhalation.	Delayed symptoms within several hours after exposure. Similar symptoms to sulfur mustard. Can produce arsenic-like effects (low blood pressure, vomiting, diarrhea).	Remove clothes that may be contaminated. Immediately wash area thoroughly, and flush eyes. Treatment is supportive. Rapid topical administration of dimercaprol may prevent effects.
Blister agents (vesicants)	Phosgene oxime	Exposure through skin, eyes, inhalation causes severe irritation.	Immediately irritating, almost unbearable pain on contact. Severe itching followed by blanching, then red rings. Hives within 24 h, followed by skin becoming brown with scab formation. Does not cause blisters. Effect on eyes and lungs similar to sulfur mustard.	Remove clothes that may be contaminated. Immediately wash area thoroughly, and flush eyes. Treatment is supportive. No antidote.

Data from Walter FG. Advanced hazmat life support provider manual. 4th edition. Tucson (AZ): University of Arizona Press; 2014; and Tomassoni AJ, Smith D. Chemical guidelines: a quick guide to the management of disasters. Yale-New Haven Health System – Center for Emergency Preparedness and Disaster Response; New Haven (CT); 2007. Available at: http://yalenewhavenhealth.org/emergency/WhatWeDo/ClinicalGuidelines.html. Accessed August 22, 2014.

Table 5
Antidotes to selected toxicants

Antidote	Rationale and Guidelines	Comments
Amyl nitrite	For cyanide poisoning to initiate care while establishing IV access for sodium nitrite and sodium thiosulfate. Nitrites induce methemoglobinemia to facilitate removal of cyanide from cytochrome oxidase. See also sodium nitrite below.	Amyl nitrite is volatile and flammable. Avoid accidental inhalation. Use caution in dosing to avoid hypoxemia from excessive methemoglobinemia. May cause hypotension.
Atropine	For organophosphate and carbamate poisoning. Blocks effects of acetylcholine excess. Potentially lifesaving. Titrate to respiratory signs and symptoms, not pupillary size. Treat only for symptoms, not potential exposure in asymptomatic patients, unless directed by a medical toxicologist/poison center. Endotracheal intubation and/or airway suction may also be indicated in severe poisoning. IV route preferred; may be administered IM.	Initial dose may be guided by severity of symptoms. If no response to initial dose, double the dose and proceed as above. Because of acetylcholinesterase inhibition total doses may be much higher than ordinary maximum doses of 2–3 mg. Reevaluate frequently. Titrate additional atropine to respiratory signs and symptoms.
Diazepam	For treatment of seizure. Raises seizure threshold. Other benzodiazepines may be substituted. Consider prophylactic use in organophosphate and hydrazine exposures.	May necessitate endotracheal intubation. Phenytoin and derivatives are not likely to terminate toxicant seizures and may worsen toxicant sodium channel blockade.
Fomepizole	For treatment of toxic alcohol ingestion. Inhibits metabolism of methanol or ethylene glycol to toxic metabolites via inhibition of alcohol dehydrogenase.	Dosing frequency must be increased during hemodialysis. Also, if last dose was >6 h from initiation of dialysis, give dose at initiation of dialysis.
Hydroxocobalamin	An alternative to the nitrite/thiosulfate treatment for cyanide poisoning. A form of vitamin B_{12} that accepts cyanide and is water soluble for renal elimination of the toxicant complex.	Initial dose is usually infused over 15 min but may be given IV push (off label) in cardiac arrest. May color mucus membranes and body fluids red. Do not infuse at the same time or site with sodium thiosulfate.
Methylene blue	A redox chemical used as a reversal agent for methemoglobinemia. Methemoglobinemia may result from many chemical exposures, and is occasionally encountered as the result of an idiosyncratic reaction to topical local anesthetics, such as benzocaine.	May cause additional methemoglobinemia, especially at high doses. Those without cardiorespiratory symptoms and/or methemoglobin <30% rarely require treatment. Contradiction: known glucose-6 phosphate dehydrogenase deficiency.

(continued on next page)

Table 5 (continued)		
Antidote	Rationale and Guidelines	Comments
Pralidoxime (2-PAM)	For organophosphate poisoning and carbamate poisoning with agents other than carbaryl. Used in conjunction with atropine. Reverses binding of organophosphate to acetylcholinesterase. Administration in the absence of poisoning may cause hypertension. IV route preferable to IM route.	Dose may be tailored to severity of poisoning. Ongoing treatment: Reevaluate frequently. Titrate additional pralidoxime in consultation with toxicologist/poison center for patients with persistent signs of poisoning.
Pyridoxine (vitamin B$_6$)	For hydrazine poisoning. Cofactor for pyridoxal phosphate facilitating antiepileptic effects of γ-aminobutyric acid. Coadminister benzodiazepine of choice.	Maximum adult dose 5 g or 70 mg/kg infused IV at 0.5 g/min until seizures terminate, then infuse remainder over 4–6 h.
Sodium nitrite	For cyanide poisoning. Causes conversion of hemoglobin/cyanohemoglobin to methemoglobin/cyanomethemoglobin, which facilitates removal of cyanide from cytochrome oxidase to improve oxidative phosphorylation and yields cyanide to thiosulfate.	May cause hypotension. One half of the initial dose may be repeated in 2 h for inadequate clinical improvement or for prophylaxis. Reduce dose if significant anemia is present. Follow immediately with sodium thiosulfate as below.
Sodium thiosulfate	For cyanide poisoning. Accepts cyanide moiety from cyanomethemoglobin to yield methemoglobin (which undergoes endogenous conversion to hemoglobin) and the less toxic thiocyanate, which undergoes renal elimination.	May cause nausea and vomiting. May use same IV catheter and vein as for sodium nitrite administration. May repeat at half the initial dose if symptoms recur or at 2 h for prophylaxis.

Abbreviations: IM, intramuscular; IV, intravenous.

Data from Yale-New Haven Health System – Center for Emergency Preparedness and Disaster Response. 2007. Available at: http://yalenewhavenhealth.org/emergency/WhatWeDo/ClinicalGuidelines.html. Accessed August 22, 2014.

Selected Specific Hazardous Industrial Chemicals

In addition to the agents discussed in the text and tables, many additional agents may be encountered by the clinician. Some notable examples are listed in **Table 6**.

SPECIAL CONSIDERATIONS

Children and pregnant women are routinely exposed to hundreds of chemicals through their environment. Only a relative few of these chemicals have been identified as harmful in small doses. Children may be especially vulnerable to the toxic effects of chemicals. Exposure to some chemicals at specific stages of development may have long-term impact on health and cognitive development. Notable examples include

Table 6

Selected hazards associated with some common industrial chemicals

Class/Agent	Examples	Selected Actions and Comments
Acrylamide	Neurotoxic; reproductive toxicity in males; developmental toxicity	Carcinogenic; also a component of tobacco smoke and high carbohydrate foods cooked at high temperature (eg, French fries)
Aniline	Methemoglobinemia	Methylene blue is antidotal
Arsine (g)	Arsine results from reaction of arsenic with an acid	Hemolysis after inhalation; may require exchange transfusion. May be generated in the etching of As-doped silicon wafers with HF in the manufacture of semiconductors
Asbestos	Crocidolite form ("blue asbestos")	Mesothelioma
Azides	NaN_3 $Pb(N_3)_2$ Organic azides	Explosophoric and toxic (similar to cyanide but without antidote); NaN_3 is used in automotive airbags and decomposes explosively to Na and $N_2(g)$
Beryllium	Inhalation of beryllium particles in aerospace and other high-tech industry	Sensitization and lung disease
Carbon disulfide		Neurotoxic at high exposure levels and with long-term exposure
Carcinogens	Numerous chemical have been identified as carcinogens. US Department of Health and Human Services released the 12th Report on Carcinogens on June 10, 2011.	The Report is available at: http://ntp.niehs.nih.gov/pubhealth/roc/roc12/index.html The 13th Report is in progress.

(continued on next page)

Table 6
(continued)

Class/Agent	Examples	Selected Actions and Comments
Formaldehyde		Dermal, gastrointestinal, immunologic, respiratory (nose to lungs) effects
		Known to be a human carcinogen
Heavy metals	Arsenic (As)	As^{+3} (inorganic) nausea, vomiting, diarrhea, abdominal pain, multisystem organ failure (liver, kidney, cardiovascular shock), neuropathy and neurotoxicity; hematopoietic effects; dermal changes with long-term exposure; carcinogenic; chelating agents include dimercaprol (BAL), dimercaptopropane sulfonate (DMPS), and succimer (DMSA)
		As^{+5} (organified) nontoxic "dietary arsenic," often as arsenobetaine or arsenocholine from shellfish and ground fish. Although some interconversion of As species occurs in vivo chelation is not usually indicated.
	Cadmium	Cardiovascular developmental, gastrointestinal, neurologic, renal, reproductive, and respiratory effects. May cause necrosis of nasal septum.
	Lead	Nausea, vomiting, headache, hypertension, anemia/basophilic red blood cell stippling; musculoskeletal effects, neurotoxic, nephrotoxic reproductive toxicity; potentially carcinogenic; chelating agents include penicillamine, BAL, ethylenediaminetetraacetic acid, and succimer
	Mercury (Hg)	Hg^0 Pulmonary toxicity via inhalation of metallic mercury vapor
		$HgCl_2$ gastrointestinal toxicity and multisystem organ failure by ingestion
		Methyl Hg, neurotoxic after dietary or other ingestion, Minamata disease
		Like other heavy metals, Hg is also nephrotoxic
Halogenated hydrocarbons (see also **Table 3**)	Carbon tetrachloride (tetrachloromethane)	Centrilobular necrosis and fatty liver secondary to interference with apolipoprotein synthesis and fatty acid oxidation
	Trichloroethylene	"Degreaser's flush" disulfiram reaction
n-Hexane		Neuro (peripheral neuropathy) and reproductive toxicity; has been abused as an inhalant

Insecticides	Carbamates	See **Table 3**
	Organochlorines	Lindane, chlordane: seizures in acute transdermal exposure/ingestions secondary to γ-aminobutyric acid antagonism; blood disorders, dizziness, headaches, endocrine effects (sex hormones)
	Organophosphates	See **Table 3**
	Pyrethrins and pyrethroids	High levels of exposure are required to produce effects and second-generation pyrethroids are more toxic than first-generation; dizziness, headache, nausea, muscle twitching, reduced energy, altered mental status, seizures and loss of consciousness; persons with hay fever may be allergic
	Anticoagulant rodenticides (warfarins and super warfarins, such as brodifacoum)	Vitamin K antagonists: monitor international normalized ratio and administer vitamin K only if international normalized ratio rises after exposure; reverse anticoagulation with fresh frozen plasma if active bleeding
Phenol		Causes burns and anesthesia on dermal contact. Decontaminate with polyethylene glycol (MW $\sim$ 300–400) if available, glycerol or isopropanol is a less desirable alternative. In all cases irrigate with copious amounts of decontamination agents or soap and water; ingestion of small amounts may be highly corrosive and lethal.
Phosphine		Exposures via inhalation of phosphine or ingestion of metallic phosphides; dermal exposure may cause systemic effects; flammable and explosive yielding dense fumes of phosphorous pentoxide (strong respiratory irritant); fishy or garlic-like odor, but odor is not sufficient to reliably warn of dangerous concentrations
		Phosphine is a respiratory tract irritant; may cause peripheral vascular collapse, cardiac arrest, heart failure, and pulmonary edema

Data from ATSDR Toxic Substances Portal. Available at: http://www.atsdr.cdc.gov/substances/toxsubstance.asp?toxid=236. Accessed July 26, 2014.

Table 7	
Potential chemical hazards by industry	
Industry	**Some Potential Hazards**
Aerospace industry	Hydrazines in fuel; epoxy, phenolic, amino, bismaleimide, styrene and polyurethane resins and dianiline hardeners; solvents; heavy metals; graphite fibers
Agriculture	Numerous herbicides and insecticides (some potentially carcinogenic); immunologic and nonimmunologic pulmonary insults, mycotoxins, infectious agents, NH_3, H_2S, CO, CO_2, ozone, methane, chlorine, SO_2, NO, NO_2, particulates; soil, air, and groundwater contaminants
Art	Heavy metals, epoxies and polymers; styrene, peroxides; exotic wood dusts; stone dusts; solvents including benzene, methanol, ketones, methylene chloride; vinyls, asbestos, acids
Firefighting	CO, CO_2, HCl, SO_2 and other acids, HCN, NO_2, NH_3, particulates, heavy metals, acrolein, acrylonitrile, benzene, benzopyrene, chlorine, formaldehyde, vinyl chloride, hydrocarbons, aromatic, and substituted hydrocarbons
Hazardous waste facilities and incinerators	Potential carcinogens, immunotoxins; metals; potential water and soil contaminants; dioxins and furans
Laboratories	Chemistry/manufacturing: numerous including cyanides, azides; Pathology: toluene, xylene, formaldehyde Biotechnology/microbiology: fungi, phenol, glutaraldehyde and other sterilants, anesthetic gases, viruses and bacteria, allergens and sensitizing agents, acids/bases, cyanogen bromide, dimethyl sulfoxide
Metalworking	Heavy metals Metal oxides, including vaporized zinc oxide (metal fume fever/smelters' ague)
Plastic manufacturing	Phenol, formaldehyde, ammonia, CO, vinyl chloride, dioxins, furans, styrene, cyanide, diisocyanate and other isocyanates, aldehydes, NO_2, hydrofluoric acid, phosgene, carbonyl fluoride, perfluoroisobutylene, HCl, acrolein, acrylonitrile; polymer fume fever (polytetrafluoroethylene decomposition); epoxy resins (contact dermatitis)
Pulp and paper manufacturing	H_2S, mercaptans, sulfides, chlorine, chlorine dioxide, hypochlorite, calcium oxide, SO_2, chloroform and other volatile organics, dioxins, polychlorinated dibenzofuran, particulates
Rubber manufacturing	Solvents, phenols, formaldehyde, ZnO, sulfur donors, peroxides, diisocyanates, organic acids, carbon black/furnace black with polycyclic aromatic hydrocarbons; thiurams and other accelerators and curing agents may be carcinogenic
Semiconductor manufacturing	Noteworthy: glycol ethers; gallium arsenide dust; gases including arsine, phosphine, and others; hydrofluoric acid. Also: nitric/acetic/hydrochloric/hydrofluoric acids; metallo-organics; diborane; silanes; photoresists; sodium/potassium hydroxide; fires/halon; chlorine, bromine trichloroboron, trifluorocarbon, tetrafluorocarbon, tetrachlorocarbon, dichloromethane, methanol, phenol, hydrazine, others
Sewer/wastewater facilities	Cleaners/disinfectants, solvents, pesticides, chlorine, ferric chloride, aluminum sulfate, laboratory reagents including KI and $K_2Cr_2O_7$, H_2S, CO, CO_2, methane, NH_3, disposed industrial waste chemicals
Shipbuilding	Asbestos, man-made mineral fibers, metals and metal oxides, nitrogen dioxide, ozone, chromates, solvents, paints, particulates, wood dust, confined spaces

Data from Sullivan JB, Krieger GR Jr, editors. Hazardous materials toxicology: clinical principles of environmental health. Baltimore (MD): Williams and Wilkins; 1992.

identified teratogens that may cause birth defects, carcinogens, and heavy metals (including lead, arsenic, and mercury). Air pollutants may impact short- and long-term respiratory health. Chemicals introduced into the food supply naturally (eg, mycotoxins) or by design (eg, pesticides) are also of concern.

Although some chemicals and their risks have been well described, insufficient data and research methodology regarding potential chemical exposure risks to developing fetuses and children remain for many common chemicals. The most conservative approach may be to assume an exposure elimination-minimization or "safety first" position regarding exposures for pregnant women and children (actually a wise approach for all). Strategies for minimizing exposure include fresh (not canned, plastic packaged, or preserved) foods in the diet; avoiding vapors from solvents and paints; and minimizing the use of over-the-counter and herbal medications, tobacco, alcohol, and even personal care products.[23] Strategies also include avoidance of exposure in the workplace through job selection; environmental controls; use of PPE; and avoidance of transferring chemicals from the workplace to home on one's person, clothing, and vehicle.

Following chemical exposures, counseling by a toxicologist, occupational medicine specialist, and/or genetic counselor or obstetrician or other specialist may provide specific information regarding risk, and it is hoped, reassurance (**Table 7**).

SUMMARY

Emergency care providers have a unique role and share the responsibility of becoming well-versed in the recognition, treatment, mitigation, and prevention of exposures to hazardous industrial chemicals.

Hazard mitigation and advanced preparation for potential chemical accidents can help to minimize risk and optimize response when events occur. Astute clinicians are invited to facilitate this work on a local and regional scale and to take an active role in antidote stewardship. Preparations should be based on local and regional hazard vulnerability analysis. Such analysis should be based on real risks associated with past chemical events (they may occur again), current chemical inventories for fixed facilities, and chemicals in transit. Risks may be offset by mitigation, including such preparations as responder education, preparation for mass decontamination, and antidote stockpiling and distribution mechanisms.

REFERENCES

1. Urbina I. Think those chemicals have been tested? New York Times 2013.
2. Auf der Heide E. Disaster response: principles of preparation and coordination. Mosby; 1989. Available at: http://sheltercentre.org/sites/default/files/CVMosby_DisasterResponsePrinciples.pdf.
3. Marshall L, Weir E, Abelsohn A, et al. Identifying and managing adverse environmental health effects: 1. Taking an exposure history [comment]. CMAJ 2002; 166(8):1049–55.
4. Thompson JN, Brodkin CA, Kyes K, et al. Use of a questionnaire to improve occupational and environmental history taking in primary care physicians. J Occup Environ Med 2000;42(12):1188–94.
5. Wisnewski AV, Xu L, Robinson E, et al. Immune sensitization to methylene diphenyl diisocyanate (MDI) resulting from skin exposure: albumin as a carrier protein connecting skin exposure to subsequent respiratory responses. J Occup Med Toxicol 2011;6:6. http://dx.doi.org/10.1186/1745-6673-6-6.

6. Madhya Pradesh Government: Bhopal gas tragedy relief and rehabilitation department, Bhopal. Available at: Mp.gov.in. Accessed August 28, 2012.

7. Dubey AK. Bhopal gas tragedy: 92% injuries termed "minor". First 14 News. Available at: http://www.first14.com/bhopal-gas-tragedy-92-injuries-termed-minor-822.html. Archived 26 June 2010 and Accessed July 12, 2014.

8. Broughton E. The Bhopal disaster and its aftermath: a review. Environ Health 2005; 4:6. http://dx.doi.org/10.1186/1476-069X-4-6 BioMed Central 10 May 2005. Available at: http://www.ncbi.nlm.nih.gov/pmc/articles/PMC1142333/. Accessed July 13, 2014.

9. Eckerman I. The Bhopal Saga- causes and consequences of the world's largest industrial disaster. Hyderabad, India: Universities Press; 2005. ISBN 81-7371-515-7.

10. US EPA Technology Transfer Network – Air toxics website. Available at: http://www.epa.gov/ttn/atw/hlthef/methylis.html. Accessed July 13, 2014.

11. Goldman RH, Peters JM. The occupational and environmental health history. JAMA 1981;246(24):2831–6.

12. Erikson K. Toxic reckoning: business faces a new kind of fear. Harv Bus Rev 1990;1:118–26.

13. Ballantyne B, Sullivan JB. Basic principles of toxicology. In: Sullivan JB, Krieger GR Jr, editors. Hazardous materials toxicology: clinical principles of environmental health. Baltimore (MD): Williams and Wilkins; 1992. p. 2–8.

14. Ballantyne B. Exposure-dose-response relationships. In: Sullivan JB, Krieger GR Jr, editors. Hazardous materials toxicology: clinical principles of environmental health. Baltimore (MD): Williams and Wilkins; 1992. p. 24–30.

15. Luckey TD. Radiation hormesis: the good, the bad, and the ugly. Dose Response 2006;4(3):169–90. http://dx.doi.org/10.2203/dose-response.06-102.Luckey.

16. Castell JV, Donato MT, Gomez-Lechon MJ. Metabolism and bioactivation of toxicants in the lung. The in vitro cellular approach. Exp Toxicol Pathol 2005;57:189–204. Available at: http://www.uv.es/jcastell/Metabolism_and_bioactivation.pdf.

17. Ioannides C, Lewis DF. Cytochromes in the bioactivation of chemicals. Curr Top Med Chem 2004;4:1767–88.

18. ATDSR taking an exposure history. Available at: http://www.atsdr.cdc.gov/csem/exphistory/docs/exposure_history.pdf. Accessed June 23, 2014.

19. OSHA. Personal protective equipment. Available at: https://www.osha.gov/Publications/osha3151.html. Accessed July 26, 2014.

20. Mofenson HC, Greensher J. The nontoxic ingestion. Pediatr Clin North Am 1970; 17(3):583–90.

21. Tomassoni AJ, Bogdan G, Sinha V, et al. Toxicologic hazard vulnerability analysis: a timely tool. Clin Toxicol 2011;49(6):600–1 [abstract: 260].

22. Dart RC, Borron SW, Caravati EM, et al. Expert consensus guidelines for stocking of antidotes in hospitals that provide emergency care. Ann Emerg Med 2009; 54(3):386–94.

23. Royal College of Obstetricians and Gynaecologists. Chemical exposures during pregnancy: dealing with potential, but unproven, risks to child health. Scientific Impact Paper No. 37. May, 2013. Available at: http://www.rcog.org.uk/files/rcog-corp/5.6.13ChemicalExposures.pdf. Accessed August 25, 2014.

Hospital Preparedness for Chemical and Radiological Disasters

Brooks L. Moore, MD*, Robert J. Geller, MD,
Charlotte Clark, CEMHP

KEYWORDS

• Hospital preparedness • Chemical injuries • Radiological injuries

KEY POINTS

• Disaster planning can be broken into 4 phases: mitigation, preparation, response, and recovery.

• Although some other types of disasters like hurricanes and tornadoes may be more frequent, chemical and radiological emergencies have the potential for major disruptions to clinical care, owing to their rarity and to their psychological impact on victims and emergency responders.

• Hospitals should prepare and train a decontamination team and set up a decontamination area complete with a shower with a separate ventilation system.

• Every hospital needs to have a variety of antidotes for toxicants in-house and should incorporate a strategy for urgent acquisition of antidotes from other sources, such as nearby hospitals and regional wholesalers. The role and abilities of the Strategic National Stockpile should be carefully evaluated before blithely delegating responsibility to the Strategic National Stockpile in their response plans.

OVERVIEW

The past 2 decades have seen a transformation of our health care system from one in which only 6% of hospitals in a survey[1] reported readiness to receive patients from a sarin exposure to one in which 99% of responders stated a readiness for both chemical and radiological event casualties.[2] Yet, for all of the focus on systemic preparation for these events, there is still widespread discomfort by individuals within the health care system to address the events. Indeed, there has been little correlation with the development of disaster plans and the competency levels of those entrusted to carry out the plans.[3,4] This article seeks to address some of these concerns. In the course of

Department of Emergency Medicine and Grady Health System, Emory University, 49 Jesse Hill Jr Drive SE, Atlanta, GA 30303, USA
* Corresponding author.
E-mail address: bmoor02@emory.edu

Emerg Med Clin N Am 33 (2015) 37–49
http://dx.doi.org/10.1016/j.emc.2014.09.005
0733-8627/15/$ – see front matter © 2015 Elsevier Inc. All rights reserved.

this article, the authors discuss disaster planning in general, with a focus on conducting a hazard-vulnerability analysis for chemical and radiological dangers. The authors article discusses what medications to stockpile for treatment of the most common chemical and radiological exposures. Finally, the authors discuss how to set up appropriate triage and treatment, focusing on establishing an effective decontamination team.

HOSPITAL PREPAREDNESS

The concept of hospital disaster preparedness in the United States extends back to Cold War preparations for nuclear casualties in the 1950s. Under the Federal Civil Defense Administration, a massive disaster response capacity was created, encompassing specialized training through medical schools, rapidly deployable hospital beds, and civilian defense shelters.[5] The system was largely dismantled in the 1970s, only to see reconstitution in various forms in following decades. The modern era of domestic preparedness began in 1986, with the Emergency Planning and Community Right-to-Know Act. It continued with the authorization of the Nunn-Lugar-Domenici National Preparedness Act, in response to the Tokyo sarin attack of 1995. Disaster planning remains a priority, albeit a small one, across many governments today.

THE DISASTER CYCLE

The first decade of the twenty-first century saw the loss of thousands of American lives to the twin horrors of terrorism and natural disaster, such as the attack on the World Trade Center in 2001 and hurricanes Katrina and Rita in 2005. In response, local, state, and federal governments once again invested heavily in the creation of disaster-ready communities. Although every disaster has its own unique characteristics, general planning for disasters can be broken down into discreet phases. These phases are mitigation, preparation, response, and recovery.[6] Although there are several aspects of preparation for chemical and radiological incidents that are unique to those events, a hospital must have a robust ability to respond to disasters in general before any expertise can be reached in these topics.

MITIGATION

The mitigation phase of disaster planning highlights those steps that can be taken to either prevent or, secondarily, minimize the effects of a disaster. This phase is frequently manifested in anticipatory means, such as preparing a building for an earthquake by installing bracing hardware or structural supports. Mitigation can also take less tangible forms, such as gathering intelligence on local hazards or establishing regulations to bring all health care entities within a given geographic area into a unified planning and response framework.

United States National Regulatory Requirements

The Joint Commission mandates that every hospital have a designated emergency manager, and an all-hazards emergency response plan.[7] Plans must address several key areas (communications, resources and assets, security and safety, staff, utilities, patients, and volunteers). The Joint Commission recommends that hospitals create specific management plans for chemical and radiological emergencies and that a specific contact person with expertise in these areas be designated.

In addition, plans must comply with the Federally sanctioned National Incident Management System (NIMS) created to allow for successful interface between agencies by creating a standard hierarchy of command. Hospital accreditation is contingent on compliance with these rules. For further discussion on the implementation of these regulations, please see www.thejointcommission.org. Compliance with the NIMS process includes the Healthcare Incident Command System (HICS) because HICS is NIMS-based with an additional health care focus, while remaining in the guidelines of the NIMS structure.

The US Occupational Safety and Health Administration (OSHA) has rules regarding the hospital workplace, including rules for the safety of workers involved in decontamination activities. OSHA states, in 29.CFR.1910, that all personnel involved in the decontamination of contaminated patients must wear approved respirators when they are in the process of decontaminating individuals.

The policy requires the use of level C and D respirators (see the article by Holland M, in this issue) in response to chemical hazards to protect the health and safety of all employees by excluding hazardous exposures where possible, and using engineering and administrative controls to minimize hazardous exposures that cannot be eliminated. In some cases, however, such controls will not reduce exposures to safe levels; the use of respiratory protection may be required.

The purpose of this respiratory protection program is to maximize the protection afforded by respirators when they are used. It establishes the procedures necessary to meet the regulatory requirements for use of respiratory protection. This program applies to all employees and contractors who may need to wear respiratory protection because of the nature of their work at the hospital. It applies to the use of all respirators, including filtering facepiece (disposable) respirators, such as the N-95 respirator, for which OSHA requires fit testing annually. The use of the level C respirator, hooded powered air purifying respirators (hooded PAPRs), is important for the more dangerous chemical situations. These respirators do not require fit testing and allow the wearer to have facial hair. The OSHA Respiratory Protection Standard, in 29 CFR 1910.134(e), also requires that all employers obtain, in writing, a medical opinion regarding an employee's ability to wear a respirator. The regulatory requirement applies regardless of whether other medical evaluations are needed under the HAZWOPER (Hazardous Waste Operations and Emergency Response) Standard. It also applies to all types of respirators (including hooded PAPRs), with the exception of filtering facepiece respirators used by the employee on a voluntary basis. An additional medical evaluation is required by paragraph 1910.134(c) (7) under certain circumstances when an increase in the employee's physical activities or the weight of the protective clothing would place an added burden on the employee.

Risk Assessment

Risk assessment begins with a hazards vulnerability analysis (HVA). Conducting an HVA allows a hospital to create an accurate hierarchy of preparatory needs. The HVA consists of ranking a hospital's risk to events by analyzing their probability; magnitude of impact on human, property, and business; and the potential mitigating steps that can be taken internally and externally. Many health care institutions follow the HVA model promulgated by the American Society of Healthcare Engineers to its members. Further detail about the performance of an appropriate HVA is beyond the scope of this article, but excellent recommendations have been published including a spreadsheet tool.[8]

The potential for chemical or radiological exposure is substantial. Each year, more than 10 billion pounds of chemicals are either under management or transported[9]; nearly 3 million radiologically active packages are mailed.[10] Although death or injury from chemical or radiological events still ranks low on the overall frequency of lethality scale, such events could have widespread impact on communities at large, given the general populace's fearful perception of these events. Likewise, given the rarity of these events, it is unlikely that community preparedness plans accurately reflect what would happen or that internal or external partners are adequately prepared for such events.[11] Contrast these likelihoods with more common scenarios, such as internal mechanical failure, hurricane, tornado, or flood, and the risk profile for chemical or radiological events remains significant.

Recognition of a chemical or radiological event may be driven by information provided or may be guided by the presence of clusters of symptoms present in patients arriving for care. These toxic syndromes, or toxidromes, are helpful, though nonspecific, hints that may help to guide further diagnostic and therapeutic maneuvers (**Table 1**).

Communications

In disasters, communications are as vital as they are vulnerable to decline. Hospital public relations should be involved in all aspects of planning for radiological and chemical events with a clear understanding of the hospital response protocols. The hospital's public relations staff should plan with local and regional officials, in advance, who will perform the role of public information officer (PIO) by coordinating and leading media relations for various event scenarios. Draft public statements covering the expected hospital-based response to a disaster should be written and vetted by the hospital emergency manager and subject-matter experts and modified to report the particulars of an event. Hospital staff other than those assigned to the media relations role must be trained to defer all media contacts back to the PIO.

Phone systems are likely to suffer from severe congestion in times of crisis and may not be usable by hospital staff. Backup communications systems, such as pagers, text messaging, or 2-way radio, should be considered; staff should be trained in their use. Local amateur radio operators may also be incorporated as a backup communications system.

Determining a hospital's true daily bed capacity, as well as surge capacity into alternate care sites, should be ascertained well in advance of a disaster. As a significant portion of patients affected by a chemical or radiological release may require admission for either treatment or monitoring, bed capacity in the emergency department and medical/surgical wards should be accurately counted. Patients with burns will require specialty care, as will patients suffering the immunosuppressive effects of chemical or radiological releases. These specialty beds should be tallied, and strong

Table 1 Some toxidromes to consider in the mass-casualty situation	
Substance	Symptoms
Acetylcholinesterase inhibitors (organophosphates, sarin, VX)	Secretions, miosis, vomiting, diarrhea, fasciculations, paralysis, seizures, coma
Asphyxiants (CO, CN, HS)	Headache, fatigue, dizziness, nausea, vomiting, dyspnea, altered mental status, syncope, coma, seizure
Irritants (pepper spray, ammonia, HF, H2SO4)	Bronchospasm, hoarseness, stridor
Radioactive material	Vomiting, delayed-onset skin manifestations
Vesicants (nitrogen mustard)	Skin and mucous membrane reaction

Abbreviations: CO, carbon monoxide; CN, cyanide; HF, hydrogen fluoride; H_2S, hydrogen sulfide; H_2SO4, sulfuric acid.

consideration should be placed on regionalizing the needs of this type of care. Memoranda of understanding should be drafted between regional receiving facilities before disasters regarding their collaboration if the patient volume for any given location proves too great. A reliable means of tracking patients between facilities should be tested and put into regular use.

PREPARATION
Staff Education

As the first point of contact for many incoming patients, the emergency department is particularly vulnerable to the hazards of secondary contamination (contamination brought into the facility on the patients). Consequently, emergency managers should train a wide array of emergency department support staff to recognize the symptoms of chemical and radiological exposure. Specifically, staff should be trained to recognize the symptoms of patients exposed to asphyxiants, acetylcholinesterase inhibitors, irritants, and vesicants.[12] Job action sheets should be created to instruct staff on the steps they should take after encountering a patient with possible chemical exposure. The names and contact information for subject-matter experts for chemical and radiological exposures should be compiled and shared with relevant individuals. Drills and refresher courses should be offered on these topics no less than once a year. Hospitals accredited by the Joint Commission in the United States are required to hold at least 2 exercises annually, one of which must extend to involve community partners. A real event may substitute for an exercise.

Decontamination Teams

Past experiences have shown that most victims present to the hospital before decontamination on the scene.[13] The Joint Commission mandates that all hospitals have the capability to respond to either internal or external chemical and radiological threats. Staffing a decontamination team can present a logistical challenge to many hospitals. Mounting a full traditional response capability in a large metropolitan hospital may require up to 40 personnel with a significant level of training in order to retain timely responsiveness,[14] which is impractical or impossible. This logistical problem has led to the exploration of other mass decontamination strategies, such as a drenching water system.[15] In order to construct a program of the appropriate size for any given institution, the scope of the operation must be taken into account. Although most incidents involve only one or 2 patients, the risk to the facility and its staff from larger events remains a concern. Most facilities will opt to create a team of providers to respond to internal disasters and to those patients who either self-transport or are brought to the hospital after decontamination.[16]

A decontamination teams should have at its core a team leader, safety officer, triage unit leader, and decontamination team members.[17] Team members should have basic training in the use of personal protective equipment (PPE) (at least to level C if they will be performing only hospital-based decontamination for patients arriving at the hospital), the proper decontamination procedure, and a broader understanding of incident command and communication. Team members who may be filling a wider role may benefit from training in the use of higher levels of PPE. There are many forms of free and fee-based instruction available to participants. Emergency managers should make appropriate efforts to conduct refresher training, retention of staff, and expansion of the team's skill base in response to the specific hazards identified in the local community.[17]

Personal Protective Equipment

The choice of PPE for a given chemical or radiological emergency is discussed fully in other chapters. Briefly, OSHA mandates 4 levels of protection when encountering potential chemical or radiological toxins:

Level A: totally encapsulating chemical suit with self-contained breathing apparatus
Level B: independent breathing apparatus with chemical-resistant outer clothing
Level C: chemical resistant clothing with air purifiers
Level D: standard work uniform designed to protect from nuisance exposures

Research has demonstrated that unless a hospital is the site of the hazardous material release or is specifically targeted as the victim of an attack, Level C PPE should be adequate for protection in most cases of exposure.[18] Untrained responders should not be allowed to wear advanced protective equipment, as this may result in unintended exposure or dangerous worker fatigue and heat stress. The individual assigned to the event team as the Safety Officer should monitor all personnel, especially those wearing PPE, for signs and symptoms of fatigue, heat stress, and other illness.

Decontamination: Showers (See Also Holland M, for Further Information on Decontamination)

Time to initial decontamination is a critical factor in limiting a patient's exposure to either chemical or radiological exposure.[19] Removal of contaminated clothing and contact with a water rinse are considered mandatory for all chemical and radiological exposures (with the possible exception of isolated gas exposures). To limit the time required to establish patient decontamination, a predesignated area of the hospital should be determined to initiate decontamination. The area should have an entrance isolated from the remainder of the hospital. It should be easily demarcated between a contaminated zone used for decontamination and a clean zone where patients are treated after decontamination. As a means of saving time and simplifying the steps needed to initiate a decontamination line, many facilities have fixed shower facilities in nearby structures, such as parking lots.[20] Planning should address the need to provide separate facilities for men and women and for the need for a strategy to decontaminate nonambulatory patients.

Treatment: Stocking Antidotes, Strategic National Stockpile Resources

Antidotes may be considered to be those pharmaceutical agents used to counteract the effects of one or more toxic compounds. For the purpose of this article, only those antidotes used in the management of chemical or radiological events are considered. More information about other antidotes is readily available.[21–23]

Every hospital should aspire to stock a sufficient amount of each antidote needed for the treatment of potential life-threatening effects of chemical or radiological events. This task is daunting, given the wide scope of possible events and the unknown number of victims that could present in a short window of time. Furthermore, many of these antidotes are expensive and have a limited shelf life, resulting in the likelihood that they will expire on the shelf, never used. Multiple assessments of antidotes stocking by hospitals in many different settings have reached the same conclusion: hospitals fail to stock all antidotes in sufficient quantities for mass disaster.[24–27]

Most hospitals, therefore, resort to a strategy of stocking only a limited supply of antidotes most likely to be needed, with a plan of how to promptly access other antidotes if needed. A reasonable benchmark used is to stock enough antidotes needed for life-sustaining therapy for high-risk events to treat 2 patients for 1 day, with a pre-determined strategy for rapid restocking, unless hazard vulnerability analysis indicates an increased risk for a specific chemical or radiological event.[28,29] Several consensus guidelines for antidote stocking have been created to guide these stocking decisions.[22,23]

At a minimum, every hospital should aim to stock the drugs shown in **Table 2** for the treatment of chemical or radiological events. Many other antidotes are desirable to stock but less essential, either because one of the aforementioned agents may be an alternative or because of the difficulty obtaining them. Further discussion of the relative merits of various antidotes may be found in the consensus guidelines[23] and by discussing these issues with the leadership of the poison center serving your community.[29]

Potassium iodide deserves special mention. Potassium iodide given promptly after substantial exposure to radioactive iodine has been demonstrated to reduce the long-term risk of thyroid cancer.[30,31] Although this is a prudent public health measure for immediate postexposure use, it is extremely difficult to maintain current stocks in each home and business in a large area; the presence of this agent in such a large number of sites poses a potential risk for accidental or intentional misuse. Because this agent is not truly an antidote used in hospital preparedness, it is not included in the aforementioned table. Other antidotes used for contamination with radioactive material like Prussian blue and calcium and zinc diethylenetriamine pentaacetic acid are covered in article by Kazzi and colleagues, in this issue.

Table 2
Suggested minimum antidote stocking

Antidote	Minimum Recommended Stocking Amount for Most Hospitals
Atropine 1 mg/mL	16 mg
Dextrose 50%	100 mL
Diazepam 5 mg/mL	40 mg
Hydroxocobalamin, plus sodium thiosulfate (or an alternative cyanide treatment)	4 Kits
Methylene blue 10 mg/mL, 10 mL ampules/vials	8 Units
Naloxone, 1 mg/mL preferred; 0.4 mg/mL alternate	16 mg
Pralidoxime, 1-g vial	4 gm
Pyridoxine, 100 mg/mL in 1- or 10-mL vials	10 gm
Succimer, 100-mg capsules	1800 mg
Prussian blue, 500 mg/capsule (binds cesium, thallium)	Ideally, it is stocked by every hospital; based on 3000 mg given orally 3 times daily, at least 12 capsules. However, given the difficulty often experienced in stocking it before an event, hospitals may wish to establish a strategy for its rapid procurement but decide not to stock it.

This table assumes stocking enough antidote for high-risk chemical or radiological events to treat 2 patients for 1 day, with a predetermined strategy for rapid restocking, unless HVA indicates an increased risk for a specific chemical or radiological event. More extensive discussion appears in published consensus documents.[29]

Even a hospital that meets these stocking benchmarks may occasionally be presented with an overwhelmingly large influx of patients requiring these agents. In the United States, 2 programs have been created to address these situations. One is the Strategic National Stockpile (SNS) and the other is the Chempack program; both programs are managed by the Centers for Disease Control and Prevention.

The SNS[32–37] aims to maintain a comprehensive stock of medical supplies to address catastrophic disasters, ranging from intravenous catheters to bandages, isolation masks, and pharmaceuticals. Some of this material is already in storage at undisclosed locations nationwide, and others are accessible as vendor-managed inventory through special arrangements with various vendors. SNS supplies are designed to be available anywhere in the continental United States within 8 to 12 hours after approval for release. SNS materials can be accessed by request of a state health official to the US Secretary of Health and Human Services or his or her designee. The immediate value of stocking of antidotes by the SNS is strictly limited because of the time frame for delivery. Therefore, local planning should incorporate the availability of antidotes determined to be needed in quantity based on the hazard vulnerability analysis.

In the circumstance of nerve agent or potent organophosphate exposure, this 8- to 12-hour time window is too long to achieve optimal outcomes of therapy. Therefore, the Chempack[32,35] program has been established as a joint federal and state program in most states. The Chempack program pre-positions antidotes needed for the treatment of organophosphate toxicity under the guidance and control of each participating state, with the goal of having these antidotes available to the entire state within 1 to 2 hours after request to the coordinating state entity.

The pharmaceuticals used in the Chempack program are federal assets. They are stored under carefully controlled temperature conditions and are, therefore, eligible for the shelf-life extension program. The drugs are checked annually for potency and purity. If they meet the current standards, the expiration date can be extended without replacing the drug. On the other hand, if the testing reveals that they do not meet new-drug standards, then they are replenished with new stock. Local government emergency management personnel determine the mechanisms for obtaining Chempacks locally. Chempacks could potentially be used, not only for organophosphate nerve agents but also for mass-casualty incidents resulting from organophosphate or carbamate pesticides. Emergency physicians should make themselves aware of the contact information for Chempack coordinators in their area.

RESPONSE
Decontamination

In general, chemical exposures occur in small quantities. The average number of patients who are transported from a chemical exposure is less than 3 per event.[3] Previously, conventional instruction emphasized the creation of a complex decontamination layout on site at hospitals before entry for treatment. Recent analysis of real-world events has demonstrated that most chemical exposures are inhalational (posing minimal exposure to responders and hospital personnel) and that the creation of such complexity poses unneeded risks to the responders.[38]

Conventional decontamination teaching suggests that disrobing removes as much as 80% of all surface contaminants and trapped gasses, depending on the individual's level of clothing at the time of the exposure.

No significant differences between long and short shower times have been noted in the one available study.[39] Experimental evidence to support a specific recommendation is limited. Based on the limited evidence and expert opinions, duration and methods of decontamination are ideally determined based on product toxicity and physical characteristics, such as water solubility, in consultation with the regional poison center and industrial toxicology experts. Practical considerations, such as mass chemical casualties, may require the use of short decontamination times. A draft national guideline for mass casualty decontamination suggests that 3 minutes is a generally adequate decontamination time.[38]

Rinsing patients with a deluge of water suffices to return most patients to precontamination levels of exposure.[15] Furthermore, deluge applications of water have been found to be sufficient to dilute most chemical contaminants to levels low enough to permit patient care without endangering hospital staff or immediately adjacent patients.[18]

Radiological decontamination follows most of the same principles of chemical decontamination. In most situations, up to 80% to 90% of surface radiological contaminants are removed by removing clothes before showering; patients should be scanned with radiation-detection equipment to note areas of contamination. After washing, patients should be resurveyed for continued radiation contamination and further cleaning strategies used until the hospital radiation safety officer deems the residual level of contamination acceptable. Unlike patients who are contaminated with toxic chemicals, decontamination should not delay the administration of life-saving interventions in patients who are contaminated with radioactive material. The diagnosis of internal contamination with radioactive material is covered in article by Kazzi and colleagues, in this issue.

In mass-casualty situations, security of the decontamination process is paramount. Victims seeking immediate treatment have the potential to transform the receiving hospital into a secondary contamination site. Hospital security agents should receive special training in conducting crowd-control operations and in initiating quick facility lockdowns.

When the volume of patients requiring medical assistance exceeds immediately available resources, triage of each patient should be performed to assist in prioritizing which patients should receive attention next. Patient triage should be performed considering both standard triage strategies and what is known or suspected about the agents involved in the event. One such strategy, patterned after the suggestions of Cone and Koenig,[4] appears in **Table 3**.

Table 3
Suggested triage criteria

Patient Category	Patient Status Based on Brief Assessment
Immediate	Difficulty breathing and responsive but immobile and incapacitated with findings consistent with chemical or radiological exposure
	Seems to be in cardiovascular shock
Urgent	Minimal respiratory distress, mobile with findings consistent with chemical or radiological exposure, and cardiovascular status stable *or*
	Incapacitated with findings apparently unrelated to the chemical or radiological exposure
Delayed	Mobile, stable cardiac and respiratory status
Expectant	Apneic after airway reposition, in cardiovascular shock

Note that no single finding should be considered as the sole basis for triage.
Adapted from Cone DC, Koenig KL. Mass casualty triage in the chemical, biological, radiological, or nuclear environment. Eur J Emerg Med 2005;12(6):294.

For victims of chemical exposure, decontamination should generally precede medical care in order to prevent contamination of hospital staff and hospital facilities. Failure to follow this prudent practice has led to staff injury and imminent closure of the emergency department itself,[40–42] which obviously would prevent care to any patients. For victims of radiological exposure, because of the lower risk of transmitting contamination when appropriate protective gear is used, initially life-saving care should precede decontamination efforts. Once decontamination has been performed and patients rendered reasonably safe of the risk of contaminating care staff, supportive care is essential. All usual care should be provided as needed for the clinical situation. Also, evaluation and treatment should be provided to address any concomitant findings that may have occurred before, during, or after exposure to the hazard. Provision of supportive care should not be delayed while awaiting the arrival of needed antidotes. Depending on the circumstances of the exposure, it is often appropriate to provide a summary of information about the agents involved for the health care personnel involved in patient care, both to reassure them about any concerns they may perceive to their own health as a result of caring for the exposed patients and to assist them in monitoring the patients for progression of illness.

Antidote administration alone will not be adequate to reverse the clinical findings caused by the exposure. Furthermore, in mass-casualty situations, sufficient amounts of antidotes to treat all affected patients are unlikely to be immediately available. In such a situation, assistance should be sought from regional poison centers and emergency management personnel to find, release, and emergently transport antidote supplies while the care personnel at the health care facility devote their attention to the patients at hand.

Recovery

The goal of all disaster management should be a return to normal activity as soon as it is safe and practical. Equipment used to manage the event should be cleaned, inspected for damage, inventoried, and returned to storage. The emergency management team should perform a detailed after-action report to describe areas of the emergency response plan that were used well and those areas that need improvement. Disaster plans should be revised, and drills should be conducted to test the revised plan.

Exposure to chemical or radiological contaminants can prove to be extremely stressful for both patients and hospital responders. Indeed, patients treated for anxiety related to chemical exposures have outnumbered patients with true chemical exposures by as much as 16 to 1.[12] It is vital that hospital planners engage with public health officials and local mental health experts to plan for both critical stress debriefing of staff[14] and long-term mental health monitoring.

Checklist for Hospital Preparedness

Several agencies have proposed checklists for hospital preparedness. A checklist that the reader may find useful appears in article by Borron of this issue, highlighting general precepts of hospital preparedness as well as specific readiness requirements for chemical and radiological events.

SUMMARY

Hospital planning for chemical or radiological events is essential. Although some other types of disasters like hurricanes and tornadoes may be more frequent, chemical and radiological emergencies have the potential for major disruptions to clinical care, owing to their rarity and to their psychological impact on victims and emergency responders.

Hospitals should prepare and train a decontamination team and set up a decontamination area, complete with a shower with its own ventilation source. Every hospital needs to have a variety of antidotes for toxicants in-house and should incorporate resupply from other sources like the SNS into their response plans.

Plans should be developed to provide care for affected patients after decontamination, addressing both their findings related to the event and those findings not directly related. Mental health support should be included in the planning, as patients and staff alike will likely need it during and after the event. Communication strategies to address concerns from patients, patients' families, and the media should be articulated, and responsibility should be assigned.

REFERENCES

1. Wetter D, Daniell W, Tresser C. Hospital preparedness for victims of chemical or biological terrorism. Am J Public Health 2001;91(5):710–6.
2. Niska R. Hospital preparedness for emergency response: United States, 2008. National Health Statistics Report. Atlanta (GA): Centers for Disease Control and Prevention; 2011. p. 37.
3. Agboola F, Mccarthy T, Biddinger PD. Impact of emergency preparedness exercise on performance. J Public Health Manag Pract 2013;19:S77–83.
4. Cone DC, Koenig KL. Mass casualty triage in the chemical, biological, radiological, or nuclear environment. Eur J Emerg Med 2005;12(6):287–302.
5. Koenig KL, Schultz CH. Disaster medicine: comprehensive principles and practices. Cambridge (MA): Cambridge University Press; 2010.
6. Brewster P. Emergency management program guidebook. VHA Center for Engineering & Occupational Safety and Health in conjunction with the VHA Emergency Management. Washington (DC): Department of Veterans Affairs, Veterans Health Administration; 2003.
7. The Joint Commission. Accreditation, health care, certification. Available at: http://www.thejointcommission.org. Accessed June 30, 2014.
8. California Hospital Association. Hazard vulnerability analysis. Available at: http://www.calhospitalprepare.org/hazard-vulnerability-analysis. Accessed July 30, 2014.
9. Chemical manufacturing. EPA. Available at: http://www.epa.gov/sectors/sectorinfo/sectorprofiles/chemical.html. Accessed June 12, 2014.
10. Fong MF, Schrader DC. Radiation disasters and emergency department preparedness. Emerg Med Clin North Am 1996;14(2):349–70.
11. Kirk M, Cisek J, Rose S. Emergency department response to hazardous materials incidents. Emerg Med Clin North Am 1994;12(2):461–81.
12. Kales SN. Acute chemical emergencies. N Engl J Med 2004;350(20):2102–4.
13. Auf der Heide E. The importance of evidence-based disaster planning. Ann Emerg Med 2006;47(1):34–49.
14. Perry R, Lindell M. Hospital planning for weapons of mass destruction incidents. J Postgrad Med 2006;52(2):116–20.
15. Houston M, Hendrickson RG. Decontamination. Crit Care Clin 2005;21(4):653–72.
16. Burgess JL, Kirk M, Borron SW, et al. Emergency department hazardous materials protocol for contaminated patients. Ann Emerg Med 1999;34(2):205–12.

17. Hick JL, Penn P, Hanfling D, et al. Establishing and training healthcare facility decontamination teams. Ann Emerg Med 2003;42(3):381–90.
18. Georgopoulos PG, Fedele P, Shade P, et al. Hospital response to chemical terrorism: personal protective equipment, training, and operations planning. Am J Ind Med 2004;46(5):432–45.
19. Clarke S, Chilcott R, Wilson J, et al. Decontamination of multiple casualties who are chemically contaminated: a challenge for acute hospitals. Prehosp Disaster Med 2008;23(2):175–81.
20. Barelli A, Biondi I, Soave M, et al. The comprehensive medical preparedness in chemical emergencies: 'the chain of chemical survival'. Eur J Emerg Med 2008; 15(2):110–8.
21. Marraffa J, Cohen V, Howland M. Antidotes for toxicological emergencies: a practical review. Am J Health Syst Pharm 2012;69(3):199–212.
22. Dart RC, Goldfrank LR, Chyka PA, et al. Combined evidence-based literature analysis and consensus guidelines for stocking of emergency antidotes in the United States. Ann Emerg Med 2000;36(2):126–32.
23. Dart RC, Borron SW, Caravati EM, et al. Expert consensus guidelines for stocking of antidotes in hospitals that provide emergency care. Ann Emerg Med 2009; 54(3):386–94.e1.
24. Abbott V, Creighton M, Hannam J, et al. Access in New Zealand to antidotes for accidental and intentional drug poisonings. J Prim Health Care 2012;4(2):100–5.
25. Thanacoody RH, Alridge G, Laing W, et al. National audit of antidote stocking in acute hospitals in the UK. Emerg Med J 2013;30(5):393–6.
26. Wiens MO, Zed PJ, Lepik KJ, et al. Adequacy of antidote stocking in British Columbia hospitals: the 2005 Antidote Stocking Study. CJEM 2006;8(6):409–16.
27. Wium CA, Hoffman BA. Antidotes and their availability in South Africa. Clin Toxicol 2009;47(1):77–80.
28. Sharp TW, Brennan RJ, Keim M, et al. Medical preparedness for a terrorist incident involving chemical or biological agents during the 1996 Atlanta Olympic Games. Ann Emerg Med 1998;32(2):214–23.
29. Johnson R, Geller RJ. Evaluating and responding to chemical emergencies: the role of poison control centers and public health labs. Available at: emergency. cdc.gov/coca/ppt/2013/01_31_13_chemical-threats_final.pdf. Accessed June 3, 2014.
30. Schneider AB, Smith JM. Potassium iodide prophylaxis: what have we learned and questions raised by the accident at the Fukushima Daiichi nuclear power plant. Thyroid 2012;22(4):344–6.
31. Reiners C, Schneider R. Potassium iodide (KI) to block the thyroid from exposure to I-131: current questions and answers to be discussed. Radiat Environ Biophys 2013;52:189–93.
32. Schwartz M, Gorman SE. Medical toxicology and public health–update on research and activities at the Centers for Disease Control and Prevention, and the Agency for Toxic Substances and Disease Registry. J Med Toxicol 2007; 3(3):139–40.
33. CDC - PHPR - Strategic National Stockpile. Available at: www.cdc.gov/phpr/stockpile/stockpile.htm. Accessed June 3, 2014.
34. Strategic National Stockpile fact sheet. Available at: www.astho.org/Programs/Preparedness/Public-Health-Emergency-Law/Emergency-Use-Authorization-Toolkit/Strategic-National-Stockpile-Fact-Sheet/. Accessed June 3, 2014.
35. Radiation emergency medical management. Available at: http://www.remm.nlm.gov/sns.htm. Accessed June 3, 2014.

36. Chemical hazards emergency management. Available at: http://chemm.nlm.nih.gov/sns.htm. Accessed June 3, 2014.
37. Technology and Medicine. OSHA best practices for hospital-based first receivers of victims from mass casualty incidents involving the release of hazardous substances. Washington, DC: Occupational Safety and Health Administration; 2004.
38. US Department of Homeland Security. Patient decontamination in a mass chemical exposure incident: national planning guidance for communities (draft of February 2014). Available at: http://www.regulations.gov/contentStreamer?objectId=0900006481676335&disposition=attachment&contentType=pdf. Accessed July 30, 2014.
39. Amlot R, Larner J, Matar H, et al. Comparative analysis of showering protocols for mass-casualty decontamination. Prehosp Disaster Med 2008;15(2):435–9.
40. Geller RJ, Singleton KL, Tarantino ML, et al. Nosocomial poisoning associated with emergency department treatment of organophosphate toxicity – Georgia, 2000. MMWR Morb Mortal Wkly Rep 2001;49:1156 Reprinted in Journal of Toxicology-Clinical Toxicology 2001;39:109–11.
41. Silverman JJ, Hart RP, Garrettson LK, et al. Posttraumatic stress disorder from pentaborane intoxication. Neuropsychiatric evaluation and short-term follow-up. JAMA 1985;254(18):2603–8.
42. Yarbrough BE, Garrettson LK, Zolet DI, et al. Severe central nervous system damage and profound acidosis in persons exposed to pentaborane. J Toxicol Clin Toxicol 1985–1986;23(7–8):519–36.

Personal Protective Equipment and Decontamination of Adults and Children

Michael G. Holland, MD[a,b,c,*], David Cawthon, PhD[c]

KEYWORDS

- Decontamination • Personal protective equipment (PPE) • Levels A, B, C, D
- HAZMAT • Chemical contamination

KEY POINTS

- Accurate identification of the chemical substances involved is the most important information necessary for proper care of the hazardous materials (HAZMAT) incident, but is often not available initially.
- Proper decontamination prevents further chemical injury, protects health care workers and prevents secondary contamination of facilities and equipment.
- Many patients will not have been decontaminated at the scene; proper triage and security must be in place to prevent contamination. Many "worried well" present without significant exposures, but can overwhelm staffing.
- Decontamination by health care workers in Level C suits is sufficient protection. Decontamination areas are located outdoors ideally to prevent hospital air becoming contaminated.
- Proper advanced planning and practice are essential for efficient performance in an emergency. Knowledgeable hospital security and efficient triage can effectively control patient flow.

PERSONAL PROTECTIVE EQUIPMENT IN HAZARDOUS MATERIALS INCIDENTS

Biological, chemical, and radiologic materials that result in adverse effects to the health and safety of exposed individuals are termed hazardous materials (HAZMAT). These substances represent significant risks to health care workers when hospitals receive patients contaminated with these materials. Therefore, hospitals and their

[a] Emergency Medicine, Upstate NY Poison Center, SUNY Upstate Medical University, Syracuse, NY, USA; [b] Center for Occupational Health, Glens Falls Hospital, Glens Falls, NY, USA; [c] Center for Toxicology and Environmental Health, L.L.C., 5120 North Shore Dr., North Little Rock, AR 72118, USA
* Corresponding author. Center for Toxicology and Environmental Health, L.L.C., 5120 North Shore Dr., North Little Rock, AR 72118.
E-mail address: mholland@cteh.com

Emerg Med Clin N Am 33 (2015) 51–68
http://dx.doi.org/10.1016/j.emc.2014.09.006
0733-8627/15/$ – see front matter © 2015 Elsevier Inc. All rights reserved.

emed.theclinics.com

workforce must be prepared to use personal protective equipment (PPE) to protect themselves when these situations arise. Federal, state, and local regulations may specify types of PPE for specific job tasks when dealing with specific HAZMAT. There are 4 key issues which must be fully understood whenever PPE is required[1]:

1. The various types of PPE
2. The basics of a "hazard assessment"
3. How to select appropriate PPE; and
4. Training in the proper use of PPE.

It is only after these 4 key issues have been adequately addressed that a properly equipped and well-trained health care staff facility can provide a safe and effective response.

TYPES OF PERSONAL PROTECTIVE EQUIPMENT

PPE are articles worn or equipment used to protect the user from harmful contaminants released into the environment. In this article, this means the PPE used by hospital personnel when decontaminating and caring for patient(s) involved in a HAZMAT incident. The main function of PPE is to provide a barrier between the user and respiratory or skin exposure to the contaminant in the environment or on the skin/clothing of contaminated patients. PPE can be listed in the following categories:

1. Respiratory protection
2. Eye and face protection
3. Hand protection
4. Foot protection; and
5. Body protection.

A specific combination of PPE from each of these categories is normally needed to properly protect the wearer from each specific contaminant.

Respiratory Protection

Respiratory equipment prevents airborne contaminants from being inhaled, and some types can also protect the eyes and face. There are 2 primary types of respirators, air purifying and supplied air respirators. Air-purifying respirators (APRs) have filters, cartridges, or canisters that trap contaminants from the air. APRs are the most common protection method for particulates and vapors, and are used in environments where there is no chance of an oxygen-deficient state. Available filters should protect against, at a minimum, organic vapors and also contain a high-efficiency particulate air cartridge for particulates.[2] Supplied air respirators provide breathable air from a clean source such as an air tank or air compressor located outside the contaminated area, and are suitable for use in an oxygen-deficient environment. Respiratory protection must only be used in compliance with the applicable Occupational Safety and Health Administration (OSHA) regulations and National Institute for Occupational Safety and Health (NIOSH) publications.

The advantages and disadvantages of various styles of respirator face pieces are discussed in the OSHA best practices document.[3] Half-face pieces allow workers to wear any appropriate eyewear that does not interfere with the respirator seal, but they provide no eye protection themselves, and contaminated air can enter the mask if the seal is broken. Full face pieces provide eye protection and a tight-fitting face piece may be able to pull filtered air into the face piece if the battery fails on a powered APR (PAPR). Loose-fitting helmet/hood face pieces provide eye and head protection, fit testing is not required, they can be worn by employees with facial hair, and they can wear their own glasses under the helmet/hood; the main disadvantage is when used with a PAPR, the hood will provide little or no protection if the battery fails. PAPRs have a motorized blower that delivers filtered air at a slight positive pressure into the face piece, reducing the chance of contaminated air reaching the user in the event of a leak.

Eye and Face Protection

OSHA requires that "eye and face protection must be provided whenever necessary to protect against chemical, environmental, radiological or mechanical irritants and hazards."[4] Liquid chemical contaminants may present hazards from splash, fumes, vapors, and mists. Solid chemical contaminants may involve airborne particles and dusts. Biological agents cause infections through eye contact. Eye protection typically takes the form of glasses, goggles, and face shields, or as part of full-face respirators.

Hand Protection

Gloves for hand protection are produced from a wide variety of both common and proprietary materials, including latex, nitrile, vinyl, polyurethane, butyl rubber, foils, and neoprene. Each material offers different ranges of protection, depending on the specific contaminant. Additionally, glove selection may need to be modified if there is a greater need for dexterity by the clinician. The appropriate type of glove necessary for each individual chemical can usually be found on the Material Safety Data Sheet/ Safety Data Sheets when available. When dealing with unknown contaminants, standard latex or latex-free clinical examination gloves covered by nitrile or similar chemical-resistant gloves should be employed.

Foot Protection

Like gloves, chemical protective overboots and boots with steel toes are available in a variety of both common and proprietary materials, including vinyl, latex, polyvinyl chloride, polyurethane, and butyl rubber. Boots tend to have thicker side walls than gloves, and therefore are likely to provide more protection than gloves made of the same material.[3]

Body Protection

Protective clothing is available in a wide variety of styles and materials. Manufacturers produce a broad spectrum of protective fabrics that protect against a wide range of chemicals in liquid, solid, or vapor form. Protective clothing is typically illustrated as chemical protective suits but aprons, sleeves, and leggings are also available, which may represent a more appropriate selection in some instances. Chemical protective suits offer protection from radionuclides that are alpha and beta emitters, but do not offer protection from gamma or neutron radiation, and thus, it is important to assess radiation levels and determine staff exposure rates.[2]

HAZARD ASSESSMENT

OSHA published a handbook titled: *Best Practices for Hospital-Based First Receivers of Victims from Mass Casualty Incidents Involving the Release of Hazardous Substances*. This document "(1) provides information to assist hospitals in selecting personal protective equipment (PPE) based on current interpretations of OSHA standards, published literature, current hospital practices, stakeholder input, and the practical limitations of currently available respiratory protective devices and (2) consolidates OSHA standards and interpretations on training needs of first receivers."[3]

"First receivers" are defined as hospital employees who work at a site remote from the location where the hazardous substance release occurred. Therefore, their exposures are limited to the substances transported to the hospital on victims' skin, hair, clothing, or personal effects. Conditions necessary for hospitals to rely on the OSHA PPE recommendations include a thorough and complete hazard vulnerability analysis and emergency management plan (EMP), which have been conducted and developed with community input, and updated within the past year. Specifically, OSHA (2005) states: "By tailoring emergency plans to reflect the reasonably predictable "worst-case" scenario under which first receivers might work, the hospital can rely on these plans to guide decisions regarding personnel training and PPE.[1,3] The Joint Commission requires an all-hazard approach to allow organizations to be flexible enough to respond to emergencies of all types, whether natural or manmade (unintentional or intentional)."

HOW TO SELECT APPROPRIATE PERSONAL PROTECTIVE EQUIPMENT

OSHA guidelines typically rely on generalized statements, indicating PPE should be of safe design and construction, and selected to protect the employee from the hazards identified in the hazard assessment. Similarly, Material Safety Data Sheets and the new format Safety Data Sheets tend to recommend "appropriate protective equipment." More specific information can also be found in selection charts available from governmental and commercial agencies. Parker[5] states: "The most specific protective information and protective material compatibility information comes from the manufacturer." The author further notes that "the financial disincentive derived from legal liability from human injury and/or death drives these industries to thoroughly study their product and disseminate information to the public."

It is important to recognize the need to select the most appropriate and not necessarily the most protective PPE, because the use of PPE itself carries significant health risks for responders and greater levels of protection confer greater potential risk, including limited visibility, reduced dexterity, restricted movement, suit breach, hyperthermia owing to reduced heat dissipation, and dehydration.[6]

Respiratory protection should be selected first because it will be needed before and at greater distances than skin protection. Typically, supplied-air respirators are required for oxygen-deficient atmospheres, contaminants with inadequate warning properties, unidentified contaminants, and immediately dangerous to life and health environments. Immediately dangerous to life and health environments can only be identified when the contaminant is known and air monitoring has identified the concentration of the contaminant. These scenarios are present at a HAZMAT scene, and are not usually an issue in the hospital setting receiving contaminated patients.

Air-purifying respirators can only be used when the contaminant has adequate warning properties (eg, odor, taste, or irritation effects) that will alert the user if the respirator malfunctions. Additionally, they can only be used for certain ranges of air contaminant concentrations. OSHA has assigned a respirator protection factor to each type of respirator based on the overall effectiveness of the respirator. Respirator protection factors are used in conjunction with published or regulatory exposure limits to determine the upper concentration limit, and maximum use concentration for which the respirator is acceptable. Many hospitals have a strong interest in PAPRs with helmet/hoods because they require no fit testing, can be worn by employees with facial hair and eyeglasses, and are generally considered to be more comfortable than other air-purifying respirators.[3] However, they are also more costly to purchase than full-face masks.

Skin protection should be chosen after respiratory protection has been determined. Skin protection is intended to prevent direct contact with chemical liquids or vapors. Specific agents that might be problematic are the vesicants, such as sulfur mustard, and the persistent nerve agents, such as VX.[2] A variety of protective fabrics are available from manufacturers. OSHA provides a list of specific examples.[3]

A general description and discussion of the levels of protection and protective gear is provided in 29 CFR 1910.120 App B and is reproduced herein.[7]

Level A Protection

Level A provides the highest level of protection available, and protects the user from liquids, vapors and gases. Level A should be used when (1) the hazardous substance has been identified and requires the highest level of protection for skin, eyes, and the respiratory system based on either the measured (or potential for) high concentration of atmospheric vapors, gases, or particulates; or the site operations and work functions involve a high potential for splash, immersion, or exposure to unexpected vapors, gases, or particulates of materials that are harmful to skin or capable of being absorbed through the skin; (2) substances with a high degree of hazard to the skin are known or suspected to be present, and skin contact is possible; or (3) operations must be conducted in confined, poorly ventilated areas, and the absence of conditions requiring Level A have not yet been determined (**Fig. 1**).

Level A equipment (to be used as appropriate)
- Positive-pressure, full-face piece, self-contained breathing apparatus (SCBA), or positive-pressure supplied air respirator with escape SCBA, approved by NIOSH.
- Totally encapsulating chemical-protective suit.
- Gloves, outer, chemical resistant.
- Gloves, inner, chemical resistant.
- Boots, chemical resistant, steel toe and shank.
- Disposable protective suit, gloves, and boots (depending on suit construction), may be worn over totally encapsulating suit.[8]

Level B Protection

Level B protection provides adequate skin protection, but is not vapor impervious like Level A. Level B should be used when (1) the type and atmospheric concentration of substances have been identified and require a high level of respiratory protection, but less skin protection, (2) the atmosphere contains less than 19.5% oxygen, or (3) the presence of incompletely identified vapors or gases is indicated by a direct-reading organic vapor detection instrument, but vapors and gases are not suspected of containing high levels of chemicals harmful to skin or capable of being absorbed through the skin. (This involves atmospheres with immediately dangerous to life and health concentrations of specific substances that present severe inhalation hazards and that do not represent a severe skin hazard; or that do not meet the criteria for use of APRs.) SCBA present time restrictions on the use of a standard tank (~20–30 minutes of operational time) and the carrying weight of tanks make them impractical for most health care personnel.[2] This level of protection, like Level A, is generally used at a HAZMAT site, and not usually needed in health care facilities dealing with contaminated patients (**Fig. 2**).

Level B equipment (to be used as appropriate)
- Positive-pressure, full-face piece SCBA, or positive-pressure supplied air respirator with escape SCBA (NIOSH approved).

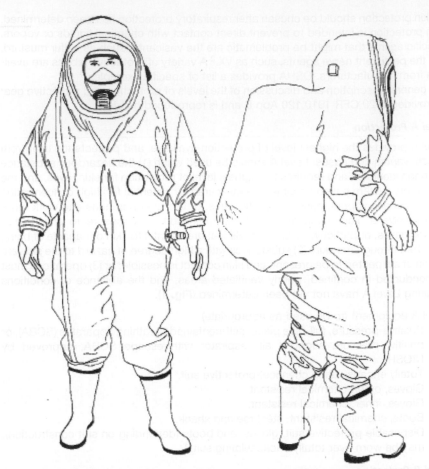

Fig. 1. Level A personal protective equipment. (*From* ATSDR. Managing Hazardous Material Incidents (MHMI). Volumes 1, 2, and 3. Agency for Toxic Substances and Disease Registry (ATSDR). Atlanta (GA): U.S. Department of Health and Human Services, Public Health Service; 2001. Available at: http://www.atsdr.cdc.gov/MHMI/index.asp. Accessed July 15, 2014).

- Hooded chemical-resistant clothing (1- or 2-piece chemical splash suit; disposable chemical-resistant overalls).
- Gloves, outer, chemical resistant.
- Gloves, inner, chemical resistant.
- Boots, outer, chemical-resistant steel toe and shank.
- Boot-covers, outer, chemical resistant (disposable).
- Face shield.[8]

Level C Protection

Level C is the most common type of PPE used in health care facilities when dealing with contaminated patients. Level C protection should be used when (1) the atmospheric contaminants, liquid splashes, or other direct contact will not adversely affect or be absorbed through any exposed skin, (2) the types of air contaminants have been identified, concentrations measured, and an APR is available that can remove the

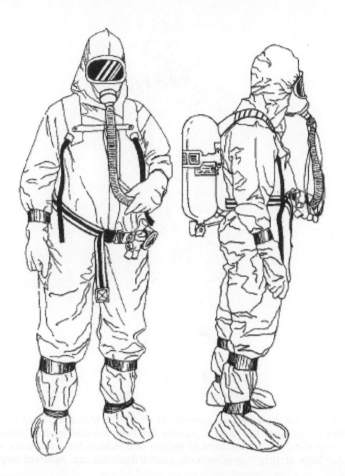

Fig. 2. Level B personal protective equipment. (*From* ATSDR. Managing Hazardous Material Incidents (MHMI). Volumes 1, 2, and 3. Agency for Toxic Substances and Disease Registry (ATSDR). Atlanta (GA): U.S. Department of Health and Human Services, Public Health Service; 2001. Available at: http://www.atsdr.cdc.gov/MHMI/index.asp. Accessed July 15, 2014).

contaminants, and (3) all criteria for the use of APRs are met. Level C PPE has generally been agreed to be adequate for most hospital decontamination scenarios, unless specific releases require increased levels of protection.[2,9] Level C PPE is also the recommended PPE for first receivers in a radiation emergency from external or internal contamination in patients being treated; however, no PPE can protect against exposure from high-energy, highly penetrating forms of ionizing radiation (ie, gamma radiation) associated with most radiation emergencies, such as at a nuclear power plant or a radiation therapy source. Level D PPE can be used in postdecontamination areas or if the risk of external contamination is low as recommended by the hospital radiation safety officer (**Fig. 3**).[10]

Level C equipment (to be used as appropriate)
- Full-face or half mask, air-purifying respirators (NIOSH approved).
- Hooded chemical-resistant clothing (chemical splash suit; disposable chemical-resistant overalls).

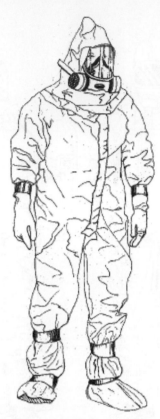

Fig. 3. Level C personal protective equipment. (*From* ATSDR. Managing Hazardous Material Incidents (MHMI). Volumes 1, 2, and 3. Agency for Toxic Substances and Disease Registry (ATSDR). Atlanta (GA): U.S. Department of Health and Human Services, Public Health Service; 2001. Available at: http://www.atsdr.cdc.gov/MHMI/index.asp. Accessed July 15, 2014).

- Gloves, outer, chemical resistant.
- Gloves, inner, chemical resistant.
- Boots, outer, chemical-resistant steel toe and shank.
- Boot covers, outer, chemical resistant (disposable).
- Face shield.[8]

Level D Protection

Level D protection should be used when (1) the atmosphere contains no known hazard, and (2) work functions preclude splashes, immersion, or the potential for unexpected inhalation of or contact with hazardous levels of any chemicals (**Fig. 4**).

Level D equipment (to be used as appropriate)
- A work uniform affording minimal protection.
- Gloves.
- Boots/shoes, chemical-resistant steel toe and shank.
- Safety glasses or chemical splash goggles.
- Face shield.

Combinations of PPE other than those described for Levels A, B, C, and D may be more appropriate and may be used to provide the proper level of protection.

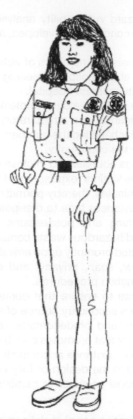

Fig. 4. Level D personal protective equipment. (*From* ATSDR. Managing Hazardous Material Incidents (MHMI). Volumes 1, 2, and 3. Agency for Toxic Substances and Disease Registry (ATSDR). Atlanta (GA): U.S. Department of Health and Human Services, Public Health Service; 2001. Available at: http://www.atsdr.cdc.gov/MHMI/index.asp. Accessed July 15, 2014).

Appropriate PPE for a decontamination team may be determined by consulting reference guidebooks, websites, database networks, telephone hotlines, or a regional Poison Control Center.[8] Appropriate dress for the decontamination team could include:

- A scrub suit
- Plastic shoe covers
- Disposable chemical protective clothing with built-in hood and booties, with hood taped at the neck
- Polyvinyl chloride gloves taped to sleeves
- Respiratory protection, as appropriate
- Multiple layers of surgical gloves, neoprene or disposable nitrile gloves, with the bottom layer taped; should be changed whenever torn; and
- Protective eyewear.[8]

OSHA defined the "Hospital Decontamination Zone" to include "any areas where the type and quantity of hazardous substance is unknown and where contaminated victims, contaminated equipment, or contaminated waste may be present." OSHA further identified 8 specific conditions necessary for hospitals to rely on the OSHA minimum PPE selections.[3]

1. Thorough and complete hazard vulnerability analysis and EMP, which consider community input, have been conducted/developed, and have been updated within the past year.
2. The EMP includes plans to assist the numbers of victims that the community anticipates might seek treatment at this hospital, keeping in mind that the vast majority of victims may self-refer to the nearest hospital.
3. Preparations specified in the EMP have been implemented (eg, employee training, equipment selection, maintenance, and a respiratory protection program).
4. The EMP includes methods for handling the numbers of ambulatory and nonambulatory victims anticipated by the community.
5. The hazardous substance was not released in close proximity to the hospital, and the elapsed time between the victims' exposure and victims' arrival at the hospital exceeds approximately 10 minutes, thereby permitting substantial levels of gases and vapors from volatile substances time to dissipate.
6. Victims' contaminated clothing and possessions are promptly removed and contained (eg, in an approved hazardous waste container that is isolated outdoors), and decontamination is initiated promptly upon arrival at the hospital. Hospital EMP includes shelter, tepid water, soap, privacy, and coverings to promote victim compliance with decontamination procedures.
7. EMP procedures are in place to ensure that contaminated medical waste and waste water do not become a secondary source of employee exposure.
8. The decontamination system and predecontamination victim waiting areas are designed and used in a manner that promotes constant fresh air circulation through the system to limit hazardous substance accumulation. Air exchange from a clean source has been considered in the design of fully enclosed systems (ie, through consultation with a professional engineer or certified industrial hygienist) and air is not recirculated.

The "hospital postdecontamination zone" is defined as an area considered uncontaminated and equipment and personnel are not expected to become contaminated in this area.[3] This zone requires seven conditions which hospital must be met to rely on the OSHA minimum PPE selections:

1. EMP is developed and followed in a way that minimizes the ED personnel's reasonably anticipated contact with contaminated victims (eg, with drills that test communication between the hospital and emergency responders at the incident site to reduce the likelihood of unanticipated victims).
2. Decontamination system (in the hospital decontamination zone) and hospital security can be activated promptly to minimize the chance that victims will enter the ED and contact unprotected staff before decontamination.
3. EMP procedures specify that unannounced victims (once identified as possibly contaminated) disrobe in the appropriate decontamination area (not the ED) and follow hospital decontamination procedures before admission (or readmission) to the ED.
4. Victims in this area were previously decontaminated by a shower with soap and water, including a minimum of 5 minutes under running water. Shower instructions are clearly presented and enforced. Shower facility encourages victim compliance (eg, shelter, tepid water, reasonable degree of privacy).
5. EMP procedures clearly specify actions ED clerks or staff will take if they suspect a patient is contaminated. For example, (1) do not physically contact the patient, (2) immediately notify supervisor and safety officer of possible hospital contamination, and (3) allow qualified personnel to isolate and decontaminate the victim.

6. The EMP requires that, if the ED becomes contaminated, that space is no longer eligible to be considered a hospital postdecontamination zone. Instead, it should be considered contaminated and all employees working in this area should use PPE as described for the hospital decontamination zone.

The US Department of Homeland Security and the US Department of Health and Human Services have posted a draft document regarding national planning guidelines for patient decontamination in a mass chemical exposure incident.[11] Readers are directed to this for further evidence-based analysis of best practices.

When used in conjunction with the OSHA Best Practices for Hospital-based First Receivers of Victims from Mass Casualty Incidents Involving the Release of Hazardous Substances the minimum PPE required for the hospital decontamination zone and hospital postdecontamination zone includes the following.

Hospital Decontamination Zone
- PAPR that provides a protection factor of 1000. The respirator must be NIOSH approved.
- Combination 99.97% high-efficiency particulate air/organic vapor/acid gas respirator cartridges (also NIOSH approved).
- Double layer protective gloves.
- Chemical-resistant suit.
- Head covering and eye/face protection (if not part of the respirator).
- Chemical-protective boots.
- Suit openings sealed with tape.

Hospital Postdecontamination Zone
- Normal work clothes and PPE, as necessary, for infection control purposes (eg, gloves, gown, and appropriate respirator).

TRAINING IN THE PROPER USE OF PERSONAL PROTECTIVE EQUIPMENT

Employees performing their duties while wearing PPE should receive training in its proper care and use, including hazards identification, orientation to the equipment, appropriate donning and doffing techniques, proper use, safety issues, and break-through times. Employees need to understand the situations in which their equipment can be safely used and those in which it cannot. Potential adverse health effects from the use of PPE include impaired vision, heat stress, dehydration, and impaired balance.[12] Responders in PPE can also be frightening to pediatric patients.[11] Regular drills and exercises "conducted to test emergency preparedness" are required by the Joint Commission that sets standards for accreditation under Emergency Management Standard EC 1.4 (Hick, 2003b).

DECONTAMINATION

Few things can be as anxiety provoking for ED personnel as being notified that a HAZMAT incident has occurred and patients with chemical, biological, or radiologic contamination will be arriving. This can be greatly diminished by educational and training programs concentrating on proper emergency response and frequent drills with mock patients to practice decontamination procedures and patient flow logistics. In this way, the required equipment will be familiar and accessible, and each ED employee will know their expected role in the incident response.

As in all medical conditions, history is the most important part; in the HAZMAT incident, the "history" is the information about the materials involved—the chemicals involved, numbers and ages of exposed individuals, signs and symptoms being expressed by exposed individuals, and any associated injuries (ie, owing to fire or explosion). Many times, initial responders will know some specifics about the materials, and more information can be obtained from the regional Poison Control Center (PCC):1-800-222-1222. Other resources are listed in the article by Kirk and Iddins elsewhere in this issue.

Generally, plain tepid water is the best solution for decontamination; it is readily available, cheap, and effective.[13] If necessary for non–water-soluble chemicals, addition of mild liquid soap (ie, baby shampoo, body wash) and gentle scrubbing with a soft sponge or cloth can improve removal. However, older recommendations for addition of bleach to solutions because of their purported ability to neutralize nerve agents are no longer current owing to adverse effects that would occur before any neutralization owing to required contact time.[14] Rarely, reactive alkali metals (elemental sodium, elemental potassium) and other chemicals can react violently with water, indicating a need for alternative solutions in these cases. An US Food and Drug Administration–approved Reactive Skin Decontamination Lotion, used for both removal and neutralization of chemical warfare agents (vesicants and organophosphorus nerve agents), has been shown to be superior to water and other conventional solutions for decontamination of these agents.[15] This product is also available in soaked pads for the decontamination of a small area. Another commercially available solution, Diphoterine, has been shown to be efficacious as well, especially for chemical splashes to the eyes.[16,17] Finally, easyDECON spray foam has been used to decontaminate the US Senate of anthrax spores, and is approved for HAZMAT and military applications, but it is only for decontamination of equipment and rooms, and so on, and is not to be used on patients for personal decontamination.[18] Some of these commercial solutions, because of their ability to neutralize or bind a chemical as well as remove it, may be preferable to outdoor water showering in very cold weather areas.

Several strategies should be used to determine which patients need decontamination, and can help to rank the priority for decontamination in a mass casualty incident. Factors to consider include the presence of the expected signs and symptoms of exposure to the particular chemical involved (ie, the "toxidrome"; see the article by Tomassoni et al elsewhere in this issue), obvious visible contamination on the person or their clothing, and the victim's geographic proximity to the release or spill.

Experience from the Tokyo Subway sarin gas attack in 1995 showed that many more patients present to the ED on their own accord, rather than the numbers brought by EMS. EDs must be prepared for this by having a plan in place to avoid having contaminated patients present unannounced and enter the ED without proper decontamination, possibly leading to contamination of the entire ED, forcing evacuation and creating an inability to use the facilities for patient care. Security personnel should be trained to recognize this possibility, and a staging area outdoors should be set up to receive and decontaminate these patients. One option would be to have a local fire department or HAZMAT team not at the HAZMAT incident site respond to the ED and set up triage and decontamination stations outside the ED. These details need to be worked out in the planning drills and practice scenarios, as described.

DECONTAMINATION AREA PREPARATION

All patients received from the chemical HAZMAT incident should be considered contaminated until proven otherwise, and therefore need to be decontaminated before entry into the ED. If the logistics or the weather requires transfer of victims from the ED to an indoor decontamination area, proper protection and isolation from the rest of the hospital must be ensured (such as plastic or paper taping of floors, covering/masking of handles, knobs, switches). The size of the decontamination area needed depends on the number of expected victims, and must be set up to accommodate that patient flow as well as the necessary ED staff and equipment. The preplanning stages and practice drills in advance of a true HAZMAT emergency will help to identify the logistics of what indoor area can serve this purpose, which must have a separate exhaust ventilation system that does not mix with the general hospital air handling system. For these reasons, outdoor areas such as ambulance entranceways to the ED are usually preferred sites for decontamination stations.[8]

EDs must also prepare for the many minimally exposed patients who arrive on their own and may not need full decontamination. An area for triage decisions regarding who needs to be decontaminated must therefore be available. Many of the "worried well" who present to EDs after HAZMAT incidents will have had exposure only to odors, gases, or vapors, and will not need decontamination.

Portable decontamination systems can be as simple as plastic garbage bags for sealing of contaminated clothing, handheld shower nozzles supplied by hoses, and showering patients who stand in portable plastic wading pools. These can be assembled and stored easily and cheaply in advance of an incident. Portable patient screens or similar visual barriers can be erected for privacy. More sophisticated, commercially available tents and decontamination systems are available.

CONTAMINATED PATIENT ENTRY

A properly trained and knowledgeable physician or nurse, wearing appropriate PPE, should perform triage upon arrival of ambulance patients to both assess patient condition as well as the degree of chemical or radiologic contamination and the need for decontamination. This initial evaluation involves removing clothing and jewelry and wiping or vacuuming away visible contamination.

Ideally, decontamination would be performed before patient transport from a HAZMAT site; however, the ability to decontaminate at the site might be limited, and all HAZMAT victims should be considered contaminated until proven otherwise (ie, only gas exposure has occurred or EMS confirms that the patient has been decontaminated). If a patient's clothing was not removed at the incident site, it should be removed before entry into the ED. This reduces further exposure to the patient and lessen the extent of contamination introduced into the ED. Contaminated clothing should be double bagged in plastic bags, sealed, and labeled. The decontamination team should bring the prepared stretcher to the ambulance, transfer the patient, and take him or her directly to the decontamination area along the predesignated route.[8]

Priority should be given to the fundamentals of emergency treatment: airway, breathing, and circulation (ABCs) simultaneous with contamination reduction by personnel in Level C PPE. Once life-threatening matters have been addressed, ED personnel can then direct their attention to thorough decontamination and thorough patient assessment. Appropriate PPE must be worn until it is deemed ED personnel are no longer at risk of secondary contamination.[8]

DECONTAMINATION PROCEDURES

Decontamination serves 2 roles: It prevents further absorption of or injury from the chemical in question, and protects the health care worker from suffering injury from exposure to a contaminated patient. This cannot be emphasized enough, because secondary contamination resulting in adverse health effects in first responders and in health care workers caring for HAZMAT victims has been reported frequently in the literature.[19–26] In addition, proper decontamination prevents off-gassing of chemicals from contaminated patients that can contaminate the hospital and render the ED inoperable.[20,25,27]

There is always the temptation to begin treatment to contaminated victims who arrive in extremis, without decontaminating the victim. However, this must be avoided unless proper protections are in place, because the first priority must be to keep the health care worker safe from becoming ill owing to secondary contamination. ABCs and emergency treatment should be performed only by ED personnel wearing appropriate PPE, and includes securing the airway, spinal precautions, controlling exsanguinating bleeding (by tourniquet or direct pressure), and use of premixed antidote autoinjectors in the case of nerve agent poisoning. Decontamination should then proceed and standard emergency care performed after decontamination has been completed.

Many patients arriving from a HAZMAT site will already have had their clothing removed by EMS personnel and already gone through decontamination procedures; they will not need to undergo repeat decontamination and can proceed directly into the ED for definitive examination and treatment.

Patients may arrive from a HAZMAT incident on foot or by private vehicle who have not undergone decontamination, and must be assumed to be contaminated. In these cases, simply removing a patient's clothing effectively removes significant portions of the contamination. Decontamination still needs to be performed, because exposed areas not covered by clothing and areas where chemicals have soaked through need to be removed.

The discussion herein of decontamination assumes victims are contaminated with liquid chemicals. However, some HAZMAT incidents may involve discharge of solid particles or powders, and many HAZMAT incidents involve only gases. Solid particles or dusts can be removed by vacuuming; battery-operated portable vacuums allow this to occur outdoors independent of power cords. In the case of exposures to gases, most victims will simply need removal from the source of the gas, and decontamination is not necessary. In instances where victims have been exposed to high concentrations of a highly water-soluble gas (eg, anhydrous ammonia), rinsing of eyes and mucous membranes may need to be performed if there is evidence of conjunctival injection or complaints of eyes burning. Rarely, high concentrations of highly water soluble gases or acid mists can also cause skin burning sensation, and therefore exposed skin should be washed in these cases.

Because most decontamination of ambulatory personnel will be in showers, decontamination with soap and water should begin with the head and proceed downward. Injury to the eyes and mucous membranes can be most devastating, and special attention should be directed to the eyes and any open wounds. Full-body showering with the soap and water, including hair, axilla, skin folds, and genital/buttocks area, effectively decontaminates the ambulatory HAZMAT victims. Supervision by same-gender hospital personnel must ensure victims do not neglect areas such as hands, feet, nails, and so on.

Generally, copious, tepid water flow adequately decontaminates most chemicals. The addition of a mild soap enhances removal of oily or non–water-soluble chemicals. Care must be made to not injure or abrade skin that may enhance absorption. This is especially true with elderly patients and young children. Also, a child's larger surface area to weight ratio allows a greater chance of systemic absorption of skin contaminants. All water run-off from the decontamination process should be collected for proper disposal and not allowed to contaminate local sewer systems.

In the nonambulatory HAZMAT victim who has suffered injuries, decontamination must proceed on a suitably designed decontamination stretcher with a surface sloped from head to toe. This allows the run-off to funnel into a drain nozzle to be captured in a drum for appropriate disposal.

Open wounds should be irrigated with copious amounts of physiologic solutions such as normal saline or Lactated ringers (plain water, being nonisotonic, can cause cellular swelling and tissue injury, but decontamination should proceed with plain water if sufficient isotonic solutions are not immediately available).

After open wounds, decontamination of the eyes and mucous membranes of the face should be undertaken next. Washing the eyes with isotonic saline is the preferred method. A frequently employed method involves attaching an oxygen nasal cannula to an IV line, and placing the cannula prongs over the bridge of the nose, directing 1 prong over the medial aspect of each eye. This allows irrigation fluid to proceed from medial to lateral, washing chemicals away from the nasal lacrimal duct. Irrigation and suctioning may be necessary for nasal and otic contamination. Moving down the body in a rostral–caudal direction, special attention must be directed toward skin fold areas such as neck, axilla, antecubital fossae, groin, popliteal region, and hands and feet. Commonly ignored or missed areas in skin decontamination are hairy areas (scalp, axillae, genitalia), skin creases and folds, and hands and feet, especially nails. Full inspection of the patient's body, including rolling the patient over to inspect the back, should be performed to ensure complete decontamination has occurred.

Decontamination of young children can be especially problematic, owing to their fear of the unknown. Families should be kept together for decontamination whenever possible. Alternatively, a nurse or attendant must stay with the child at all times for reassurance.[28]

After completion of decontamination, the victim will need to exit the decontamination area without recontamination and without spreading contamination. Once transferred to a clean area from the decontamination area, standard ED management of the patient's conditions can proceed, with hospital admission as indicated. Generally, the asymptomatic patient can be discharged home, providing no late effects from the chemical exposure are expected.

DECONTAMINATION AFTER RADIOLOGIC INCIDENTS

Radiologic contamination can occur as a result of a nuclear reactor accident, detonation of a thermonuclear weapon, or detonation of a radiologic dispersion device (or "dirty bomb"). Depending on the type of accident (unshielded fission vs coolant failure and meltdown/explosion) exposures at a nuclear reactor incident can be restricted to penetrating high-energy radiation (ie, gamma rays) in the case of unshielded fission exposure, or exposure can involve both high-energy waves and radionuclide particles in the case of a meltdown or explosion. Victims in the first scenario would not need decontamination, but the second would. This is why an accurate history of the incident is critical to offering efficient and effective response. By contrast, nuclear weapons involve fallout, and the very nature of an radiologic dispersion device (radionuclides placed in or on a conventional explosive such as dynamite, and exploded with the intent to disperse radioactive particles over a designated target site) will involve radiologic contamination of victims.

Health care facilities routinely involved with drills and emergency response to a local nuclear facility will often have a supply of PPE that is designated for radiation decontamination known as "Anti-C's". However, standard Level C PPE, like that described herein for chemical decontamination, is also acceptable PPE to be utilized to avoid exposure and contamination of health care workers when caring for victims of a radiologic disaster. Like chemically exposed patients, those without life- or limb-threatening injuries should be appropriately decontaminated before ED entry.

The sequence for chemical decontamination outlined herein should also be used for the radiologically contaminated victim: Removal of clothing and jewelry (and double bagging and sealing them), followed by showering with water at high volume with low pressure, with gentle scrubbing as needed, in a rostral–caudal direction. As long as ED personnel are wearing proper PPE (Level D or C), emergent attention to the ABCs can proceed, followed by decontamination. After decontamination, standard medical care and full patient surveys can proceed.[29] The bagged belongings and wash run-off need special considerations for storage and disposal, however, owing to the radioactivity. Open wounds need special attention with radionuclide exposures, especially with alpha emitters, because once they are internalized, these isotopes have a greater potential to cause adverse health effects than gamma or beta emitters (see the article by Kazzi et al, elsewhere in this issue).

It is posited that most patients in the radiologic contamination scenarios will not have heavy enough radiation contamination from radionuclides to place health care workers at a significant health risk from their brief exposures to these patients when encountered before decontamination. Unless heavy, generalized radiologic contamination is demonstrated by Geiger–Müller surveys, most victims can be safely spot decontaminated by health care workers in level D PPE. Only the most heavily contaminated patients require full-body decontamination by health care workers using Level C PPE. Workers must also be reminded that victims of acute radiation sickness owing to massive gamma irradiation are not themselves radioactive and do not pose any risk to caregivers (just like a patient receiving radiation therapy for cancer is not a radiation risk to others). Only patients contaminated by radioisotopes pose a secondary contamination risk to ED staff. Radiation detectors (Geiger–Müller meters and similar devices), which are usually available in most hospitals that perform nuclear medicine studies, can be used to ensure proper decontamination of radionuclides from a patient, a luxury that is not available to ensure complete decontamination from a chemical spill.

SUMMARY

Accurate identification of the chemicals substances involved is the most important information necessary for proper care of the HAZMAT incident, but is often not available initially. Protection of the health and safety of the health care worker and maintaining the integrity of the hospital and ED must be the first priority in a HAZMAT incident, and is in the best interest in public health, to be able to properly care for the expected victims. Decontamination for both chemical and nuclear HAZMAT incidents are handled in a similar fashion by hospital personnel: Level C PPE is sufficient for worker protection, and decontamination using high-flow, low-pressure, tepid water, with a mild liquid soap if needed, washing from head to toe. Wounds and eyes should be decontaminated with physiologic solutions, and special attention must be directed to hairy areas and skin folds and hands and feet. Containment of run-off water must be assured, because this is considered hazardous waste. Emergent management of life- and limb-threatening conditions must only be performed by health care workers in proper PPE; once full decontamination is completed, standard evaluation and treatment can begin. Efficient patient flow will occur when proper protocols are followed and mock-up scenarios and drills have been practiced regularly by appropriate staff.

REFERENCES

1. Occupational Safety and Health Administration. Personal protective equipment. Washington, DC: Occupational Safety and Health Administration; 2003. OSHA 3151–12R.
2. Hick JL, Hanfling D, Burstein JL, et al. Protective equipment for health care facility decontamination personnel: regulations, risks, and recommendations. Ann Emerg Med 2003;42(3):370–80.
3. Occupational Safety and Health Administration. Best practices for hospital-based first receivers of victims from mass casualty incidents involving the release of hazardous substances. Washington, DC: Occupational Safety and Health Administration; 2005. OSHA 3249-08N.
4. Occupational Safety and Health Administration. Eye and face protection. Washington, DC: Occupational Safety and Health Administration; 2014. Available at: https://www.osha.gov/SLTC/eyefaceprotection/index.html.
5. Parker JS. Hazardous materials personal protective equipment options for the Fort Thomas, Kentucky Fire Department. Cincinnati (OH): University of Cincinnati; 2009. Available at: http://ceas.uc.edu/content/dam/aero/docs/fire/Papers/Personal_Protective_Equipment.pdf.
6. Yeung RS, Chan JT, Lee LL, et al. The use of personal protective equipment in Hazmat incidents. Hong Kong J Emerg Med 2002;9(3):171–6.
7. Available at: https://www.osha.gov/pls/oshaweb/owadisp.show_document?p_table=STANDARDS&;p_id=9767. Accessed July 28, 2014.
8. Agency for Toxic Substances and Disease Registry. Managing hazardous material incidents (MHMI). Volumes 1, 2, and 3. Agency for toxic substances and disease registry (ATSDR). Atlanta (GA): US Department of Health and Human Services, Public Health Service; 2001. Available at: http://www.atsdr.cdc.gov/MHMI/index.asp. Accessed July 15, 2014.
9. Daugherty EL. Health care worker protection in mass casualty respiratory failure: infection control, decontamination, and personal protective equipment. Respir Care 2008;53(2):201–12 [discussion: 212–4].
10. DHHS REMM. Radiation Emergency Medical Management: Guidance on Diagnosis and Treatment for Healthcare Providers. Available at: http://www.remm.nlm.gov/radiation_ppe.htm. Accessed July 28, 2014
11. DHS/DHHS. (Draft Document). Patient decontamination in a mass chemical exposure incident: national planning guidance for communities. Available at: http://www.regulations.gov/#!documentDetail;D=DHS-2014-0012-0002.
12. Hick JL, Penn P, Hanfling D, et al. Establishing and training health care facility decontamination teams. Ann Emerg Med 2003;42(3):381–90.
13. Brent J. Water-based solutions are the best decontaminating fluids for dermal corrosive exposures: a mini review. Clin Toxicol 2013;51(8):731–6.
14. Wormser U, Brodsky B, Sintov A. Skin toxicokinetics of mustard gas in the guinea pig: effect of hypochlorite and safety aspects. Arch Toxicol 2002;76(9):517–22.
15. Schwartz MD, Hurst CG, Kirk MA, et al. Reactive skin decontamination lotion (RSDL) for the decontamination of chemical warfare agent (CWA) dermal exposure. Curr Pharm Biotechnol 2012;13(10):1971–9.
16. Nehles J, Hall AH, Blomet J, et al. Diphoterine for emergent decontamination of skin/eye chemical splashes: 24 cases. Cutan Ocul Toxicol 2006;25(4):249–58.
17. Donoghue AM. Diphoterine® for alkali splashes to the skin. Clin Toxicol (Phila) 2014;52(2):148.

18. Available at: http://www.easydecon.com/easydecon/index.html. Accessed October 11, 2014.
19. Merrit N, Anderson M. Case review malathion overdose: when one patient creates a departmental hazard. J Emerg Nurs 1989;15(6):463–5.
20. Huff S. Lessons learned from hazardous materials incidents. Emerg Care Q 1991; 7(3):17–22.
21. Nozaki H, Hori S, Shinozawa Y, et al. Secondary exposure of medical staff to sarin vapor in the emergency room. Intensive Care Med 1995;21(12):1032–5.
22. Okumura T, Suzuki K, Fukuda A, et al. The Tokyo subway sarin attack: Disaster management, Part 2: hospital response. Acad Emerg Med 1998;5(6):618–24.
23. Geller RJ, Singleton KL, Tarantino ML, et al. Nosocomial poisoning associated with emergency department treatment of organophosphate toxicity-Georgia, 2000. Clin Toxicol 2001;39(1):109–11.
24. Zeitz P, Berkowitz Z, Orr MF, et al. Frequency and type of injuries in responders of hazardous substances emergency events, 1996 to 1998. J Occup Environ Med 2000;42(11):1115–20.
25. Horton DK, Orr M, Tsongas T, et al. Secondary contamination of medical personnel, equipment, and facilities resulting from hazardous materials events, 2003-2006. Disaster Med Public Health Prep 2008;2(2):104–13.
26. Scanlon J. Chemically contaminated casualties: different problems and possible solutions. Am J Disaster Med 2010;5(2):95–105.
27. Burgess JL. Hospital evacuations due to hazardous materials incidents. Am J Emerg Med 1999;17(1):50–2.
28. Heon D, Foltin G. Principles of pediatric decontamination. Clin Pediatr Emerg Med 2009;10(3):186–94.
29. Yamamoto LG. Risks and management of radiation exposure. Pediatr Emerg Care 2013;29(9):1016–26.

Resources for Toxicologic and Radiologic Information and Assistance

Mark Kirk, MD[a], Carol J. Iddins, MD[b],*

KEYWORDS

- Resources • Chemical • Radiological • Nuclear detonation • Competencies
- Risk assessment

KEY POINTS

- Information management is crucial to effective emergency response during a large-scale chemical or radiologic/nuclear incident.
- The emergency medicine physician should know what potential chemical and radiological/nuclear hazards are present locally and regionally; a basic awareness is paramount.
- Emergency physicians must competently amass information elements most critical to know during a crisis, choosing an appropriate resource to rapidly find reliable information.
- Identifying single point of entry information resources (information leverage points) to many other robust and reliable resources is a helpful strategy for information access during overwhelming large-scale chemical or radiological/nuclear incidents.
- Information needs will vary over time in an emergency response. Early on, situational awareness is paramount. As the event evolves, information needs to be focused, guiding critical decisions about managing mass casualties, protective actions for first receivers, and aligning and mobilizing patient care resources. Rapid-access 24/7 telephone consultation services should be considered first line for attaining human health effects and treatment information about suspected/identified toxicants (chemical or radiological), especially in the early phases of an incident, to provide the best care possible.

Funding Sources: None (M. Kirk); ORAU (C.J. Iddins).
Conflict of Interest: None.
Declarations and Disclaimers: See last page of the article.
[a] Chemical Defense Program, Health Threats Resilience Division, Office of Health Affairs, US Department of Homeland Security, 245 Murray Lane, SW, Mailstop: 0315, Washington, DC 20528, USA; [b] U.S. DOE, Radiation Emergency Assistance Center/Training Site, ORISE, ORAU, PO Box 117, MS 39, Oak Ridge, TN 37831, USA
* Corresponding author.
E-mail address: carol.iddins@orau.org

INTRODUCTION

Information management is crucial to effective emergency response during a large-scale chemical or radiation/nuclear (CRN) incident. The ability to rapidly acquire key information, share it with others, and use that information to make critical decisions and take life-saving actions is a core competency for individual responders (especially emergency physicians) and for every response agency within the community's entire emergency response network. However, Auf der Heide[1] identifies information management as one of the most common problems during all types of mass casualty incidents, and it is often cited as a "lesson learned" in after-action reviews.

In a published account of the 1995 Tokyo subway sarin attack, Okumura and colleagues[2] highlighted the hospital's challenges in responding to an incident causing hundreds of people to arrive at the hospital, many carrying residual contamination, exhibiting effects of a toxic exposure and many ill, requiring specific antidotal therapy. Applicable to all types of disasters, Okamura divided the hospital's challenges into 3 categories: (1) hardware problems (structural problems pertaining to the hospital facilities); (2) software problems (preparedness problems pertaining to disaster plans and response capabilities); and (3) transmission problems (information management problems).Those challenges he termed transmission problems included the need for early information about the offending agent, expert medical information, including emergency guidelines for treatment and standardization of care, and surveillance for long-term care.

During a large-scale CRN emergency response, all key decision-makers from the emergency medical technician first responder to first receivers, emergency physician (EP), hospital incident commander, fire chief, and the city's emergency manager will find themselves in an ambiguous, complex, and uncertain situation requiring critical decisions be made rapidly. In these situations, the amount of information flowing to the decision-maker is often not the problem; instead it is the quality of that information. Copious information flowing in, but not reliable or useful for making key decisions, conceals those crucial pieces of information that will lead to decisions resulting in desirable outcomes. For the EP, one of the most useful competencies is to become an expert at managing information, and the EP can best accomplish this by understanding critical information needs, knowing where to quickly access the most reliable information, and separating the information useful for decision-making from the "noise." The authors intend to provide information to increase understanding about information elements most critical to know during a CRN incident and to gain the ability to choose an appropriate resource, rapidly acquiring reliable information. In addition, a helpful strategy for information access during such overwhelming scenarios is identifying (ideally during the preplanning phase) information resources that serve as leverage points. These information leverage points are single points of entry to many other robust and reliable resources, and are highlighted here. The intention of this article is to provide a concise, condensed, and useful collection of resources and assistance for the EP physician from the standpoint of the provider "in the trenches" delivering care and the EP who may be the Director interacting with the Hospital Incident Commander for CRN incidents. Rather than provide an endless list of resources, the authors attempt to compartmentalize the various resources along an acute (up to 12 hours after incident for these purposes) and prolonged timeline (definitive care/recovery). The following are basic competencies in information management for the EM physician when handling a large-scale CRN incident:

1. Planning information (pre-event actions, hazard vulnerability analysis [HVA], education and training, drills and exercises)

2. Incident management information (local resources with information for situational awareness [SA] and managing resources)
   • Protection (protective action guidelines [PAG]; evacuation; staff personal protective equipment [PPE]; decontamination [decon]; hospital [force] protection)
   • Crisis communication/risk communications (messaging for shelter/evacuation/communication/community reception centers [CRC]/alternative treatment facilities)
   • Psychological first aid (PFA)
   • Supplies, equipment, and medications
3. Toxicant management (subject matter experts/triage/risks to physician, staff, patients, and facility; and patient management)
4. Definitive care/disposition (admission, transfer; discharge)
5. Recovery management (decedents/Community Reception Center/cleanup)

CHEMICAL INCIDENT PREPLANNING

Two important areas information resources greatly assist with preplanning are (1) recognizing, in advance, the most probable chemical threats to the community that the EP may face, and (2) developing competencies through education and training for effectively responding to high-impact chemical scenarios.

HAZARD VULNERABILITY ANALYSIS AND RISK ASSESSMENT

Effective preplanning should include an investigation (hazard vulnerability analysis/risk assessment), identifying those chemicals with the greatest potential to affect large numbers of people if released in an accident or used as chemical weapons of opportunity.[3] A list of priority chemicals should be identified, especially focusing on those possessing high inherent toxicity and having the ability to readily become airborne allowing dispersion away from the point of origin. In addition, priority should be given to those chemicals manufactured, transported, or stored in quantities large enough to deliver dangerous concentrations to nearby large populations. It is a realistic expectation for first responders and first receivers to have knowledge and training for response to chemical events based on community-specific chemicals greatest risks.[4,5]

Most communities have Local Emergency Planning Committees (LEPCs) or community-wide emergency response interagency coalitions. Joining a community planning committee is an excellent way for an EP to become involved in community planning and learn about the unique local chemical risks.[6]

CHEMICAL INCIDENT EDUCATION AND TRAINING

The EP and the emergency department (ED) staff must maintain competencies in mass casualty triage and critical care for handling chemical incidents. Many formats (eg, Web-based, didactic, and hands-on training) are available for acquiring these skills. Because performing specific skills is essential for successful response to a chemical incident, hands-on and discussion-based training courses are encouraged, either through a formal course or local training and exercises. EPs, searching for courses to attend or take on-line, should make certain the goals and objectives align with competencies of emergency medicine practice before investing precious time and money.

Several hands-on courses are specifically designed to prepare health care providers for responding to chemical emergencies. The Federal Emergency Management Agency (FEMA) Center for Domestic Preparedness (CDP) in Anniston, Alabama offers courses for mass casualty incident management and specific courses focused on

Chemical Biological Radiological Nuclear and Explosive (CBRNE) and Hazmat incidents (eg, Hospital Emergency Response Training for Mass Casualty Incidents).[7] The US Army Medical Research Institute of Chemical Defense's Chemical Casualty Care Division (USAMRICD) offers the Hospital Management of Chemical, Biological, Radiological, Nuclear and Explosive Incidents Course (HM-CBRNE) and the Field Management of Chemical and Biological Casualties Course.[8]

Other didactic and facilitated discussion courses are designed for health care providers to gain knowledge about how to recognize and treat victims exposed to toxic substances. The American Academy of Clinical Toxicology cosponsors the Advanced Hazmat Life Support (AHLS) Course, and the American College of Medical Toxicology offers a course entitled Chemical Agents of Opportunity for Terrorism: TICS & TIMs.[9,10] The National Disaster Life Support offers several courses teaching principles for all hazards, but includes skills applicable to chemical incidents (eg, decontamination).[11]

Training on quick access to the most reliable information is available through the National Library of Medicine Special Information Services (NLM SIS). In a webinar entitled "Packing Your Digital Go-Bag: Essential Disaster Health Information on Your Mobile Device," the NLM discusses key resources that first responders and first receivers can access through the Web or load onto their mobile devices.[12]

INCIDENT MANAGEMENT INFORMATION

Incident relevant information can be divided into 2 distinct kinds: (1) situational awareness of the incident reported from the scene or from a coordinating center, driving emergency response actions (eg, protection of staff); and (2) expert medical information guiding treatment of patients. Early in an emergency response, information delivered to the EP should provide awareness of the situation, size it up, provide details, and allow the EP to gear up for a potentially large-scale, resource-taxing event. As an event evolves, information needs to change, now requiring sharply focused, detailed information, guiding critical decisions about managing mass casualties entering the ED, protective actions for the first receivers, and aligning and mobilizing patient care resources such as decontamination teams or antidote stockpiles. Finally, detailed, tactical information guides each caregiver's actions such as triaging, treating, and deciding disposition of patients.

SITUATIONAL AWARENESS

During the initial phase of response to a large-scale chemical incident, the EP needs information to gain clarity of the situation to:

- Gain knowledge of expected injuries and likely clinical patterns
- Gather enough details to take appropriate actions
- Gain understanding of the magnitude to forecast near-term future needs

Information related to situational awareness, particular in the first few hours, will come from local information sources such as patient descriptions, emergency medical services reporting, emergency response centers, incident command communications, or even the media. Reliable reporting of on-scene size-ups and updates will occur by building key relationships, in advance, with the most trustworthy local sources. Examples of trustworthy local resources include:

- On-scene reports from first responders or the incident commander
- Reports from community emergency management coordination points
- Regional poison centers

Each incident is unique, and situational awareness information should be delivered to the ED as quickly as possible (ideally before any patients arrive from the scene of the incident). As an incident unfolds, more detailed information may follow such as confirmed chemical identification, plume modeling results, critical resource needs, and epidemiology of victims. The EP must be flexible, adapting to new information as it arrives.

PERSONAL PROTECTIVE EQUIPMENT AND DECONTAMINATION

First receiver PPE selection and training requires extensive pre-event planning, training, and regular practice to attain skills (see article by Holland and Cawthon elsewhere in this issue for important resource recommendations). Recommended information resources useful before an incident include:

- Occupational Safety and Health Administration (OSHA)[5]: Best practices for hospital-based first receivers of victims from mass casualty incidents involving the release of hazardous substances
- Hick and colleagues[13]: Protective equipment for health care facility decontamination personnel: regulations, risks, and recommendations

During an incident, additional factors to consider in the selection of PPE are available through situational awareness information and include the suspected substance, toxicity of the substance, potential routes of exposure, degree of contact, and the specific task assigned to the treatment team.

Recommended information resources during an incident include:

- Regional Poison Centers
- Wireless Information System for Emergency Responders (WISER)[14]
- Emergency Response Guidebook: *A Guidebook for First Responders During the Initial Phase of a Dangerous Goods/Hazardous Materials Transportation Incident*[15]
- National Institute for Occupational Safety and Health (NIOSH) *Pocket Guide to Chemical Hazards*[16]

Patient decontamination is a medical intervention and is complementary to other life-saving interventions. The decision to perform mass decontamination is one of the most important decisions made during the emergency response to a large-scale chemical incident. Often it must be made with limited information to guide that decision. The reader is referred to the article on important resource recommendations elsewhere in this issue.

This decision-making process must be underpinned by preplanning based on applicable regulations (OSHA), standards (NIOSH), evidence-based guidance (Department of Homeland Security [DHS]/Department of Health and Human Services [DHHS]) and best practices.

Recommended information resources before an incident include:

- Patient Decontamination in a Mass Chemical Exposure Incident: National Planning Guidance for Communities; US Department of Homeland Security and Department of Health and Human Services, draft, 2014.[17]
- OSHA[5]: Best practices for hospital-based first receivers of victims from mass casualty incidents involving the release of hazardous substances.
- Hick and colleagues[18]: Establishing and training health care facility decontamination teams
- Guidelines for Mass Casualty Decontamination during a Hazmat/Weapon of Mass Destruction Incident. Volumes I & II.[19]

Recommended information resources during an incident include:

- WISER[14]
- Emergency Response Guidebook: *A Guidebook for First Responders During the Initial Phase of a Dangerous Goods/Hazardous Materials Transportation Incident*[15]
- NIOSH *Pocket Guide to Chemical Hazards*[16]
- Best practices and guidelines for CBR mass personnel decontamination (second edition)[20]

TOXICANT MANAGEMENT

To provide the best care, clinicians must rapidly access reliable information regarding specific aspects of the suspected/identified chemicals, and especially the human health effects and treatment. Information can be rapidly accessed through several resources, including 24/7 telephone or bedside consultation resources, Internet-accessible sites, or electronic or paper-based references. During a large-scale chemical incident, the EP may not have access to Web-based resources or reference texts. A helpful strategy for information access during such overwhelming scenarios is identifying (ideally during the preplanning phase) information resources that serve as leverage points. These information leverage points are easily accessible, single points of entry to reliable information. Therefore, learning how to access 24/7 telephone resources can serve as leverage points and can offload the burden of time often required to use other reference resources. The rapid-access consultation services should be considered first-line resources for toxicant management during an incident.

RAPID ACCESS TO CONSULTATION (TELEPHONE HOT-LINE RESOURCES)

In response to the Tokyo subway sarin attack in 1994, physicians identified the lack of an efficient chemical disaster information network as one of the most significant problems with communications.[2] It was suggested that poison information centers should act as regional mediators of all toxicologic information, and that all community response components (eg,. police, fire departments, and hospitals) need to form an information network. The regional poison centers' abilities to acquire and disseminate information in a crisis makes it a critical information resource in this communications network.[2,21]

The Institute of Medicine's 2004 report, Forging a Poison Prevention and Control System, supports those suggestions and recommends:[22]

Poison control centers can play an important role in preparedness and response to acts of bioterrorism, chemical terrorism, or other public health emergencies. The efforts involved in the rapidly evolving, present day building of capacity in the areas of bioterrorism and chemical terrorism preparedness and response is likely to strengthen the ability of centers to respond to natural disasters and other threats to public health.[22]

The report further recommends that poison centers, during a community response, can: provide assistance with early recognition and notification of bioterrorism and chemical terrorism events; coordinate antidote distribution and guide appropriate antidote use; assist health care professionals with management of exposed patients and rescue personnel; disseminate threat and preventive/therapeutic information to the public; and provide consultative support to public health and law enforcement authorities.

The American Association of Poison Control Centers lists 55 regional poison centers available 24 hours a day, 7 days a week at 1-800-222-1222.[23]

In addition, medical toxicologists are available throughout the country, most commonly at academic centers, and can provide bedside consultation with case management, assist with obtaining and interpreting specialty toxicology lab tests, and identify other public health assets as needed. These actors should be integrated into the response through preplanning, and contacted early in the incident to enlist their expertise. Often a medical toxicologist can be contacted through the regional poison center for telephone consultation if not available for bedside care. During preplanning, toxicologists can be located through the American College of Medical Toxicology or Agency for Toxic Substance and Disease Registry's regional toxicology network.[24,25]

One leverage point of gaining access to many public health resources is contacting the state or local health department,[26] which investigates environmental hazards, answers monitoring questions, and can refer to other contacts and agencies as needed.

The US Army Medical Research Institute of Chemical Defense/Chemical Casualty Care Division (MRICD) has a staff of subject matter experts that is available for consultation on medical aspects of chemical warfare agents and for analysis of biological specimens for possible exposure to chemical agents.[27]

Other telephone-accessible resources exist for large-scale incidents, but their focus is not specific to human health aspects. CHEMTREC is a 24/7 resource designed to provide emergency responders and others with response information and access to a network of experts. The US Coast Guard's National Response Center (NRC) is the federal government's communication center, and serves as the sole point of contact for reporting all hazardous substances releases and oil spills.

ON-LINE RESOURCES

On-line resources are available and can provide rapid, focused information useful for toxicant management. Many are readily accessible through the Web or can be downloaded to a personal computer or mobile device. The EP loses valuable time attempting to search for data during an emergency response unless already familiar with the benefits of each resource and has developed the ability to navigate through it quickly, accessing the essential information needed to make sound decisions.

The National Library of Medicine provides several very useful resources and is a leverage point for gaining access to many useful sites.[28]

WISER is designed for use by emergency responders during a hazardous material incident, and provides a quick overview of specific chemicals including substance identification support, physical characteristics, PPE recommendations, health effects, and treatment overview.[14] For the EP, one of the most valuable aspects of WISER is excerpting information from many important references such as NIOSH, Emergency Response Guide, Poisindex, and Meditext. It also provides links to the original reference sources. It is not designed specifically for the EP but can be a quick reference during an incident.

Chemical Hazards Emergency Medical Management (CHEMM) is another resource offered by the NLM, specifically designed for the EP and medical first responders to use during a mass casualty chemical incident.[29] CHEMM complements the basic information in WISER, providing more detailed information on health effects and medical treatment. WISER and CHEMM used together provides the EP with a comprehensive resource from which to gather a great deal of important information very quickly. In addition, CHEMM serves as a leverage point to many other valuable resources.

CHEMM Intelligent Syndromes Tool (CHEMM-IST) is a decision support tool intended to aid recognition of toxidromes by entering a few key patient observations.[30] For first responders and first receivers, recognizing a toxidrome serves as a detection tool for realizing a potential hazardous chemical exposure, leading staff to take protective actions and administer empiric treatments. This decision support tool can be accessed at the CHEMM Web site.

The NLM SIS supplies a variety of environmental health databases that are potentially beneficial during a large-scale chemical incident.[31] TOXNET (TOXicology Data NETwork) is a group of databases covering chemicals and drugs, diseases and the environment, environmental health, occupational safety and health, poisoning, risk assessment and regulations, and toxicology. In addition to Hazardous Substance Data Bank (HSDB), TOXLINE, and ChemIDplus found in TOXNET, NLM has evaluated and made accessible on their Web site many other resources of potential benefit (many as mobile apps) in emergency and disaster situations.

The Agency for Toxic Substances and Disease Registry (ATSDR) Medical Management Guidelines for Chemical Agents contains an overview of human health effects and treatment recommendations for specific agents, and can serve as a rapid immediate training for the front-line care providers.[32,33]

DIAGNOSTICS

During a large-scale chemical incident, point-of-care testing and hospital laboratory diagnostics guide local clinical decision-making. Often these public health emergencies will require additional resources to confirm the causative agent involved. Specialized analytical toxicology testing is beyond the capabilities of nearly all hospital laboratories. The Centers for Disease Control and Prevention (CDC) Laboratory Response Network (LRN) is an integrated network of laboratories designed to respond quickly to biological and chemical threats, and other high-priority public health emergencies.[34,35] The LRN is composed of more than 150 local, state, and federal public health, food testing, veterinary diagnostic, and environmental testing laboratories providing the laboratory infrastructure and capacity to respond to biological and chemical terrorism, and other public health emergencies. The state or local health department can serve as the access point to the LRN laboratories and provide clear guidance, obtaining samples and packaging clinical samples for transport or accessed at the CDC emergency preparedness and response Web site.[34]

ANTIDOTES

The EP needs to quickly identify antidotes and specific treatments necessary to treat suspected poisoning by recognizing toxidromes, interpreting diagnostic tests, or responding to on-scene investigations relayed from the scene. Many of the resources already outlined are useful for determining pharmaceutical needs. The regional poison center or hospital pharmacy may be most helpful assisting with identifying caches of pharmaceuticals beyond those immediately available on site.

CRISIS COMMUNICATION AND MESSAGING

Delivering information and reassurance during a crisis provides people with accurate information, and tends to alleviate anxiety that stems from rumor and misinformation. Information can be regarded as an antidote to fear, because those who have more knowledge regarding the risks of exposure improve their attitudes toward those exposures.[36,37] Many of the resources outlined herein are useful for providing information that will guide risk communication messaging. A helpful resource in assisting crisis and risk communication training is the CDC's Crisis and Emergency Risk Communication Quick Guide.[38]

DISPOSITION

During a large-scale incident, health care resources may be strained. First receivers are often challenged to evaluate and treat the surge of patients arriving. Caregivers can also manage the surge by rapidly and safely discharging such patients with mild or minimal exposures. Providing these discharged patients with appropriate discharge information can alleviate fears and future concerns about their health. This information is best derived from authoritative sources such as public health officials, poison centers, medical toxicologists, or various on-line resources such as:

- ATSDR Medical Management Guidelines for Chemical Agents contains a Patient Information Sheet providing answers to commonly asked questions specific to an acute exposure to specific chemicals.[32] In addition, a Follow-up Instructions page is included for providing tailored follow-up care for every patient.
- ATSDR's Toxicology FAQs for Chemical Agents[39]

Follow-up and medical surveillance may be crucial to the care of community casualties. Making sure all patients have a means to follow up is crucial. This tracking is most often coordinated by the local or state health department's epidemiologists.

ADDITIONAL RESPONSE RESOURCES TO AUGMENT THE COMMUNITY RESPONSE

Although the early stages of response to a large-scale chemical incident depend on local resources and capabilities, eventually other specialized regional, state, and federal teams will respond. It is not likely the role of the EP to mobilize these resources. However, it is useful for the EP to be aware of specialized teams that may arrive to augment the community response capabilities or bring highly technical resources, such as the National Guard's Weapons of Mass Destruction Civil Support Teams (WMD-CST) and CBRNE-enhanced Response Force Packages (CERFP) teams; the US Marine Corps' Chemical Biological Incident Response Force (CBIRF) team; the DHS Metropolitan Medical Response System (MMRS) Grant Program; the US Environmental Protection Agency's National Decontamination Team; and the Federal Bureau of Investigation's Hazardous Materials Response Unit (HMRU)/Hazardous Evidence Response Team Unit (HERTU).[40–44]

PLANNING INFORMATION FOR RADIOLOGICAL/NUCLEAR INCIDENTS
Hazard Vulnerability Analysis and Risk Assessment

The EP should know which hazards are present locally and regionally. The hospital emergency response plan should have a comprehensive risk assessment for the area (nuclear power plant, national laboratory) and incorporate the players from these locations into their planning (http://www.calhospitalprepare.org/hazard-vulnerability-analysis).[45]

For radiological/nuclear (R/N) incidents, one method of identifying the most common radioisotopes of concern is to break them down into the areas where they are often used or the source of incidents, sometimes known as the University Five, Military Five, and Industrial Three (**Table 1**).[46] These radioisotopes may be further categorized according to their primary type of hazard to humans: external contamination (skin, eye), internal contamination, and exposure. The multiagency document, Planning Guidance

Table 1
Categories of radioisotopes

Category	Radioisotope	Primary Hazard
University Five	Carbon 14 (^{14}C)	May be internal, negligible external
	Phosphorous 32 (^{32}P)	External and internal
	Iodine 125 (^{125}I)	Internal (thyroid)
	Iodine 131 (^{131}I)	Internal (thyroid)
	Californium 252 (^{252}Cf)	Internal (neutron activation)
Military Five	Tritium (^{3}H)	Internal (and absorption through skin)[a]
(and potentially	Uranium 235 (^{235}U)	Internal
the Department	Uranium 238 (^{238}U)	Internal
of Energy)	Plutonium 239 (^{239}Pu)	Internal
	Americium 241 (^{241}Am)	Internal
	Iodine 131 and 129 are often included	Internal (thyroid)
Industrial Three	Iridium 192 (^{192}Ir)	Exposure
	Cobalt 60 (^{60}Co)	Exposure
	Cesium 137 (^{137}Cs)	Exposure

[a] http://ehs.uky.edu/radiation/isotopes/tritium.html.[48]

Data from Radiation Emergency Assistance Center/Training Site. Available at: http://orise.orau. gov/files/reacts/medical-aspects-of-radiation-incidents.pdf. p. 29. Accessed June 15, 2014.

for Response to a Nuclear Detonation, was developed in response to the National Planning Scenario for a Detonation of an Improvised Nuclear Device (IND) and may be accessed at http://www.epa.gov/radiation/docs/er/planning-guidance-for-response-to-nuclear-detonation-2-edition-final.pdf. Accessed October 14 2014.[47] This document is an excellent resource to review and download/print as a planning/response tool.

Education and Training

Most injuries will be the same as occur from conventional explosive/blast incidents with an IND (or RDD). There are caveats to this when dealing with R/N incidents. The treatment of life-threatening trauma/burns/medical illnesses will still be the number 1 priority; the caveats come into play with the handling of contamination (internal and/or external) and exposures (irradiation), or both. Further complicating this is the combined radiation injury (CRI), that is, the presence of a burn/trauma with a radiation injury/illness. These casualties have a much worse prognosis, and with an IND scenario with scarce resources may be initially triaged into expectant categories.[49] The main formats for education on R/N incidents include numerous Web-based training (WBT) courses that provide Continuous Education (CE) credit and live courses that provide CE (both didactic and with hands-on training) (see the article on checklists for hazardous materials emergency preparedness elsewhere in this issue). There are also training courses that address the awareness level of nonhospital personnel for R/N incidents. There are 3 live, educational centers directed toward medical providers caring for R/N illnesses and injuries; 2 of these provide Accreditation Council for Continuing Medical Education (ACCME) Category 1 credit:

- The Armed Forces Radiobiology Research Institute (AFRRI) offers a 3-day Medical Effects of Ionizing Radiation (MEIR) course that is didactic-based with table-top exercises and a hands-on laboratory handling of RADIAC or radioactivity, detection, indication, and computation equipment (http://www.usuhs.edu/afrri/outreach/meir/meir.htm, accessed 18 June 2014).[50]

- The FEMA CDP in Anniston, Alabama offers a Hospital Emergency Response Training for Mass Casualty Incidents (HERT) 3-day course that "prepares health-care personnel to conduct a safe and effective emergency medical response to a mass-casualty incident" as well as a prehospital and a decision-making course.[51] The CDP does not offer ACCME credit at this time.
- The Radiation Emergency Assistance Center/Training Site (REAC/TS) in Oak Ridge, Tennessee offers physicians (health care providers, emergency planners, public health) a basic Radiation Emergency Medicine (REM) 3-and-a-half-day course. The course includes: didactics; handling radiation detection instrumentation laboratory; a decontamination demonstration; a drill in which participants receive and handle live, moulaged "patients" in a hospital setting; and decontaminating wounds with transferable, liquid radioactive contamination. In this process, the participants learn about and use proper PPE, survey for contamination, "treat" the patients' injuries, and decontaminate the patients. For physicians desiring a higher level of learning, the Advanced Radiation Medicine (ARM) 4-and-a-half-day course offers the world's leading experts in radiation medicine didactic-format, interactive, and hands-on exercises.[52]

Additional training that should be done in advance includes the FEMA WBT courses: IS-100.HCb Introduction to the Incident Command System (ICS 100) for Healthcare/Hospitals, IS-200.HCa Applying ICS to Healthcare Organizations, and many other offerings available at their Web site.[53]

Drills and Exercises

There are numerous formats for keeping skills sharp with drills and exercises. These formats should exercise all hazard responses and focus on identified risks specific to the local and regional area. The US Department of Veteran's Affairs (VA) collaborated with the Oak Ridge Institute for Science and Education (ORISE) to develop a tool named Exercise Builder: Hospital, which standardizes all aspects of their preparedness, exercise, response, and after-action reports for all of the hospitals within the system.[54]

The reader is also referred to the article on hospital preparedness for chemical and radiological disasters elsewhere in this issue.

INCIDENT MANAGEMENT INFORMATION
Local Resources

In the first 12 hours after an incident (and likely up to 72 hours), the response effort will be local (**Box 1**). The first receiver or EP should request the support of the radiation safety officer (RSO), medical physicist, nuclear medicine, or radiology department staff who may have experience in radiation. Nuclear medicine scanners such as the thyroid probe or the gamma camera used in positron emission tomography scanners can be adapted for use in the measurement of contamination with radioactive material. The EP and ED director need to be aware of the local assets, resources, and various agreements within the local area and region. The Local Emergency Planning Committee should be incorporated into the hospital's emergency operations plan. A listing of agencies that will be mobilized to provide assistance (but will not likely be available in the first 12 hours) may be found under the Resources section. The Medical Reserve Corps (MRC), a civilian citizen volunteer group, is another asset that may be available locally.[55] A few state MRC teams (Ohio, Florida, Georgia, and Mississippi) have a partner program, the Radiation Response Volunteer Corps (RRVC), which includes individuals with professional background and training in radiation.[56] Many

---

Box 1

Chemical and radiological/nuclear emergency speed-dial on-call resources

Chemical Emergency Speed Dial: 24/7 On-Call Resources

- Regional Poison Center: 1-800-222-1222 (any chemical emergency)
- Chemtrec: 1-800-424-9300 (hazardous material spills)
- National Response Center: 1-800-424-8802 (major oil or chemical release)
- Local and State Health Departments (report unusual illness, suspected epidemics, obtain epidemiologic and laboratory support):
  - Local Health Departments: _____. For a map with directory for your locality go to: http://www.naccho.org/about/lhd/
  - State Health Departments: _____. For a map with directory for your state go to: http://www.cdc.gov/mmwr/international/relres.html

Radiological/Nuclear Emergency Speed Dial: 24/7 On-Call Resources

1. Radiation Emergency Assistance Center/Training Site (REAC/TS): 865-576-1005 ask for REAC/TS
2. The Regional Poison Control Center: 1-800-222-1222
3. AFRRI Emergency Operations Center (for military and civilian command and control centers): 301-295-0530
4. CDC Emergency Operations Center: 770-488-7100
5. State Radiological Health: _____. For a map with directory for your state go to: http://www.crcpd.org/Map/default.aspx.

---

cities have built coalitions among the hospital systems for mechanisms of aid that would be the initial means of help. The state emergency management agency will provide assistance and resources but may take longer than the initial 12 hours.

Real-time 24/7 assistance for radiological injuries/illnesses advice and consultation, triage and treatment recommendations, and dose estimates may be obtained from REAC/TS by calling (865) 576-1005 (http://orise.orau.gov/reacts/). The regional Poison Center (1-800-222-1222) is also available for real-time information 24/7 regarding toxicologic emergencies (http://www.acmt.net/physician_resources.html). The CDC has an Emergency Operations Center 24/7 in case of an emergency: (770)-488-7100. Numerous sources regarding personal protective equipment, radiological terms, triage, and treatment (see the article by Holland, Cawthon and Borron elsewhere in this issue) are available. Additional sources for radiological protection may be provided by the Conference on Radiological Control Program Directors (CRCPD) and the state radiological health/public health departments.[57] An easy-to-use map directory may be found at http://www.crcpd.org/Map/default.aspx.

Being aware of the state-based radiological health resources ahead of time is important for a successful response during an incident.

Situational Awareness

Within 6 to 10 hours, the Department of Energy (DOE) and National Nuclear Security Administration (NNSA) Federal Radiological Monitoring and Assessment Center (FRMAC) may have a Consequence Management Response Team (CMRT) anywhere in the United States, once requested by the DHS and state and local agencies to respond to an R/N incident.[58] The CMRT would provide radiological emergency response professionals within the Department of Energy's national laboratories to support the Aerial Measuring System (AMS), Radiological Assessment Program (RAP), REAC/TS and the National Atmospheric Release Advisory Center (NARAC). These teams supplement the FRMAC to provide: medical advice and consultation for radiation injuries/illnesses; radiation monitoring; radiological analysis and data assessments; and atmospheric transport modeling.[58]

Atmospheric plume modeling with HotSpot, free downloadable software provided by NARAC, will help give the EP guidance for sheltering and evacuation, and may provide some information to assist with dose estimation (casualty location with atmospheric variables).[59] This tool helps the EP to plug in variables (wind speed/direction and shielding), and will give a plume direction model and estimation of percentage of types of injuries, fatalities, with timing and distance data sheet, all based on computer modeling. It is recommended for the EP to download and become familiar with the tool in advance as part of the planning process. This tool may be accessed at the NARAC site on the Lawrence Livermore National Laboratory (LLNL) Web site: https://narac.llnl.gov/.

Protection

The planning and education steps are the ideal time for knowing how to protect the patient, the health care providers, and the facility. For "Just In Time (JIT)" information, the CDC has some excellent videos that cover required PPE, handling casualties, and decedent care (see Recovery section), and are accessible at http://www.bt.cdc.gov/radiation.[60,61] Other resources for medical management, radiation basics, decontamination, and dose magnitude estimation (determining if you have a problem) are available from REAC/TS by accessing their Web site (under Resources and see Treatment Algorithm section) or by calling the on-call team. The DHHS Radiation Emergency Medical Management (REMM) Web site also provides useful clinical information and is available as a downloadable app.[62] AFRRI has many available resources and has the Biodosimetry Assessment Tool (BAT) and First Responders Radiological Assessment Tool (FRAT), which should be downloaded in advance to help with patient triage.[63]

Protective Action Guidelines

PAGs exist to reduce or eliminate the threat of adverse health effects following an R/N incident.[64] Initial guidelines may change with time as more information is gathered. These recommendations should be communicated in Emergency Messaging forms that use all available avenues of communication.

Crisis Communications and Messaging

These messages may include recommendations to "Get Inside" shelter or "Stay Inside" a shelter to evacuate to another area; and may include "Stay Tuned" for more information regarding changing conditions and safe places for shelter; where to find safe food and water; where to receive medications; or how to decontaminate individuals and animals (pets or livestock).[65]

Psychological

Numerous texts, articles, and multimedia have explored the fear out of proportion to R/N incidents when compared with biological or chemical incidents.[66] Many articles have discussed radiation being "the most dreaded of all hazards."[67] EM physicians will need to be aware of various tools to assess the mental health of patients and provide initial care. Psychological First Aid is one of several tools used for this purpose.[68]

The article elsewhere in this issue on psychological aspects of chemical and radiological disasters explores these and other psychological issues surrounding R/N incidents.

Supplies, Equipment, and Medications

The hospital emergency operations plan should describe types and quantities of supplies, equipment, and medications to have on hand to sustain operations for 72 to 96 hours until assistance arrives from other areas/agencies. The CDC Strategic National Stockpile (SNS) has push packages containing medications, supplies, and equipment that will take up to 12 hours to mobilize after the deployment decision is made.[69] The request goes from the local level to the state level. The state governor then requests the deployment from CDC or DHHS. These agencies will then make the deployment decision. Medical countermeasures that are specific for radiation injuries and contamination with some radioactive material are also available in the SNS.

Toxicant Management

If external contamination is present, it will need to be removed once the patient is stabilized to reduce the dose risk to the patient, the health care providers, and the facility. The EP should follow the facility decontamination plan (see the article elsewhere in this issue on personnel protection and decontamination of adults and children). Internal contamination will require rapid administration of countermeasures for certain radionuclides and begin 24-hour collection of bioexcreta (see the article by Kazzi, Buzzell, Bertelli and Christensen elsewhere in this issue on assessment and management of internal contamination with radioactive materials). Another consideration is collection of peripheral blood to be sent for chromosomal aberration testing. Currently, the United States has one operational cytogenetic biodosimetry laboratory capable of doing these tests at REAC/TS in Oak Ridge, Tennessee.[70]

Treatment of radiological illnesses/injuries in the first 12 hours after an incident consists of supportive care; decontamination; treatment of internal contamination; colony-stimulating factors for suspected, impending bone marrow damage (hematopoietic acute radiation syndrome); and comfort care/hospice for a very high, unsurvivable dose. The first 12 hours will allow the physician to use few parameters to estimate dose and therefore, triage the patient for admission to a specific service, discharge home to follow-up or with hospice, or refer for definitive care such as a burn, trauma, or bone marrow treatment center (see Disposition/Definitive Care Management section). Resources for these tools are available in many planning documents and on many Web sites (see the article by Borron elsewhere in this issue on checklists for hazardous materials emergency preparedness). The time to onset of emesis, lymphocyte depletion rate (based on at least 2 absolute lymphocyte counts), temperature, and patient history (location/shielding, and so forth) will likely be among the few initial parameters available within the first 12 hours.[71,72] If there is a loss of use of electrical and cellular equipment, triage may become very rudimentary (**Table 2**). The time to emesis has been criticized for not being the most sensitive or specific parameter. However, if there are no technological adjuncts (electricity, computers, cellular phones), this may be the EM physician's only real parameter.

The AFRRI BAT and FRAT program (see Incident Management Information, Protection section), RADPRO calculator, and RADAR Exposure Calculator are all tools to help the physician triage the patient.[73-75] There are other complex triage tables that are based on computer modeling using the lymphocyte depletion table, along with numerous other inputs that may be helpful.[76]

Table 2
Estimated dose using 2 parameters available in first 12 hours

Dose (Gy)	Time to Emesis (h)	% with Emesis	Lymphocyte Count at 12 h ($\times 10^9$/L)
1		19	2.30
2	4.63	35	2.16
3	2.62	54	2.03
4	1.74	72	1.90
5	1.27	86	1.79
6	0.99	94	1.68
7	0.79	98	1.58
8	0.66	99	1.48
9	0.56	100	1.39
$\geq$10	0.48	100	1.31

Data from Waselenko JK, MacVittie TJ, Blakely WF, et al. Medical management of the acute radiation syndrome: recommendations of the strategic National Stockpile Radiation Working Group. Ann Intern Med 2004;140:1037–51.

DISPOSITION AND DEFINITIVE CARE

The EP may need to initiate the medical countermeasures for internal contamination for certain radionuclides. The EP will need to have an estimate of the patient's dose to properly triage and treat the patient; this is also necessary for ultimate disposition of the patient. The multiagency Planning Guidance for Nuclear Detonation is an excellent resource for the EP, and has triage recommendations and treatment information (see the article by Borron elsewhere in this issue on checklists for hazardous materials emergency preparedness).[77]

RECOVERY MANAGEMENT

Recovery management information should be included in the planning stage. There are resources for R/N incidents that may help both the EP and the ED Director along the timeline of the incident. The CDC CRC is a tool for helping to monitor the population, including those with minor injuries.[78] A CRC would be set up off-site from the scene and from the hospital; this could help divert the surge of anxious individuals who will seek reassurance at the closest medical facility. A virtual CRC is available for training purposes.[79] Additional recovery management resources for handling of decedents from the ED and hospital will also be needed.[80,81] The local Medical Examiner/Coroner (ME/C) will be in charge of these issues assisted by the local mortuary directors. Further along the disaster timeline, once more assistance is mobilized, the Disaster Mortuary Operations Response Team (DMORT) can help in mass fatality incidents.[82]

ENVIRONMENT, FOOD, AND HEALTH

An important part of the recovery process will be minimizing contamination of milk, food and water supplies. The Advisory Team for Environment, Food, and Health has representatives from the US Department of Agriculture (USDA), the Environmental Protection Agency (EPA), the CDC, and the Food and Drug Administration (FDA).[83] The Advisory Team is a radiological emergency response asset that provides protective action recommendations to federal, state, tribal, and local agencies. There will also need to be guidance for relocation, return, and cleanup, all provided by the Advisory Team. Contact the CDC emergency operations center at 770-488-7100. The Advisory Team will also be activated whenever the FRMAC is activated.

SUMMARY AND DISCUSSION

The resources for CRN toxicologic incidents are vast. Most of the information accessed in this article is from the Internet and is best used in a digital format, as the URLs are included. All disasters affect communications, and in the event of cellular phone, Internet, or electrical power outages, it is strongly recommended that the physician already has a hard copy of those resources critical to decision-making. The ability to manage these resources and information will have a large impact on the success of handling these incidents.

DECLARATIONS AND DISCLAIMERS

The opinions expressed herein are those of the author and are not necessarily those of the US Government (USG) or the DHS. Neither the USG nor the DHS, nor any of their employees, makes any warranty, expressed or implied, or assumes any legal liability or responsibility for the accuracy, completeness or usefulness of the information contained herein or represents that its use would not infringe on privately owned rights (M. Kirk); This work was performed under Contract # DEAC05-06OR23100 between Oak Ridge Associated Universities (ORAU) and the US Department of Energy (USDOE). REAC/TS is a program of the Oak Ridge Institute for Science & Education (ORISE), which is operated for the US Department of Energy (DOE) by ORAU. The opinions expressed herein are those of the author and are not necessarily those of the US Government (USG), the US DOE, ORAU, or sponsoring institutions of ORAU. Neither the USG nor the DOE, nor any of their employees, makes any warranty, expressed or implied, or assumes any legal liability or responsibility for the accuracy, completeness, or usefulness of the information contained herein or represents that its use would not infringe on privately owned rights (C.J. Iddins).

REFERENCES

1. Auf der Heide E. The importance of evidence-based disaster planning. Ann Emerg Med 2006;47(1):34–49.
2. Okumura T, Suzuki K, Fukuda A, et al. The Tokyo subway sarin attack: disaster management, part 2: hospital response. Acad Emerg Med 1998;5(6):618–24.
3. Hauschild VD, Bratt GM. Prioritizing industrial chemical hazards. J Toxicol Environ Health A 2005;68(11–12):857–76.
4. Fricker R, Jacobson J, Davis L. RAND issue paper: measuring and evaluating local preparedness for a chemical or biological terrorist attack. RAND Corporation; 2002. Arlington, Virginia. Available at: http://www.rand.org/pubs/issue_papers/IP217. html. Accessed July 17, 2014.
5. OSHA Best practices for hospital-based first receivers of victims from mass casualty incidents involving the release of hazardous substances. Occupational Safety and Health Administration, United States Department of Labor; 2005. Available at: https://www.osha.gov/dts/osta/bestpractices/firstreceivers_hospital.pdf.
6. Local Emergency Planning Committees. Available at: http://www2.epa.gov/epcra/ local-emergency-planning-committees. Accessed July 17, 2014.
7. Center for Domestic Preparedness. Available at: https://cdp.dhs.gov/. Accessed July 17, 2014.

8. US Army Medical Research Institute of Chemical Defense's Chemical Casualty Care Division (USAMRICD). Available at: http://ccc.apgea.army.mil/default.htm. Accessed July 17, 2014.

9. Advanced HAZMAT Life support course. Available at: http://www.ahls.org/ahls/ecs/main/ahls_home.html. Accessed July 31, 2014.

10. American College of Medical Toxicology Chemical Agents of Opportunity Course. Available at: http://acmt.net/Chemical_Agents_of_Opportunity.html. Accessed July 17, 2014.

11. National Disaster Life Support Course. Available at: http://www.ndlsf.org/index. php/courses/adls. Accessed July 31, 2014.

12. National Library of Medicine's Special Information Services: Disaster course digital go bag. Available at: http://disaster.nlm.nih.gov/dimrc/disastercourse_digitalgobag.html. Accessed July 17, 2014.

13. Hick JL, Hanfling D, Burstein JL, et al. Protective equipment for health care facility decontamination personnel: regulations, risks, and recommendations. Ann Emerg Med 2003;42(3):370–80.

14. Wireless information system for emergency responders (WISER). Available at: http://wiser.nlm.nih.gov/. Accessed July 17, 2014.

15. Emergency response guidebook: a guidebook for first responders during the initial phase of a dangerous goods/hazardous materials transportation incident. United States Department of Transportation, Transport Canada, & Secretariat of Communications and Transport of Mexico; 2012. Available at: http://www.phmsa.dot.gov/hazmat/library/erg.

16. NIOSH pocket guide to chemical hazards. United States Department of Health and Human Services, Centers for Disease Control and Prevention, National Institute for Occupational Safety and Health; 2010. Available at: http://www.cdc.gov/niosh/npg/.

17. Leary AD, Schwartz MD, Kirk MA, et al. Evidence-based patient decontamination: an integral component of mass exposure chemical incident planning and response. Disaster Med Public Health Prep 2014;8(3):260–6.

18. Hick JL, Penn P, Hanfling D, et al. Establishing and training health care facility decontamination teams. Ann Emerg Med 2003;42(3):381–90.

19. Lake W, Divarco S, Schulze P, et al. In: Guidelines for mass casualty decontamination during a HAZMAT/Weapon of mass destruction incident, vols. I & II. United States Army Chemical, Biological, Radiological and Nuclear School, & United States Army Edgewood Chemical Biological Center, & Dartmouth University, Geisel School of Medicine; 2013.

20. Best practices and guidelines for CBR mass personnel decontamination. United States Department of Defense, Technical Support Working Group. Washington (DC): Government Printing office; 2004.

21. Martin-Gill C, Baer AB, Holstege CP, et al. Poison centers as information resources for volunteer EMS in a suspected chemical exposure. J Emerg Med 2007;32(4):397–403.

22. Institute of Medicine Committee on Poison Prevention and Control. Forging a poison prevention and control system. Washington, DC: National Academies Press (US); 2004.

23. Regional Poison Centers. Available at: http://www.aapcc.org/centers/. Accessed July 31, 2014.

24. American College of Medical Toxicology directory of inpatient medical toxicology services. Available at: http://acmt.net/Directory_of_Inpatient_Medical_Toxicology_Services.html. Accessed July 31, 2014.

25. American College of Medical Toxicology & Agency for Toxic Substance and Disease Registry Consultation Network. Available at: http://acmt.net/ATSDR_Consultation_Network.html. Accessed July 31, 2014.

26. Directory for Local and City Health Departments. Available at: http://www.naccho.org/topics/emergency/. Accessed July 31, 2014.

27. Medical Research Institute of Chemical Defense consultation services. Available at: http://chemdef.apgea.army.mil/Default.aspx. Accessed July 31, 2014.

28. NLM-SIS. Special Information Services—environmental health and toxicology. Available at: http://sis.nlm.nih.gov/enviro.html. Accessed July 31, 2014.

29. Chemical hazards emergency medical managment. Available at: http://chemm.nlm.nih.gov/. Accessed July 31, 2014.

30. CHEMM-Intelligent Syndrome Tool. Available at: http://chemm.nlm.nih.gov/chemmist.htm. Accessed July 31, 2014.

31. NLM environmental health and toxicology. Available at: http://sis.nlm.nih.gov/enviro.html. Accessed July 31, 2014.

32. ATSDR medical management guidelines. Available at: http://www.atsdr.cdc.gov/MMG/index.asp. Accessed July 31, 2014.

33. Poisindex. Available at: http://micromedex.com/. Accessed July 31, 2014.

34. CDC Clinical Laboratory Response Network. Available at: http://emergency.cdc.gov/chemical/lab.asp. Accessed July 31, 2014.

35. CDC Chempack. Available at: http://chemm.nlm.nih.gov/chempack.htm. Accessed July 31, 2014.

36. Pastel RH. Collective behaviors: mass panic and outbreaks of multiple unexplained symptoms. Mil Med 2001;166(12 Suppl):44–6.

37. Sandman P, Lanard J. Crisis communication: guidelines for action. American Industrial Hygiene Association; 2004. Available at: http://www.psandman.com/handouts/AIHA-DVD.htm. Accessed July 17, 2014.

38. CDC's crisis and emergency risk communication quick guide. Available at: http://www.bt.cdc.gov/cerc/. Accessed July 31, 2014.

39. ATSDR's toxicology FAQs for chemical agents. Available at: http://www.atsdr.cdc.gov/toxfaqs/index.asp. Accessed July 31, 2014.

40. U.S. Marine Corps fields the Chemical Biological Incident Response Force (CBIRF) team. Available at: http://www.cbirf.marines.mil/. Accessed July 31, 2014.

41. CBRNE-enhanced response force packages (CERFP) teams. Available at: http://www.army.mil/aps/08/information_papers/transform/ARNG_CERFP.html. Accessed July 31, 2014.

42. National Guard Bureau Civil Support Team—WMD. Available at: http://www.army.mil/aps/08/information_papers/transform/ARNG_Civil_Support_Teams.html. Accessed July 31, 2014.

43. EPA National Decontamination Team. Available at: http://www.epa.gov/OEM/index.htm. Accessed July 31, 2014.

44. Federal Bureau of Investigation fields the Hazardous Materials Response Unit (HMRU)/Hazardous Evidence Response Team Unit (HERTU). Available at: http://www.fbi.gov/about-us/investigate/terrorism/terrorism. Accessed July 31, 2014.

45. California Hospital Association, 2011. Available at: http://www.calhospitalprepare.org/hazard-vulnerability-analysis. Accessed June 15, 2014.

46. Radiation Emergency Assistance Center/Training Site. Available at: http://orise.orau.gov/files/reacts/medical-aspects-of-radiation-incidents.pdf. p. 29. Accessed June 15, 2014.

47. Lawrence Livermore National Laboratory, 2010. Available at: https://responder. llnl.gov/data/assets/docs/publications/Planning_Guidance_for_Response_to_a_ Nuclear_Detonation-2nd_Edition_FINAL.pdf. p. 10, 15. Accessed July 17, 2014.

48. University of Kentucky, Radiation Safety, 2014. Available at: http://ehs.uky.edu/ radiation/isotopes/tritium.html. Accessed June 27, 2014.

49. Lawrence Livermore National Laboratory, 2010. Available at: https://responder. llnl.gov/data/assets/docs/publications/Planning_Guidance_for_Response_to_a_ Nuclear_Detonation-2nd_Edition_FINAL.pdf. p. 80–1, 88–90, 92. Accessed July 17, 2014.

50. Uniformed Services University of the Health Sciences. Available at: http://www. usuhs.edu/afrri/outreach/meir/meir.htm. Accessed June 18, 2014.

51. Federal Emergency Management Agency. Available at: https://cdp.dhs.gov/pdf/ cdp-course-list.pdf. Accessed June 18, 2014.

52. Oak Ridge Institute for Science and Education. Available at: http://orise.orau.gov/ reacts/capabilities/continuing-medical-education/default.aspx. Accessed June 18, 2014.

53. Federal Emergency Management Agency. Available at: https://training.fema.gov/ IS/crslist.aspx?all=true. Accessed June 19, 2014.

54. Oak Ridge Institute for Science and Education. Available at: http://orise.orau.gov/ national-security-emergency-management/difference/training-and-technology-support/va-technology-support.aspx. Accessed June 18, 2014.

55. Office of the Surgeon General/Office of the Assistant Secretary for Health. Available at: https://www.medicalreservecorps.gov/HomePage. Accessed July 17, 2014.

56. Office of the Surgeon General/Office of the Assistant Secretary for Health. Available at: https://www.medicalreservecorps.gov/MrcUnits/UnitDetails/2375. Accessed July 17, 2014.

57. Conference of Radiation Control Program Directors. Available at: http://www. crcpd.org/Map/default.aspx. Accessed July 18, 2014.

58. National Nuclear Security Administration, Department of Energy. Available at: http://www.nnsa.energy.gov/aboutus/ourprograms/emergencyoperationscounter terrorism/respondingtoemergencies-0-1. Accessed June 18, 2014.

59. Lawrence Livermore National Laboratory, 2012. Available at: https://narac.llnl.gov/. Accessed June 18, 2014.

60. The Centers for Disease Control and Prevention. Available at: http://www.bt.cdc. gov/radiation. Accessed June 18, 2014.

61. Oak Ridge Institute for Science and Education. Available at: http://orise.orau.gov/ reacts/. Accessed June 28, 2014.

62. Department of Health and Human Services. Available at: http://www.remm.nlm. gov/. Accessed July 18, 2014.

63. Uniformed Services University for the Health Sciences. Available at: http://www. usuhs.edu/afrri/outreach/biodostools.htm. Accessed June 18, 2014.

64. Environmental Protection Agency. Available at: http://www.epa.gov/radiation/ docs/er/ogt_manual_doe_hs_0001_2_24_2009.pdf. Accessed June 15, 2014.

65. The Centers for Disease Control and Prevention. Available at: http://www.bt.cdc. gov/radiation/stayinside.asp. Accessed June 28, 2014.

66. Becker SM. Emergency communication and information issues in terrorist events involving radioactive materials. Biosecur Bioterror 2004;2:197–8.

67. Dodgen D, Norwood A, Becker SM, et al. Social,psychological, and behavioral responses to a nuclear detonation in a US city: implications for health care planning and delivery. Disaster Med Public Health Prep 2011;5(Suppl 1):S55.

68. Office of the Surgeon General/Assistant Secretary for Health. Available at: https://www.medicalreservecorps.gov/File/Promising_Practices_Toolkit/Guidance_Documents/Emergency_Preparedness_Response/MRC_PFA_04-02-08.pdf. Accessed June 18, 2014.

69. Centers for Disease Control and Prevention. Available at: http://www.cdc.gov/phpr/documents/DSNS_fact_sheet.pdf. Accessed June 19, 2014.

70. Oak Ridge Institute of Science and Education. Available at: http://orise.orau.gov/reacts/capabilities/cytogenetic-biodosimetry/default.aspx. Accessed June 29, 2014.

71. Oak Ridge Institute of Science and Education. Available at: http://orise.orau.gov/files/reacts/medical-aspects-of-radiation-incidents.pdf. p. 39. Accessed June 19, 2014.

72. Oak Ridge Institute for Science and Education. Available at: http://orise.orau.gov/files/reacts/triage.pdf. p. 1–3. Accessed June 28, 2014.

73. Uniformed Services University for the Health Sciences. Available at: http://www.usuhs.edu/afrri/outreach/biodostools.htm. Accessed June 28, 2014.

74. Rad pro calculator. Available at: http://www.radprocalculator.com/. Accessed June 19, 2014.

75. Stabin M. Available at: http://www.doseinfo-radar.com/ExposureCalculator.html. Accessed June 19, 2014.

76. Environmental Protection Agency. Available at: http://www.epa.gov/radiation/docs/er/planning-guidance-for-response-to-nuclear-detonation-2-edition-final.pdf. Accessed June 28, 2014.

77. Lawrence Livermore National Laboratory, 2010. Available at: https://responder.llnl.gov/data/assets/docs/publications/Planning_Guidance_for_Response_to_a_Nuclear_Detonation-2nd_Edition_FINAL.pdf. p. 88–92.

78. Centers for Disease Control and Prevention. Available at: http://emergency.cdc.gov/radiation/pdf/population-monitoring-guide.pdf. Accessed June 18, 2015.

79. The Centers for Disease Control and Prevention. Available at: http://www.bt.cdc.gov/radiation/crc/simulation.asp. Accessed July 28, 2014.

80. The Centers for Disease Control and Prevention. Available at: http://www.bt.cdc.gov/radiation/pdf/radiation-decedent-guidelines.pdf. Accessed June 16, 2014.

81. Oak Ridge Associated Universities. Available at: http://www.orau.gov/rsb/radioactivedecedents/. Accessed June 16, 2014.

82. United States Department of Health and Human Services, 2014. Available at: http://www.phe.gov/Preparedness/responders/ndms/teams/Pages/dmort.aspx. Accessed June 28, 2014.

83. Conference of Radiation Control Program Directors. Available at: http://www.crcpd.org/ATeam/Ateam.htm. Accessed June 16, 2014.

Asphyxiants

Stephen W. Borron, MD, MS[a],*, Vikhyat S. Bebarta, MD[b]

KEYWORDS

- Asphyxiants • Cyanide • Hydrogen sulfide • Carbon monoxide • Hydrazoic acid
- Azide • Methemoglobinemia • Antidote

KEY POINTS

- Asphyxiants deprive the body of needed oxygen via displacement (simple asphyxiants) or by interfering with transport or use of oxygen within tissues and organs (systemic asphyxiants).
- Asphyxiants may be gases, liquids, or solids and may enter the body by multiple routes.
- Bedside clinical diagnosis is essential, because confirmatory tests are often delayed or unavailable.
- The asphyxiant toxidrome, supported by a careful history and search for distinguishing clinical features, helps to narrow the differential diagnosis.
- Aggressive supportive care is often lifesaving in these poisonings.
- Early use of appropriate antidotal therapy is effective against severe carbon monoxide, cyanide, and opioid poisonings and toxicant-induced methemoglobinemia.

INTRODUCTION

Asphyxia is defined as impaired or absent exchange of oxygen and carbon dioxide on a ventilatory basis; combined hypercapnia and hypoxia or anoxia. Stedman's further defines an asphyxiant as "anything, especially a gas that produces asphyxia."[1] Although people tend to think of highly, toxic gases when discussing asphyxiation, it is particularly important for the emergency physician to keep in mind that asphyxiants may be gases, liquids, or solids, and can potentially enter the body not only by inhalation but also by skin absorption, ingestion, or injection. The speed of onset of symptoms is determined not only by the substance's inherent toxicity and physical characteristics, such as water solubility, but by its propensity for metabolism to toxic

The opinions and comments of the authors do not reflect official policy, position, or product endorsement of the Department of the Air Force, Department of Defense, or US Government.
Disclosures: None.
[a] Paul L. Foster School of Medicine, West Texas Regional Poison Center, Texas Tech University Health Sciences Center at El Paso, 4801 Alberta Avenue, Suite B3200, El Paso, TX 79905, USA;
[b] Department of Emergency Medicine, San Antonio Military Medical Center, San Antonio, TX 78234, USA
* Corresponding author.
E-mail address: stephen.borron@ttuhsc.edu

Emerg Med Clin N Am 33 (2015) 89–115
http://dx.doi.org/10.1016/j.emc.2014.09.014
0733-8627/15/$ – see front matter © 2015 Elsevier Inc. All rights reserved.

byproducts. Thus, although inhalation of hydrogen sulfide gas in high concentrations may result in immediate knockdown and apnea, symptoms of asphyxia after ingestion of sodium azide may lag by an hour or so,[2] and symptoms of cyanide poisoning after ingestion of acetonitrile by half a day or more.[3] Failure to recognize the role of active metabolism of cyanogens to cyanide or of dichloromethane to carbon monoxide (CO) may contribute to avoidable deaths.

Mechanisms of Asphyxia

Asphyxia may occur through several mechanisms. First, oxygen in inspired air may be replaced by other gases, depriving the body of sufficient atmospheric oxygen. Such gases need not have intrinsic toxicity. Even inhalation of inert gases, such as helium or argon, may lead to death.[4] The condition of (near) death resulting from inadequate atmospheric oxygen is referred to as simple asphyxia. Another form of simple asphyxia results from inability of oxygen to reach the pulmonary capillaries for exchange with carbon dioxide. This condition may occur after exposure to irritant or corrosive gases resulting in upper airway obstruction, bronchospasm, pulmonary edema, or hemorrhage. See the article by Tovar and Leikin in this issue.

In contrast, systemic asphyxia results from exposure to a compound that directly impairs either transport of oxygen via hemoglobin (CO, methemoglobin inducers) or interferes with the efficient use of oxygen at the tissue level via inhibition of oxidative phosphorylation (azides, CO, cyanides, sulfides; **Fig. 1**). There have been significant advances in recent years in understanding of the inhibition of cytochrome-c oxidase by CO, hydrogen cyanide, hydrogen sulfide, and nitric oxide (NO). Physiologic roles for these compounds, as well as their toxicity, have been described by Cooper and Brown.[5]

CIRCUMSTANCES
Unintentional

The circumstances leading to asphyxia are manifold. Most cases are unintentional. CO is the leading cause of unintentional poisoning deaths in the United States.[6] Household exposures to CO may derive from defective furnaces, improper indoor use of generators, and charcoal cooking devices, among others. On average, there are 430 non–fire-related CO deaths per year in the United States.[7] The number of injuries attributable to CO is far greater. Some 68,316 CO exposures were reported to poison centers during 2000 to 2009. Of these, 36,691 people required treatment in a health care facility, with 9625 having moderate to major effects.[6] Industry is responsible for a concerning number of unintentional deaths from asphyxiation. On average, 22 workers die on the job each year from CO poisoning in the United States.[8] Many additional workers seek care in emergency departments after CO exposures.

Another source of industrial asphyxiation is improper confined space entry. The Occupational Safety and Health Administration describe confined spaces as areas not necessarily designed for continuous occupancy, with limited or restricted means for entry or exit. Confined spaces include, but are not limited to, tanks, vessels, silos, storage bins, hoppers, vaults, pits, manholes, tunnels, equipment housings, ductwork, and pipelines.[9] Such areas by their nature are conducive to depletion of atmospheric oxygen (with occupancy) and concentration of gases that are lighter (silo) or heavier (sewer) than air. Notorious industrial multiple casualty incidents involving asphyxiant gases have been reported. A synopsis of federal and state confined space incident investigations can be found at the Web site of the National Chemical Safety Program and in a review by Dorevitch and colleagues.[10,11]

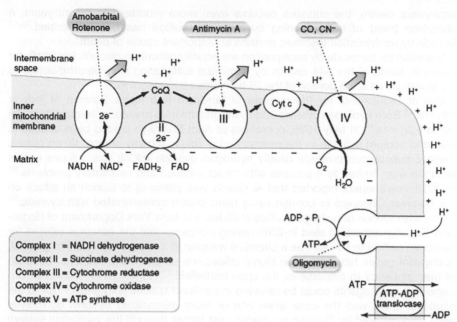

Complex I = NADH dehydrogenase
Complex II = Succinate dehydrogenase
Complex III = Cytochrome reductase
Complex IV = Cytochrome oxidase
Complex V = ATP synthase

Fig. 1. Electron transport and its inhibition. Overview of oxidative phosphorylation in the inner mitochondrial membrane. Electron flow (*thick arrows*) through complexes I, III, and IV provides energy to pump H$^+$ ions from the matrix to the intermembrane space (*thick arrows*) against the proton electrochemical gradient. The downhill movement of H$^+$ ions back into the matrix provides the energy for ATP synthesis by means of complex V. Preferential export of ATP from the matrix by ATP-ADP translocase (an antiport) maintains a high ADP/ATP ratio in the matrix. Inhibitors block electron flow through the indicated complexes (*dashed arrows*); as a result, ATP synthesis also ceases. CN, cyanide; CoQ, coenzyme Q; Cyt c, cytochrome-c; FAD, flavin adenine dinucleotide; FADH2, flavin adenine dinucleotide, reduced form; NAD, nicotinamide adenine dinucleotide; NADH, nicotinamide adenine dinucleotide, reduced form. (*From* Pelley JW, Goljan EF. Generation of energy from dietary fuels. In: Pelley JW, editor. Rapid review biochemistry. Philadelphia: Elsevier/Mosby; 2011; with permission.)

Inhalation of products of combustion (fire smoke) is responsible for the largest number of asphyxiant deaths and injuries. The Federal Emergency Management Administration reports that 2450 persons lost their lives and 13,900 were injured in some 364,500 residential building fires occurring in 2011.[12] Structure fires may lead to asphyxia from combined exposures to CO, cyanide, obstruction of alveoli by soot, and a variety of irritant gases and vapors. Although deaths from smoke inhalation are gradually declining, the rate of injuries has remained steady.

Intentional

Asphyxiant poisoning remains a common form of suicide, although related statistics are unclear, because some incidents are classified by vital statistics experts as suffocation and others as poisoning. In 2010, suffocation (which includes people putting plastic bags filled with helium over their heads) was responsible for 9493 deaths, second only to firearms as a method of suicide. Suicide by poisoning (which includes death by CO), was a close third at 6599 deaths.[13] With the uncertainty surrounding autoerotic suffocation,[14] inhalant abuse,[15] or self-poisoning by opioids (arguably an asphyxiant death), the statistics become even more muddled. In recent years, a disturbing trend of self-poisoning by hydrogen sulfide has been described.[16,17] Suicide by asphyxiation therefore remains an important cause of death.

Statistics for homicide by asphyxiation are equally difficult to discern. For 2010, for example, some of the 544 deaths by homicidal suffocation may be attributable to asphyxiation, as are a portion of the 79 homicides by poisoning.[13]

Use of asphyxiants for the purpose of terrorism is a major concern of federal officials.[18] Both hydrogen cyanide and cyanogen chloride are recognized as chemical warfare agents.[19] In May 1995, operatives of Aum Shinrikyo placed bags of sulfuric acid and sodium cyanide in the restroom of a Tokyo subway station. When mixed, these 2 substances produce deadly hydrogen cyanide (HCN) gas. Injuries in this instance were limited to 4 patients with throat irritation and respiratory problems.[20] In 2012, newspapers reported that Al Qaeda was planning to launch an attack on the Summer Olympics in London using hand cream contaminated with cyanide.[21] As a consequence of hydrogen sulfide suicides, the New York Department of Homeland Security issued an alert in 2008 raising concerns that the potential existed for hydrogen sulfide to be used as a chemical weapon in a terrorist attack.[22] In general, asphyxiant gases have not been highly efficacious as chemical weapons, because of their tendency to disperse on the open battlefield.[23] Nonetheless, there are concerns that such agents could be released in confined spaces with greater risk to the exposed. Such was the case when one or more aerosolized fentanyl derivatives were disseminated by Russian counterterrorist forces through the ventilation system in an opera house in 2002. Although the exact circumstances remain unclear, 125 hostages experienced fatal asphyxia caused by the diffusion of these opioids in an attempt to terminate a hostage situation.[24,25]

To reiterate, asphyxiants need not be in gaseous form to create havoc. In 1978, more than 900 followers of Jim Jones died in a murder/suicide incident involving cyanide-laced Kool-Aid at the People's Temple in Jonestown, Guyana. In 1982, Tylenol capsules were laced with cyanide, causing numerous deaths in the Chicago area. With little imagination and minimal resources, a terrorist group could incite significant societal disruption by targeting open foods in self-serve restaurants in several cities and contaminating them with a potent systemic asphyxiant like potassium cyanide. Although terroristic intentions have not been established in this case, an incident involving presumably intentional contamination, with sodium azide, of iced tea in a restaurant has been reported[26,27] (discussed elsewhere in this issue).

Imagined

In addition, not all apparent collective asphyxiant poisonings are what they seem. Nordt and colleagues[28] describe an event involving 22 patients initially thought to have CO poisoning. Subsequent testing revealed this to be a case of mass sociogenic illness. As the investigators point out, this is a diagnosis of exclusion.

AGENTS OF TOXICITY
Simple Asphyxiants

Virtually any gas not described as a systemic asphyxiant may cause simple asphyxia. Many are physiologically inert, such as nitrogen, helium, argon, and the other noble gases. Others, such as carbon dioxide, Freon, methane, and propane, have some physiologic effects. Nonetheless, in most cases, significant injury or death is thought to occur primarily through oxygen deprivation.

Carbon dioxide, in addition to acting as a simple asphyxiant, has physiologic effects depending on its concentration in air. As the concentration increases, the individual's respiratory rate and heart rate increase. Cardiac arrhythmias and alteration in consciousness may occur. Concentrations greater than 10% may lead to seizures, coma, and death.[29] Carbon dioxide poisoning may also be a contributor to deaths often initially assumed to be caused by hydrogen sulfide,[30] and has been implicated in mass casualty incidents.[31]

In addition to their roles in intentional inhalant abuse,[15] hydrocarbons and fluorocarbons are responsible for industrial incidents, including deaths.[11,32]

Systemic Asphyxiants

Azides

Azides are used as detonators for car airbags, primers, shell detonators, broad-spectrum biocides, and laboratory reagents.[33,34] Azides that are commonly available include sodium azide (NaN_3), lead azide ($Pb[N_3]_2$), and hydrazoic acid (HN_3); HN_3 is formed when sodium azide comes into contact with sulfuric acid. A systematic review of sodium azide exposures found that most industrial exposures occurred by inhalation, whereas laboratory exposures and suicide attempts typically involved ingestion.[33]

Carbon monoxide

Each year, nearly 500 Americans die from unintentional CO poisoning, about 15,000 visit the emergency department, and more than 4000 are hospitalized because of CO poisoning.[6,35] Mass exposures to CO are occasionally reported.[36] In the workplace, approximately 22 deaths each year are recorded to have been caused by unintentional non–fire-related CO poisoning. In most cases, motor vehicles are the exposure source, followed by heaters and generators.[8] Another source of both industrial and home hobbyist exposure includes dichloromethane (also known as methylene chloride), a common ingredient of paint strippers that is metabolized to CO.[37,38]

Cyanides and cyanogens

Cyanides pose risks from intentional exposures, occupational exposures, structural fires, and as a terrorist threat. The National Poison Center Data System annually reports more deaths from cyanide in the United States than from methanol, digoxin, and pesticides combined.[39] Ingestion of cyanide is more common than is generally supposed and is potentially deadly. Mastication and ingestion of seeds of the *Prunus* species (apricots, bitter almonds, choke cherry, peaches) can release amygdalin, which is biotransformed by β-D-glucosidase to cyanide, glucose, and aldehyde.[40] Laetrile, a semisynthetic congener of amygdalin, sold in health food stores as vitamin B_{17}, as a putative but unproven treatment of cancer, has similar potential for cyanide toxicity.[41,42] Collective deaths caused by hydrogen cyanide poisoning have occurred in industry.[43] Cyanogenic (cyanide-producing) industrial solvents, such as acetonitrile and propionitrile, have limited inherent toxicity, but are biotransformed via cytochrome P450 to release cyanide (**Box 1**).[3,44–46] Although structural fires comprise the most common cyanide exposures, another major concern for cyanide toxicity comes from its use as a terrorism weapon. At least 6 European cyanide terrorist plots and 2 US plots have been foiled in recent years.[47]

Smoke inhalation

Fire smoke contains multiple products of combustion, including multiple toxic gases, chief among them CO, cyanide, and carbon dioxide, as well as irritant vapors and soot

Box 1 Common cyanides and cyanogens	
Substance	**Characteristics and Uses**
Acetonitrile, CH_3CN	Common laboratory reagent and solvent. Slowly metabolized to cyanide in the body. Multiple pediatric deaths in past caused by household use as artificial fingernail remover; fewer suicidal and industrial poisonings[3,44,46,53–58]
Acrylonitrile, CH_2CHCN	Used in the manufacture of plastics, adhesives, and rubber. Slowly metabolized to cyanide in the body. Also has inherent toxicity unrelated to cyanide metabolism[59–61]
Calcium cyanide, $Ca(CN)_2$	Water-soluble salt converted to HCN by addition of water or acid. Used as cement stabilizer, fumigant
Cyanogen, NCCN	Colorless gas, heavier than air, soluble in water. Used for welding, cutting metals, rocket propellant. Potential rapid onset of toxicity[62]
Cyanogen bromide, CNBr	Heavy, extremely irritant gas metabolized to cyanide. Used as a fumigant[62]
Cyanogen chloride, CNCl	Heavy, extremely irritant gas metabolized to cyanide. Used as a fumigant. Prohibited chemical warfare agent[62]
Gold cyanide, AuCN	Poorly water-soluble cyanide salt. Delayed onset of toxicity after ingestion[63,64]
Hydrogen cyanide, HCN	Gas or volatile liquid used in electroplating, metallurgy. Common component of fire smoke. Susceptible to use in terrorism. Prohibited chemical warfare agent[49–52,65–67]
Mercuric cyanide, $Hg(CN)_2$	Poorly water-soluble cyanide salt; bactericide, disinfectant. Delayed onset of toxicity after ingestion. Mercury poisoning also possible[68,69]
Potassium cyanide, KCN	Water-soluble salt converted to HCN by addition of water or acid. Used in electroplating, mining, metallurgy[70–73]
Propionitrile, CH_3CH_2CN	Used as solvent, chemical intermediate. Slowly metabolized to cyanide in the body[45,74]
Silver cyanide, AgCN	Poorly water-soluble cyanide salt. Delayed onset of toxicity after ingestion. Used for silver plating[75]
Sodium cyanide, NaCN	Water-soluble salt converted to HCN by addition of water or acid. Used in electroplating, mining, metallurgy[76–78]

comprising a deadly asphyxiant mixture. The National Fire Protection Association reports that 1,375,000 fires occurred in the United States in 2012, resulting in 16,500 civilian injuries and 2855 civilian deaths. Analyses of death certificates from 2003 to 2007 indicate that 51% of fire deaths were attributable to smoke inhalation only, with an additional 23% of deaths caused by smoke inhalation and burns. Burns alone have been responsible for only 25% of deaths in recent years.[48] Of the deaths that occur immediately after exposure or that are caused by cardiac arrest, a substantial number are attributable to cyanide or combined cyanide and CO toxicity.[49–52]

Hydrogen sulfide
Hydrogen sulfide is produced from decomposition of sulfur-containing organic material and is a reagent and/or byproduct of several industrial processes. It is found in sour crude oil and petroleum workers are commonly exposed to it. The boom in natural gas production by hydraulic fracturing has raised concerns about increased releases of hydrogen sulfide.[79] Hydrogen sulfide is also produced in sulfur springs, caves, and other underground fields of natural gas. It is often present in compost pits and sewers. Hydrogen sulfide has been responsible for numerous deaths in and around manure

pits.[80] It can also be released from combining household chemicals with toilet bowl cleaners.[81] This form of so-called cookbook chemistry has been a mechanism for suicide in Japan and other countries[16,17,82] and has raised concerns for potential terrorist use.

Methemoglobin-inducing substances

Like CO, methemoglobinemia decreases the oxygen-carrying capacity of hemoglobin. By oxidizing the iron in hemoglobin to the ferric state, methemoglobin inducers render hemoglobin incapable of carrying oxygen, which is instead replaced by water. A small percentage of hemoglobin is normally in the form of methemoglobin (1%–3%). This amount is well tolerated. However, as the percentage of methemoglobin increases and the oxygen saturation decreases, symptoms ensue, depending in part on the underlying health of the person exposed. A large number of compounds have been reported to induce methemoglobinemia, including prescription and nonprescription drugs and industrial chemicals. A nonexhaustive list of methemoglobin-inducing compounds is given in **Table 1**. The pathophysiology of methemoglobin formation is described by Percy and colleagues.[83] A comprehensive review of occupational methemoglobinemia has been given by Bradberry.[84]

Opioids

Opiates and opioids easily meet the definition of an asphyxiant because they impair exchange of oxygen and carbon dioxide on a ventilatory basis, although before the use of fentanyl derivatives by Russian Special Forces in the 2002 Dubrovka theater incident in Moscow, few authorities would have classified them under the rubric of hazardous materials or agents of opportunity for chemical terrorism. Nonetheless, this catastrophic decision resulted in the deaths of 125 hostages.[24] Although speculation remains regarding the exact combination of agents used by the Special Forces, the Russian Ministry of Health admitted several days later that a derivative of fentanyl was used to neutralize the terrorists.[25] Riches and colleagues[24] were able to definitively identify carfentanil and remifentanil in extracts of clothing from casualties of the assault. If they can be used for the purpose of counterterrorism, these readily accessible agents might be equally suited for purposes of terrorism, particularly given their demonstrated lethality.

CLINICAL MANIFESTATIONS
General

Timely historical details are often lacking in cases of asphyxiation, particularly in mass casualty events, so clinicians must rely on toxic syndromes (toxidromes) for rapid decision making. Numerous descriptions exist for the asphyxiant toxidrome. Markel and colleagues[85] identified 4 toxidromes applicable to toxicologic mass casualty events, one of which is an asphyxiant toxidrome, comprising headache, fatigue, dizziness, nausea, anxiety, dyspnea, altered mental status, cardiac ischemia, syncope, coma, and seizures. Kunisaki and Godwin[86] described 2 asphyxiant toxidromes. The simple asphyxiant toxidrome consists of shortness of breath, altered mental status, seizures, and coma. The toxidrome for systemic asphyxiants includes the signs and symptoms listed previously, in addition to metabolic acidosis, cardiovascular collapse, and shock.[86] Although toxidromes (**Box 2**) are helpful to direct the clinician to initial management, the clinical manifestations produced by individual compounds are often unique; asphyxiants do not always follow the rules. Physicians should be aware of subtle distinctions in presentations. Pertinent details of the exposure, a directed physical examination, and selected point-of-care testing, may help astute

Table 1
Substances reported to induce clinically relevant methemoglobinemia

Substance	Category	References
5,6-Methylenedioxy-2-aminoindane, 2-aminoindane	Amphetamine analogues, substances of abuse	148
Aluminum phosphide	Pesticide	149–151
Amyl nitrite, butyl nitrite, iso-amyl nitrite	Medication, substances of abuse	152–154
Aniline	Dyestuff	155
Arginine alpha-ketoglutarate	Dietary supplement, NO booster	156
Automobile exhaust (nitrogen oxides)	Automobile exhaust	157,158
Benzocaine	Medication, local anesthetic	97,159–161
Chlorate salts	Matches, explosives	91,162,163
Cocaine	Medication, substance of abuse	164
Copper sulfate	Pesticide	165
Dapsone	Medication	161,166–169
Dinitrophenol	Dye, chemical intermediate	91
Holi colors	Synthetic dyes	170–172
Indoxacarb	Pesticide	173,174
Lidocaine	Medication, local anesthetic	175
Linuron	Herbicide	155
Mephedrone	Substance of abuse	107
Metaflumizone	Pesticide	176
Methylene blue	Medication, antidote	177,178
Metoclopramide	Medication, antiemetic	179,180
NO	Medication, cellular messenger	181
Nitrobenzene	Organic solvent	91,182
Nitroethane	Organic solvent	182
Phenazopyridine	Medication, urinary anesthetic	183
Phenylenediamine	Dye	91
Prilocaine	Medication, local anesthetic	184,185
Primaquine	Medication, antiinfective	161
Recombinant urate oxidase	Medication, antihyperuricemic	186
Sodium nitrite	Medication, preservative	187–189
Sulfamethoxazole-trimethoprim	Medication, antiinfective	190,191
Tetracaine	Medication, local anesthetic	192
Toluidine	Medication, dye	91
Trinitrotoluene	Explosive	91
Zinc phosphide	Pesticide	151

emergency medicine physicians to narrow the differential diagnosis, further facilitating the choice of treatment options, specifically antidotes.

Specific

Table 2 shows some of the differences in presentations of poisonings by the various asphyxiants. The reported variability comes from review articles and case series and is not intended to be definitive, but may be useful in narrowing the differential diagnosis.

Box 2				
The asphyxiant toxidrome				
Severity and Time	Central Nervous System	Cardiovascular System	Respiratory System	Gastrointestinal System
↓	Headache and fatigue	Tachycardia	Dyspnea	Nausea and vomiting
	Dizziness	Hypertension	Tachypnea	—
	Altered mental status	Myocardial ischemia	Bradypnea	—
	Syncope	Hypotension	Apnea	—
	Seizures	Bradycardia	—	—
	Coma	Cardiovascular collapse	—	—

Azides

Other than as a component of airbags, azides are not a common household product. Poisonings are likely to occur in laboratories by ingestion and in industry by inhalation.[33] Regardless of the route of exposure, the most commonly reported health effect is hypotension. Although it is counterintuitive, hypotension occurring early (less than 1 hour) is considered to indicate a pharmacologic response predicting a benign outcome. Patients with late hypotension (greater than 1 hour) are considered at high risk of death. Hypotension lasting more than 1 hour has been reported as uniformly lethal. Severe signs and symptoms included altered mental status, seizure, coma, arrhythmias, tachypnea, pulmonary edema, metabolic acidosis, and cardiorespiratory arrest.[33] Patients have survived high-dose exposures with only supportive care.[87] There are no known effective antidotes to azide.[88]

Carbon monoxide

Baud[89] reviewed cases and series of CO and cyanide poisonings with the goal of identifying differences in their clinical presentations. He emphasized the frequent muddling of clinical descriptions in the literature of what should be appreciated as 3 distinct forms of CO poisoning: (1) pure CO, such as from faulty propane and butane heaters and furnaces; (2) automobile exhaust; and (3) smoke inhalation. He then performed comparisons of non–fire-related CO (excluding automobile exhaust) and non–fire-related cyanide poisonings. Baud[89] found that, although there are significant similarities between pure CO and pure cyanide poisonings, particularly in milder poisonings, there are also some substantial differences that are emphasized in poisonings of greater severity. For example, transient loss of consciousness and/or improvement in mental status with oxygen administration alone is common with even severe CO poisoning. Transient loss of consciousness was not found in his review of cyanide poisoning. Dilated pupils were found to be very rare in CO poisoning but frequent in cyanide-induced coma. Seizures were noted also to be more frequent in cyanide poisonings. He also pointed out differences in the cardiovascular effects of the 2 agents: CO rarely presents with hypotension or bradycardia. In contrast, cyanide poisoning begins with early and transient tachycardia and hypertension followed by tachycardia and hypotension, and finally by bradycardia and hypotension preceding cardiac arrest. In addition, there are significant differences in the respiratory effects of these 2 toxicants. The most common effect on breathing in pure CO poisoning is an increase in frequency, whereas severe cyanide poisoning starts with tachypnea but ultimately leads to bradypnea and even central apnea.[89]

Table 2
Signs and symptoms of acute severe asphyxiant poisoning[a]

Signs/Symptoms	Azides	Carbon Monoxide[b]	Cyanide	Hydrogen Sulfide	Methemoglobin Inducers
Symptoms					
Vision trouble, temporary	++	++			
Signs					
Apnea	+++	+	+++	+++	
Cyanosis	+++	+	+	+++	+++
Hypertension			+++		
Hypotension	+++	+	+++	+++	+++
Knockdown/ precipitous collapse	+++	+	+++	+++	+
Lacrimation/ red eye	+	−		+++	
Loss of consciousness, transient	+++	++	−	+++	
Odor, breath or body			++	+++	+++
Pulmonary edema	++		+	+++	
Seizures	+++	++	+++	+	+++
Diagnostic Studies					
Lactic acidosis	+++	++ Usually ≤6 mmol/L in "pure" CO poisoning[b]	+++ Usually ≥8 mmol/L in "pure" CN poisoning	+++	+
Methemoglobin	+	−[b]	−[b]	+	+++ Usually >30%. Impaired consciousness and seizures at concentrations >60%. >80% is life-threatening.
Selected References	33,91	89,90,115,193	89,142,194	96,195,196	84,91

−, Not Reported or limited data.

+, Rarely Reported.

++, Occasionally Reported.

+++, Frequently Reported.

[a] All asphyxiants share the capacity to induce signs and symptoms of hypoxia, including dizziness and headache, coma, chest pain, dyspnea, and gastrointestinal signs. The role of this table is to point out some distinguishing features of various asphyxiants, to aid in their identification.

[b] Excludes smoke inhalation.

The importance of the source of CO, as pointed out by Baud,[89] is elegantly shown by the study of Chou and colleagues,[90] who compared presentations of 150 children, 90 with CO poisoning (from CO sources 1 and 2 listed earlier), and 60 with smoke inhalation (CO source 3). The differences in clinical findings are astounding (**Table 3**). Although carboxyhemoglobin levels did not differ significantly between the two groups, there was no mortality or respiratory arrests in the CO group. In contrast, the smoke inhalation group had 20% mortality and 68.5% incidence of respiratory arrest. It is therefore inappropriate to group smoke inhalation with CO poisoning of other sources. Additional toxicants are clearly at work in smoke inhalation. There is growing evidence that cyanide contributes to smoke inhalation morbidity and mortality.[49–52] The combination of soot in the mouth, nose, or secretions with altered level of consciousness in a fire involving a confined space strongly suggests cyanide as a contributing toxicant.[49,50] A plasma lactate level greater than 10 mmol/L in the setting of smoke inhalation is an even more sensitive sign of the presence of significant exposure to cyanide.[49]

Cyanide

Cyanide poisoning should be suspected in the setting of sudden collapse of laboratory and health care workers,[91,92] textile workers[71] and jewelers.[71,93] Bradypnea and/or central apnea occurring suddenly after collapse should also suggest the possibility of cyanide poisoning.[89] A plasma lactate level greater than or equal to 8 mmol/L in the setting of clinical suspicion of pure cyanide poisoning is both sensitive and specific.[94]

Hydrogen sulfide

Hydrogen sulfide is easily identified by its smell of rotten eggs, detection of which is diminished with prolonged exposure (olfactory fatigue). It is also an irritant to the

Table 3
Clinical and laboratory findings among 150 children with exposure to CO without or with accompanying smoke inhalation. Although carboxyhemoglobin levels are similar, clinical findings and outcomes are markedly different, showing that smoke inhalation is not simply CO poisoning

Measure	Category of Poisoning		
	CO Alone	CO + Smoke	P
Death (n, %)	81, 0	53, 20.3	<.001
Initial GCS (n, mean)	17, 14.7	18, 6.7	<.001
Depressed MS in ED (n, %)	83, 13.6	57, 76.3	<.001
Initial pH (n, mean)	43, 7.4	44, 7.2	<.001
Respiratory arrest (n, %)	80, 0	54, 68.5	<.001
Cardiac arrest (n, %)	80, 0	54, 25.9	<.001
Median time to ED (n, min)	27, 40	10, 25	.04
Median time to HBO (n, min)	69, 70	47, 50	.23
Mean COHb level (n, % ± SD)	85, 23.5 ± 11.53	59, 27.6 ± 16.25	.07

n in each row is the sample available for analysis.
Abbreviations: COHb, carboxyhemoglobin; ED, emergency department; GCS, Glasgow coma score; HBO, hyperbaric oxygen therapy; MS, mental status; SD, standard deviation.
From Chou KJ, Fisher JL, Silver EJ. Characteristics and outcome of children with carbon monoxide poisoning with and without smoke exposure referred for hyperbaric oxygen therapy. Pediatr Emerg Care 2000;16(3):152. Table 1; with permission.

eyes and mucous membranes. Hydrogen sulfide is most closely associated with the phenomenon of knockdown, which may occur immediately after high-dose exposure.[95,96] Workplace monitoring of hydrogen sulfide concentrations in ambient air may also simplify the diagnosis.

Toxicant-induced methemoglobinemia

Cyanosis is the hallmark of significant methemoglobinemia, caused by the production of chocolate-brown blood. The cyanosis is distinct for 2 reasons: it does not improve substantially with adequate oxygenation and ventilation, and the degree of cyanosis may be marked without accompanying respiratory distress. A quick bedside test placing venous blood from the cyanotic patient alongside venous blood from a nonpoisoned patient on a piece of filter paper may reveal the chocolate-brown color. Bedside pulse co-oximetry by specialized devices such as the Rad-57 may be useful[97,98]; laboratory-based co-oximetry provides a definitive answer.

MANAGEMENT

The general management of asphyxiant exposures requires rapid bedside decision making, aided by limited diagnostic studies, principally performed at the point of care. Definitive identification of substances other than CO is almost never available in a clinically relevant timeframe.

Supportive care starts with essential airway management and supplementation of oxygenation. Adequate ventilation and oxygenation may be lifesaving in serious asphyxiant exposure, even in the absence of specific antidotes.[99] Secure the patient's airway with endotracheal intubation and provide mechanical ventilation if the patient is comatose or unable to protect the airway. Treat shock initially with crystalloid infusion. If there is not a rapid hemodynamic response, administer direct vasopressors such as norepinephrine, epinephrine, or phenylephrine. Address cardiac dysrhythmias first with oxygenation and ventilation, and secondarily with antidysrhythmic drug administration in accordance with advanced cardiac life support guidelines. If seizures occur, immediately obtain a blood glucose measurement at the point of care. Treat refractory seizures with benzodiazepines, barbiturates, propofol, and/or specific antidotes. Correct acidemia promptly with parenteral bicarbonate or hyperventilation. Several of the asphyxiants are weak acids. Acidemia favors the nonionized state of these compounds, which allows absorption across membranes including the blood-brain barrier.[100] Therefore, target a blood arterial pH of 7.45 to 7.5 in these patients. Persistent acidemia may require extracorporeal therapies. Administer specific antidotes as indicated, without waiting for confirmation of poisoning.

Diagnostic Studies

Place asphyxiated patients on a cardiac monitor. Obtain a 12-lead electrocardiogram to detect signs of myocardial ischemia or alterations in electrolytes, such as hyperkalemia or hypocalcemia. ST segment elevation on the electrocardiogram may predict subsequent hypotension.[101] Pulse oximetry may be impossible to interpret in the setting of asphyxiant poisoning, depending on the exposure and the pulse oximeter. Conventional pulse oximetry measures total hemoglobin, oxyhemoglobin, and deoxyhemoglobin, providing an estimate of oxygen saturation based on the ratio of oxyhemoglobin to total hemoglobin.[102] Methemoglobin cannot be detected by conventional pulse oximetry and measurements of hypoxemia may not be accurate.[103] Carboxyhemoglobinemia has been shown to falsely increase displayed oxygen saturation on conventional pulse oximetry.[104] Cyanide poisoning results in an increase in oxyhemoglobin saturation, which may lead to unwarranted reassurance. In short, conventional pulse oximetry has a limited role in asphyxiant poisoning management.

The recent development of pulse co-oximetry, which measures 12 rather than 2 wavelengths of light, permits transcutaneous measurement not only of oxyhemoglobin, deoxyhemoglobin, and total hemoglobin but also of carboxyhemoglobin and methemoglobin. Initial enthusiasm for the device[102,105] has been tempered by other recent studies that have raised concerns about inaccuracy of methemoglobin detection in the presence of hypoxia.[103,106] Although pulse co-oximetry offers advantages compared with conventional pulse oximetry, undue dependence on these devices is not encouraged. When in doubt, co-oximetry by laboratory analysis is advised.[103,107,108]

Blood Gases with Co-oximetry

Severe metabolic acidosis is a constant feature in the setting of cyanide[94] and sodium azide poisonings.[2,33,88,109–111] In the absence of respiratory distress or hemodynamic instability, significant alterations in acid-base balance are rare in CO poisoning.[89] The value of arterial blood gases in CO poisoning has previously been questioned.[112,113] A venous blood gas test with co-oximetry is appropriate in most cases of CO poisoning. In cyanide poisoning, simultaneous arterial and venous blood gases may reveal a narrowed arterial-venous oxygen saturation difference, which suggests inhibition of oxidative phosphorylation.[114]

Lactate

Plasma lactate level is more mildly increased in even severe CO poisoning compared with cyanide poisoning.[94,115] In the setting of suspected pure cyanide poisoning, a plasma lactate level greater than or equal to 8 mmol/L is a sensitive and specific finding suggesting cyanide poisoning.[94] In the setting of smoke inhalation, a plasma lactate level greater than 10 mmol/L strongly suggests cyanide poisoning.[49] Azide poisonings and hydrogen sulfide poisonings are also frequently associated with lactic acidosis, although predictive values of lactate have not been established for these two poisonings.

Laboratory and Point-of-care Confirmation of Poisoning

As previously mentioned, laboratory confirmation of asphyxiant poisoning is elusive. Confirmation of methemoglobinemia and carboxyhemoglobinemia by co-oximetry is obtainable in most major hospitals. Blood cyanide is a reference laboratory study that may not yield results for days.

Antidotes

Specific antidotes comprise an important adjunct to aggressive supportive care in poisoning. Baud and colleagues[116] defined an antidote as, "a drug whose mechanisms of action have been determined, which is able to modify either the toxicokinetics or the toxicodynamics of the poison and whose administration to the poisoned patient reliably induces a significant benefit." With the possible exception of chemical mass casualties, in whom the use of an antidote autoinjector may gain time to perform other lifesaving procedures, the administration of an antidote should almost never be the treatment of first intention. Rather, antidotes should be given after institution of, or concurrently with, supportive care measures. A list of commonly available antidotes for asphyxiant poisonings is shown in **Table 4**. A more comprehensive list of antidotes that should be stocked by hospitals is provided by Dart and colleagues.[117] However, many hospitals stock inadequate amounts of antidotes, because of cost and other

Table 4
Antidotes to consider for selected asphyxiants

Antidote	Initial Adult	Pediatric Doses	Azides	CO	Cyanides and Nitriles	Fire Smoke Inhalation (CO/CN)	Hydrogen Sulfide
Hydroxocobalamin	5g IV/IO over 15 min	70 mg/kg IV/IO over 15 min	T[2]	No	Yes	Yes	T[131]
Oxygen	Normobaric at 100% by mask or hyperbaric at 3 ATA for 1 h	same as adult	Yes	Yes	Yes	Yes	Yes
Sodium nitrite	300 mg IV/IO over >5 min	0.2 mL/kg (6 mg/kg) IV/IO over >5 min	No	No	Yes	Yes[a]	Yes
Sodium thiosulfate	12.5 g of 25% solution IV/IO slowly	1 mL/kg (250 mg/kg) IV/IO slowly	No	No	Yes	Yes[b]	No

Availability of an antidote does not constitute an indication for its use. Study the indications, contraindications, and adverse effects carefully before use; consult with a regional poison center or medical toxicologist if in doubt. Hyperbaric oxygen therapy remains controversial for all poisonings; consult a regional poison center or medical toxicologist for advice.

Abbreviations: ATA, atmospheres absolute; IO, intraosseous; IV, intravenous; T, of theoretic benefit.

[a] Caution: not generally recommended; considered by some clinicians to be relatively contraindicated in this setting. Induces methemoglobinemia, which may worsen CO-associated and CN-associated tissue hypoxia.

[b] Limited data for sodium thiosulfate used alone for this indication. Considered safe.

considerations. Gasco and colleagues[118] reported that, among 286 US hospital pharmacy managers, only 38 of 234 (16%) hospitals had sufficient stocking of cyanide antidotes. The shortage of cyanide antidotes may explain in part why they are rarely used even when cyanide poisoning is suspected.[39] In contrast, hydroxocobalamin has been subject to increasing use since its introduction in 2006. There is a widely held perception that it is safer than the previous cyanide antidote kit,[119] which may increase the otherwise low use of antidotal therapy for cyanide toxicity by providers.[39]

Oxygen

Administer high-flow oxygen to all patients with asphyxiant poisoning by tight-fitting nonrebreather mask, if respirations are sufficient, or via endotracheal tube. Elimination of respiratory toxicants by adequate ventilation is elemental in their management. In many cases of CO poisoning, administration of normobaric oxygen may be all that is needed (**Fig. 2**). Hyperbaric oxygen therapy has been advocated for poisoning by CO, cyanide, and hydrogen sulfide, and in toxicant-induced methemoglobinemia.[120–123] Its use remains controversial and a review of the pros and cons is beyond the scope of this article. The decision to use hyperbaric oxygen in asphyxiant poisoning should be determined from local norms, patient condition, and nearby availability of a suitable chamber. Administration of oxygen in the setting of inhibition of oxidative phosphorylation should theoretically be superfluous (the cells cannot use the oxygen that is already transported to the mitochondria) but oxygen administration is empirically beneficial in this setting nonetheless. Both experimental studies and clinical cases have shown a direct benefit of oxygen in cyanide poisoning.

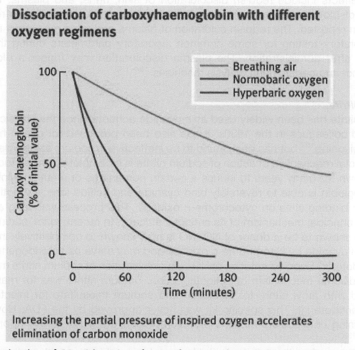

Dissociation of carboxyhaemoglobin with different oxygen regimens

Increasing the partial pressure of inspired oxygen accelerates elimination of carbon monoxide

Fig. 2. Elimination of CO with various forms of oxygen therapy. (*From* Bateman DM. Carbon monoxide. Medicine 2012;40:116; with permission.)

Hydroxocobalamin

Hydroxocobalamin (vitamin B_{12a}) has been in use in Europe as a cyanide antidote since the 1980s and was approved as a cyanide antidote (Cyanokit) by the US Food and Drug Administration (FDA) in 2006. It rapidly and essentially irreversibly binds with the cyanide anion to form cyanocobalamin (vitamin B_{12}), a compound of low toxicity that is eliminated in the urine. In addition, it acts as a scavenger of NO, increasing blood pressure, which is a desired effect in a severely hypotensive patient.[124,125]

No randomized clinical trials of human efficacy of any cyanide antidote have been undertaken. Published experience with hydroxocobalamin has included case reports and series,[49,70,126] an open-labeled clinical trial in smoke inhalation,[50] a human safety evaluation,[127] and a placebo-controlled good-laboratory-practice trial in beagle dogs.[128] Several large-animal studies have evaluated hydroxocobalamin in clinically relevant cyanide models of toxicity following its approval by the FDA. Hydroxocobalamin was as effective as sodium thiosulfate/sodium nitrite in critically ill subjects.[129] In addition, hydroxocobalamin alone was superior to sodium thiosulfate alone (92% vs 0% survival).[124] Hydroxocobalamin produced a survival of 73% in cyanide-induced cardiac arrest and the effect was seen when infused over less than 5 minutes in critically ill subjects in several swine models of cyanide toxicity.[124,129,130] Hydroxocobalamin use has also been reported for hydrogen sulfide toxicity in a case report and in an animal model, with limited results.[131,132] It may be administered intravenously (IV) or intraosseously with similar outcomes and no additional adverse events.[133] The initial dose in suspected cyanide poisoning is 5 g IV over 15 minutes in adults and may be repeated, based on response, not to exceed 15 g total. The dose in children is 70 mg/kg IV over 15 minutes (off-label use). It is category C in pregnancy. Common adverse effects include reddish discoloration of skin, urine, and plasma; transient increase of blood pressure; and reversible acneiform rash. Rare allergic reactions have been reported. The reddish coloration of plasma and urine may result in unreliable laboratory testing for some common laboratory parameters during the 24 to 48 hours after administration. The plasma discoloration may trigger a blood-leak alarm, hindering certain hemodialysis machines.[134-136]

Sodium nitrite

Sodium nitrite has been widely used as a cyanide antidote since the classic work of Chen and colleagues in the 1930s. It has also been proposed for use in hydrogen sulfide poisoning[137] but has been found to be ineffective in sodium azide poisoning.[88] The antidotal mechanism of action of sodium nitrite is incompletely understood. It has been known for many years to induce a certain percentage of methemoglobinemia. Methemoglobin is able to reversibly bind cyanide and sulfide ions, extracting them from their binding sites on cytochrome-c oxidase. This process was long assumed to be the principal mechanism of its antidotal efficacy. In recent years, sodium nitrite has been shown to be a donor of NO. NO is now known to competitively inhibit the binding of cyanide by cytochrome-c oxidase and may serve as an endogenous cyanide antidote.[138] Supplementation of NO by administration of sodium nitrite may serve as an additional mechanism of antidotal action. Sodium nitrite was for many years packaged with amyl nitrite for inhalation and sodium thiosulfate for injection as a cyanide antidote kit. This specific kit was never approved by the FDA. However, a kit containing only sodium nitrite and sodium thiosulfate was recently approved by the FDA.[139]

The efficacy of sodium nitrite, both alone and in combination with sodium thiosulfate, has been well established in animal models. Human experience has been limited to case reports and series, but these also strongly suggest its efficacy. The initial dose of sodium nitrite is 300 mg by slow intravenous injection in adults. The pediatric dose is 6 mg/kg IV at 2.5 to 5 mL/min, not to exceed 300 mg. It is category C in pregnancy. Principal side effects include hypotension[57,140] and excess methemoglobinemia.[73] Although measureable methemoglobinemia greater than 10% is uncommon,[141] cyanmethemoglobin (which also does not carry oxygen) is not detected by co-oximetry, therefore the amount of methemoglobin after treatment with sodium nitrite in the setting of cyanide poisoning may be grossly underrepresented. Thus, the practice of following serial methemoglobin levels as a means of assessing sodium nitrate therapy should be strongly discouraged. The presence of any measurable (unbound) methemoglobin after sodium nitrate therapy indicates that available cyanide has been bound and that no additional nitrate therapy is likely to be beneficial. Because sodium nitrite induces a degree of methemoglobinemia (which does not carry oxygen), most toxicologists do not recommend it use in treatment of cyanide poisoning in the setting of smoke inhalation, which results in multiple forms of hypoxia.[142]

Sodium thiosulfate

Thiosulfate sulfurtransferase (previously known as rhodanese), is an endogenous enzymatic converter of cyanide to less toxic thiocyanate found in the liver. This enzyme is effective at detoxifying cyanide, but is quickly depleted of sulfane sulfur. Sodium thiosulfate serves as a substrate for the enzyme and therefore as an effective antidote. As mentioned earlier, sodium thiosulfate has historically been packaged and used along with sodium nitrite. There are limited studies of its efficacy used alone. It has been stated that sodium thiosulfate is a slow-acting antidote,[143] although this assertion has been questioned.[144,145] The dose of sodium thiosulfate is 50 mL of a 25% solution (12.5 g) by slow intravenous bolus or infusion in adults. The pediatric dose is 1 mL/kg body weight of the 25% solution, not to exceed 12.5 g. It is category C in pregnancy. Sodium thiosulfate may be of benefit in cyanide poisoning caused by smoke inhalation,[144] but recent data in a pig model suggest that sodium thiosulfate alone is not an effective antidote.[124,146] Unlike sodium nitrite, sodium thiosulfate does not interfere with oxygenation and has minimal side effects. Although sodium nitrite has been proposed as an antidote for sulfide poisoning, sodium thiosulfate is of no theoretic benefit.

Methylene blue

Methylene blue is the antidote of choice for treatment of excessive or symptomatic toxicant-induced methemoglobinemia. Methylene blue reduces methemoglobin, in the presence of adequate NADPH (nicotine adenine dinucleotide phosphate) and the enzyme methemoglobin reductase, to hemoglobin. Methylene blue is converted in the process to leucomethylene blue. Because methylene blue is eliminated in the urine, it is contraindicated in renal failure. It is also contraindicated in G6PD (glucose-6-phosphate dehydrogenase) deficiency, in which inadequate NADPH is available and hemolysis may occur. Treatment with methylene blue is generally recommended when there are significant symptoms of hypoxia or when the methemoglobin concentration is more than 30%.[84] The recommended dose of methylene blue for children and adults is 1 to 2 mg/kg body weight given IV over 5 minutes. It is pregnancy category C. Other important adverse effects of methylene blue therapy include formation of methemoglobin at high doses, fecal and urine discoloration, and interference with co-oximetry.[147]

Naloxone

Emergency physicians are familiar with naloxone for opioid poisonings, thus its use is not further described here except to encourage emergency planners to consider sufficient stocking of naloxone to deal with a terrorist event such as that reported in the Russian theater incident.

SUMMARY

Asphyxiants are responsible for a large number of deaths and serious injuries each year. Smoke inhalation poses the greatest threat from the point of view of incidence, exacting substantial morbidity and mortality. Long referred to as CO poisoning, it is now appreciated that smoke inhalation is a complex form of asphyxiation involving not only CO but cyanide, volatile organic compounds, carbon dioxide, and soot, all of which affect oxygenation and ventilation. CO in its pure form is another frequently encountered asphyxiant, both in the home in the workplace. Another common form of asphyxiation is caused by toxicants that induce methemoglobinemia, including many drugs and industrial compounds. Rarer are poisonings by azides and hydrogen sulfide, but they continue to take an important toll in agricultural and industrial settings. The treatment of all of these poisonings is, first and foremost, aggressive supportive therapy with oxygen, mechanical ventilation, crystalloids, and when necessary vasopressors. Specific antidotes can be lifesaving, but serve as adjuncts to supportive care. It is incumbent on emergency physicians to recognize these poisonings quickly and to act quickly. The asphyxiant toxidrome, aided by careful history and examination, leads emergency physicians in the appropriate treatment direction.

REFERENCES

1. Stedman TL. Stedman's medical dictionary. 28th edition. Philadelphia: Lippincott Williams & Wilkins; 1853–1938. p. 2169.
2. Lopacinski B, Kolacinski Z, Winnicka R. Sodium azide–clinical course of the poisoning and treatment. Przegl Lek 2007;64(4–5):326–30 [in Polish].
3. Mueller M, Borland C. Delayed cyanide poisoning following acetonitrile ingestion. Postgrad Med J 1997;73(859):299–300.
4. Musshoff F, Hagemeier L, Kirschbaum K, et al. Two cases of suicide by asphyxiation due to helium and argon. Forensic Sci Int 2012;223(1–3):e27–30.
5. Cooper CE, Brown GC. The inhibition of mitochondrial cytochrome oxidase by the gases carbon monoxide, nitric oxide, hydrogen cyanide and hydrogen sulfide: chemical mechanism and physiological significance. J Bioenerg Biomembr 2008;40(5):533–9.
6. Centers for Disease Control. Carbon monoxide exposures–United States, 2000–2009. MMWR Morb Mortal Wkly Rep 2011;60(30):1014–7.
7. Xu J. CDC quick stats: average annual number of deaths and death rates from unintentional, non–fire-related carbon monoxide poisoning,*† by sex and age group — United States, 1999–2010. MMWR Morb Mortal Wkly Rep 2014; 63(3):65.
8. Henn SA, Bell JL, Sussell AL, et al. Occupational carbon monoxide fatalities in the US from unintentional non-fire related exposures, 1992–2008. Am J Ind Med 2013;56(11):1280–9.
9. Safety and health topics: confined spaces. Washington, DC: United States Department of Labor, Occupational Safety & Health Administration; 2014 [cited July 21, 2014]. Available at: https://www.osha.gov/SLTC/confinedspaces/index.html.
10. Chemical accident investigation reports from National Institute for Occupational Safety and Health College Station. TX: National Chemical Safety Program; 2014. Available at: http://ncsp.tamu.edu/reports/CDC/cdcList.htm. Accessed July 21, 2014.

11. Dorevitch S, Forst L, Conroy L, et al. Toxic inhalation fatalities of US construction workers, 1990 to 1999. J Occup Environ Med 2002;44(7):657–62.
12. Residential and nonresidential building fire estimates. Emmitsburg (MD): United States Fire Administration; 2014. Available at: http://www.usfa.fema.gov/statistics/estimates/index.shtm. Accessed July 21, 2014.
13. Murphy SL, Xu J, Kochanek KD. Deaths: final data for 2010. National vital statistics reports: from the Centers for Disease Control and Prevention, National Center for Health Statistics, National Vital Statistics System 2013;61(4):1–117.
14. Sauvageau A, Racette S. Autoerotic deaths in the literature from 1954 to 2004: a review. J Forensic Sci 2006;51(1):140–6.
15. Anderson CE, Loomis GA. Recognition and prevention of inhalant abuse. Am Fam Physician 2003;68(5):869–74.
16. Bott E, Dodd M. Suicide by hydrogen sulfide inhalation. Am J Forensic Med Pathol 2013;34(1):23–5.
17. Kamijo Y, Takai M, Fujita Y, et al. A multicenter retrospective survey on a suicide trend using hydrogen sulfide in Japan. Clin Toxicol 2013;51(5):425–8.
18. Keim ME. Terrorism involving cyanide: the prospect of improving preparedness in the prehospital setting. Prehosp Disaster Med 2006;21(2):s56–60.
19. United States chemical weapons convention: schedule 3 chemicals. Washington, DC: Bureau of Industry and Security; 2014. Available at: http://www.cwc.gov/index_chemicals_sch3.html. Accessed July 21, 2014.
20. Chronology of Aum Shinrikyo's CBW activities Monterey, CA Monterey Institute of International Studies. 2001. Available at: cns.miis.edu/reports/pdfs/aum_chrn.pdf. Accessed July 21, 2014.
21. London 2012 Olympics: terrorists 'plotting cyanide poison hand cream attack'. London: The Telegraph; 2012. Available at: http://www.telegraph.co.uk/sport/olympics/news/9166546/London-2012-Olympics-terrorists-plotting-cyanide-poison-hand-cream-attack.html. Accessed July 21, 2014.
22. Hydrogen sulfide: a potential first responder hazard. Albany (NY): New York State Office of Homeland Security, New York State Office of Homeland Security; 2008. Report No.
23. Barriot P, Bismuth C, editors. Treating victims of weapons of mass destruction: medical, legal and strategic aspects. West Sussex (United Kingdom): John Wiley; 2008.
24. Riches JR, Read RW, Black RM, et al. Analysis of clothing and urine from Moscow theatre siege casualties reveals carfentanil and remifentanil use. J Anal Toxicol 2012;36(9):647–56.
25. Wax PM, Becker CE, Curry SC. Unexpected "gas" casualties in Moscow: a medical toxicology perspective. Ann Emerg Med 2003;41(5):700–5.
26. Schwarz ES, Wax PM, Kleinschmidt KC, et al. Multiple poisonings with sodium azide at a local restaurant. J Emerg Med 2014;46(4):491–4.
27. Centers for Disease Control. Sodium azide poisoning at a restaurant - Dallas County, Texas, 2010. MMWR Morb Mortal Wkly Rep 2012;61(25):457–60.
28. Nordt SP, Minns A, Carstairs S, et al. Mass sociogenic illness initially reported as carbon monoxide poisoning. J Emerg Med 2012;42(2):159–61.
29. Langford NJ. Carbon dioxide poisoning. Toxicol Rev 2005;24(4):229–35.
30. Zaba C, Marcinkowski JT, Wojtyla A, et al. Acute collective gas poisoning at work in a manure storage tank. Ann Agric Environ Med 2011;18(2):448–51.
31. Halpern P, Raskin Y, Sorkine P, et al. Exposure to extremely high concentrations of carbon dioxide: a clinical description of a mass casualty incident. Ann Emerg Med 2004;43(2):196–9.

32. Keown D. Asphyxiation fatality exposure from chlorodifluoromethane. J Occup Environ Hyg 2013;10(3):D40–1.
33. Chang S, Lamm SH. Human health effects of sodium azide exposure: a literature review and analysis. Int J Toxicol 2003;22(3):175–86.
34. National Library of Medicine. Hazardous substances data bank (HSDB). Bethesda (MD): National Institutes of Health, US National Library of Medicine; 2014. Available at: http://toxnet.nlm.nih.gov/newtoxnet/hsdb.htm. Accessed August 1, 2014.
35. Centers for Disease Control. Carbon monoxide FAQs. Atlanta (Georgia): Centers for Disease Control and Prevention; 2013. Available at: http://www.cdc.gov/co/faqs.htm. Accessed July 31, 2014.
36. Klasner AE, Smith SR, Thompson MW, et al. Carbon monoxide mass exposure in a pediatric population. Acad Emerg Med 1998;5(10):992–6.
37. Macisaac J, Harrison R, Krishnaswami J, et al. Fatalities due to dichloromethane in paint strippers: a continuing problem. Am J Ind Med 2013;56(8):907–10.
38. Centers for Disease Control. Fatal exposure to methylene chloride among bathtub refinishers - United States, 2000–2011. MMWR Morb Mortal Wkly Rep 2012;61(7):119–22.
39. Bebarta VS, Pitotti RL, Borys DJ, et al. Seven years of cyanide ingestions in the USA: critically ill patients are common, but antidote use is not. Emerg Med J 2011;28(2):155–8.
40. Pentore R, Venneri A, Nichelli P. Accidental choke-cherry poisoning: early symptoms and neurological sequelae of an unusual case of cyanide intoxication. Ital J Neurol Sci 1996;17(3):233–5.
41. Milazzo S, Ernst E, Lejeune S, et al. Laetrile treatment for cancer. Cochrane Database Syst Rev 2011;(11):CD005476.
42. O'Brien B, Quigg C, Leong T. Severe cyanide toxicity from 'vitamin supplements'. Eur J Emerg Med 2005;12(5):257–8.
43. OSHA. Inspection: 104009105-Bastian Plating Company, Inc. Washington, DC: United States Department of Labor; 1988. Available at: https://www.osha.gov/pls/imis/establishment.inspection_detail?id=104009105. Accessed August 6, 2014.
44. Muraki K, Inoue Y, Ohta I, et al. Massive rhabdomyolysis and acute renal failure after acetonitrile exposure. Intern Med 2001;40(9):936–9.
45. Scolnick B, Hamel D, Woolf AD. Successful treatment of life-threatening propionitrile exposure with sodium nitrite/sodium thiosulfate followed by hyperbaric oxygen. J Occup Med 1993;35(6):577–80.
46. Swanson JR, Krasselt WG. An acetonitrile-related death. J Forensic Sci 1994; 39(1):271–9.
47. Cornish P. The CBRN system: assessing the threat of terrorist use of chemical, biological, radiological and nuclear weapons in the United Kingdom. London: Chatham House; 2007. p. 40.
48. Hall JR. Fatal effects of fire. Quincy (MA): National Fire Protection Association, Fire Analysis and Research Division; 2011. Report No.: NFPA Index No. 1598 Contract No.: NFPA Index No. 1598.
49. Baud FJ, Barriot P, Toffis V, et al. Elevated blood cyanide concentrations in victims of smoke inhalation. N Engl J Med 1991;325(25):1761–6.
50. Borron SW, Baud FJ, Barriot P, et al. Prospective study of hydroxocobalamin for acute cyanide poisoning in smoke inhalation. Ann Emerg Med 2007;49(6):794–801 e1–2.
51. Grabowska T, Skowronek R, Nowicka J, et al. Prevalence of hydrogen cyanide and carboxyhaemoglobin in victims of smoke inhalation during enclosed-space fires: a combined toxicological risk. Clin Toxicol 2012;50(8):759–63.

52. Stamyr K, Thelander G, Ernstgard L, et al. Swedish forensic data 1992–2009 suggest hydrogen cyanide as an important cause of death in fire victims. Inhal Toxicol 2012;24(3):194–9.
53. Caravati EM, Litovitz TL. Pediatric cyanide intoxication and death from an acetonitrile-containing cosmetic. JAMA 1988;260(23):3470–3.
54. Geller RJ, Ekins BR, Iknoian RC. Cyanide toxicity from acetonitrile-containing false nail remover. Am J Emerg Med 1991;9(3):268–70.
55. Kurt TL, Day LC, Reed WG, et al. Cyanide poisoning from glue-on nail remover. Am J Emerg Med 1991;9(3):271–2.
56. Rainey PM, Roberts WL. Diagnosis and misdiagnosis of poisoning with the cyanide precursor acetonitrile: nail polish remover or nail glue remover? Am J Emerg Med 1993;11(2):104–8.
57. Turchen SG, Manoguerra AS, Whitney C. Severe cyanide poisoning from the ingestion of an acetonitrile-containing cosmetic. Am J Emerg Med 1991;9(3):264–7.
58. Zavotsky KE, Mentler P, Gronczewski C, et al. 52-year-old acyanotic man with severe hypoxia and profound metabolic acidosis following an industry chemical exposure. J Emerg Nurs 2004;30(2):113–6.
59. Thier R, Lewalter J, Bolt HM. Species differences in acrylonitrile metabolism and toxicity between experimental animals and humans based on observations in human accidental poisonings. Arch Toxicol 2000;74(4–5):184–9.
60. Vogel RA, Kirkendall WM. Acrylonitrile (vinyl cyanide) poisoning: a case report. Tex Med 1984;80(5):48–51.
61. Buchter A, Peter H. Clinical toxicology of acrylonitrile. G Ital Med Lav 1984;6(3–4):83–6.
62. Chemical casualties. Cyanogen agents. J R Army Med Corps 2002;148(4):383–6.
63. Goodhart GL. Patient treated with antidote kit and hyperbaric oxygen survives cyanide poisoning. South Med J 1994;87(8):814–6.
64. Wright IH, Vesey CJ. Acute poisoning with gold cyanide. Anaesthesia 1986;41(9):936–9.
65. Magnusson R, Nyholm S, Astot C. Analysis of hydrogen cyanide in air in a case of attempted cyanide poisoning. Forensic Sci Int 2012;222(1–3):e7–12.
66. Musshoff F, Kirschbaum KM, Madea B. An uncommon case of a suicide with inhalation of hydrogen cyanide. Forensic Sci Int 2011;204(1–3):e4–7.
67. Lam KK, Lau FL. An incident of hydrogen cyanide poisoning. Am J Emerg Med 2000;18(2):172–5.
68. Labat L, Dumestre-Toulet V, Goulle JP, et al. A fatal case of mercuric cyanide poisoning. Forensic Sci Int 2004;143(2–3):215–7.
69. Benaissa ML, Hantson P, Bismuth C, et al. Mercury oxycyanide and mercuric cyanide poisoning: two cases. Intensive Care Med 1995;21(12):1051–3.
70. Borron SW, Baud FJ, Megarbane B, et al. Hydroxocobalamin for severe acute cyanide poisoning by ingestion or inhalation. Am J Emerg Med 2007;25(5):551–8.
71. Coentrao L, Moura D. Acute cyanide poisoning among jewelry and textile industry workers. Am J Emerg Med 2011;29(1):78–81.
72. Fortin JL, Waroux S, Giocanti JP, et al. Hydroxocobalamin for poisoning caused by ingestion of potassium cyanide: a case study. J Emerg Med 2010;39(3):320–4.
73. Peddy SB, Rigby MR, Shaffner DH. Acute cyanide poisoning. Pediatr Crit Care Med 2006;7(1):79–82.

74. Bismuth C, Baud FJ, Djeghout H, et al. Cyanide poisoning from propionitrile exposure. J Emerg Med 1987;5(3):191–5.
75. Blanc P, Hogan M, Mallin K, et al. Cyanide intoxication among silver-reclaiming workers. JAMA 1985;253(3):367–71.
76. Yan P, Huang G, Li D, et al. Homicide due to intravenous metallic mercury injection followed by sodium cyanide injection. Am J Forensic Med Pathol 2012;33(3): 273–5.
77. Amizet L, Pruvot G, Remy S, et al. Occupational cyanide poisoning. BMJ Case Rep 2011;2011. pii:bcr0920114865.
78. Holstege CP, Forrester JD, Borek HA, et al. A case of cyanide poisoning and the use of arterial blood gas analysis to direct therapy. Hosp Pract 2010;38(4):69–74.
79. Song L, Morris J, Hasemeyer D. Fracking boom leaves Texans under a toxic cloud. Bloomberg News 2014.
80. National Institute for Occupational Safety and Health. Preventing deaths of farm workers in manure pits. Cincinnati (OH): National Institute for Occupational Safety and Health; 1990.
81. Truscott A. Suicide fad threatens neighbours, rescuers. Can Med Assoc J 2008; 179(4):312–3.
82. Maebashi K, Iwadate K, Sakai K, et al. Toxicological analysis of 17 autopsy cases of hydrogen sulfide poisoning resulting from the inhalation of intentionally generated hydrogen sulfide gas. Forensic Sci Int 2011;207(1–3):91–5.
83. Percy MJ, McFerran NV, Lappin TR. Disorders of oxidised haemoglobin. Blood Rev 2005;19(2):61–8.
84. Bradberry SM. Occupational methaemoglobinaemia. Mechanisms of production, features, diagnosis and management including the use of methylene blue. Toxicol Rev 2003;22(1):13–27.
85. Markel G, Krivoy A, Rotman E, et al. Medical management of toxicological mass casualty events. Isr Med Assoc J 2008;10(11):761–6.
86. Kunisaki T, Godwin SA. Smoke inhalation. In: Adams JG, Barton ED, Collings JL, et al, editors. Emergency medicine. 2nd edition. Philadelphia: Elsevier; 2013. p. 1178–81.
87. Watanabe K, Hirasawa H, Oda S, et al. A case of survival following high-dose sodium azide poisoning. Clin Toxicol 2007;45(7):810–1.
88. Klein-Schwartz W, Gorman RL, Oderda GM, et al. Three fatal sodium azide poisonings. Med Toxicol Adverse Drug Exp 1989;4(3):219–27.
89. Baud FJ. Cyanide: critical issues in diagnosis and treatment. Hum Exp Toxicol 2007;26(3):191–201.
90. Chou KJ, Fisher JL, Silver EJ. Characteristics and outcome of children with carbon monoxide poisoning with and without smoke exposure referred for hyperbaric oxygen therapy. Pediatr Emerg Care 2000;16(3):151–5.
91. Binder L, Fredrickson L. Poisonings in laboratory personnel and health care professionals. Am J Emerg Med 1991;9(1):11–5.
92. Grellner W, Kukuk M, Glenewinkel F. About suicide methods of physicians, medical personnel and related professions. Arch Kriminol 1998;201(3–4): 65–72 [in German].
93. Garlich FM, Alsop JA, Anderson DL, et al. Poisoning and suicide by cyanide jewelry cleaner in the US Hmong community: a case series. Clin Toxicol 2012; 50(2):136–40.
94. Baud FJ, Borron SW, Megarbane B, et al. Value of lactic acidosis in the assessment of the severity of acute cyanide poisoning. Crit Care Med 2002;30(9): 2044–50.

95. Gabbay DS, De Roos F, Perrone J. Twenty-foot fall averts fatality from massive hydrogen sulfide exposure. J Emerg Med 2001;20(2):141–4.
96. Guidotti TL. Hydrogen sulfide: advances in understanding human toxicity. Int J Toxicol 2010;29(6):569–81.
97. Annabi EH, Barker SJ. Severe methemoglobinemia detected by pulse oximetry. Anesth Analg 2009;108(3):898–9.
98. Barker SJ. New sensors should improve Masimo SpMet error found by Feiner et al. Anesth Analg 2010;111(1):241 [author reply: 241].
99. Bismuth C, Cantineau JP, Pontal P, et al. Cyanide poisoning. Priority to symptomatic treatment. 25 cases. Presse Med 1984;13(41):2493–7 [in French].
100. Djerad A, Monier C, Houze P, et al. Effects of respiratory acidosis and alkalosis on the distribution of cyanide into the rat brain. Toxicol Sci 2001;61(2):273–82.
101. Muncy TA, Bebarta VS, Varney SM, et al. Acute electrocardiographic ST segment elevation may predict hypotension in a swine model of severe cyanide toxicity. J Med Toxicol 2012;8(3):285–90.
102. Barker SJ, Badal JJ. The measurement of dyshemoglobins and total hemoglobin by pulse oximetry. Curr Opin Anaesthesiol 2008;21(6):805–10.
103. Feiner JR, Bickler PE, Mannheimer PD. Accuracy of methemoglobin detection by pulse CO-oximetry during hypoxia. Anesth Analg 2010;111(1):143–8.
104. Hampson NB. Pulse oximetry in severe carbon monoxide poisoning. Chest 1998;114(4):1036–41.
105. Hampson NB. Noninvasive pulse CO-oximetry expedites evaluation and management of patients with carbon monoxide poisoning. Am J Emerg Med 2012;30(9):2021–4.
106. Shamir MY, Avramovich A, Smaka T. The current status of continuous noninvasive measurement of total, carboxy, and methemoglobin concentration. Anesth Analg 2012;114(5):972–8.
107. Ahmed N, Hoy BP, McInerney J. Methaemoglobinaemia due to mephedrone ('snow'). BMJ Case Rep 2010;2010. pii:bcr0420102879.
108. Weaver LK, Churchill SK, Deru K, et al. False positive rate of carbon monoxide saturation by pulse oximetry of emergency department patients. Respir Care 2013;58(2):232–40.
109. Emmett EA, Ricking JA. Fatal self-administration of sodium azide. Ann Intern Med 1975;83(2):224–6.
110. Abrams J, el-Mallakh RS, Meyer R. Suicidal sodium azide ingestion. Ann Emerg Med 1987;16(12):1378–80.
111. Albertson TE, Reed S, Siefkin A. A case of fatal sodium azide ingestion. J Toxicol Clin Toxicol 1986;24(4):339–51.
112. Myers RA, Britten JS. Are arterial blood gases of value in treatment decisions for carbon monoxide poisoning? Crit Care Med 1989;17(2):139–42.
113. Lebby TI, Zalenski R, Hryhorczuk DO, et al. The usefulness of the arterial blood gas in pure carbon monoxide poisoning. Vet Hum Toxicol 1989;31(2):138–40.
114. Johnson RP, Mellors JW. Arteriolization of venous blood gases: a clue to the diagnosis of cyanide poisoning. J Emerg Med 1988;6(5):401–4.
115. Benaissa ML, Megarbane B, Borron SW, et al. Is elevated plasma lactate a useful marker in the evaluation of pure carbon monoxide poisoning? Intensive Care Med 2003;29(8):1372–5.
116. Baud FJ, Borron SW, Bismuth C. Modifying toxicokinetics with antidotes. Toxicol Lett 1995;82–83:785–93.

117. Dart R, Borron S, Caravati E, et al. Expert consensus guidelines for stocking of antidotes in hospitals that provide emergency care. Ann Emerg Med 2009;54: 386–94.e1.
118. Gasco L, Rosbolt MB, Bebarta VS. Insufficient stocking of cyanide antidotes in US hospitals that provide emergency care. J Pharmacol Pharmacother 2013; 4(2):95–102.
119. Streitz MJ, Bebarta VS, Borys DJ, et al. Patterns of cyanide antidote use since regulatory approval of hydroxocobalamin in the United States. Am J Ther 2014; 21(4):244–9.
120. Weaver LK. Hyperbaric oxygen therapy for carbon monoxide poisoning. Undersea Hyperb Med 2014;41(4):339–54.
121. Lawson-Smith P, Jansen EC, Hyldegaard O. Cyanide intoxication as part of smoke inhalation–a review on diagnosis and treatment from the emergency perspective. Scand J Trauma Resusc Emerg Med 2011;19:14.
122. Lindenmann J, Matzi V, Anegg U, et al. Hyperbaric oxygen in the treatment of hydrogen sulphide intoxication. Acta Anaesthesiol Scand 2010;54(6):784–5.
123. Lindenmann J, Matzi V, Kaufmann P, et al. Hyperbaric oxygenation in the treatment of life-threatening isobutyl nitrite-induced methemoglobinemia–a case report. Inhal Toxicol 2006;18(13):1047–9.
124. Bebarta VS, Pitotti RL, Dixon P, et al. Hydroxocobalamin versus sodium thiosulfate for the treatment of acute cyanide toxicity in a swine (*Sus scrofa*) model. Ann Emerg Med 2012;59(6):532–9.
125. Gerth K, Ehring T, Braendle M, et al. Nitric oxide scavenging by hydroxocobalamin may account for its hemodynamic profile. Clin Toxicol 2006;44(Suppl 1):29–36.
126. Fortin JL, Giocanti JP, Ruttimann M, et al. Prehospital administration of hydroxocobalamin for smoke inhalation-associated cyanide poisoning: 8 years of experience in the Paris Fire Brigade. Clin Toxicol 2006;44(Suppl 1):37–44.
127. Uhl W, Nolting A, Golor G, et al. Safety of hydroxocobalamin in healthy volunteers in a randomized, placebo-controlled study. Clin Toxicol 2006;44(Suppl 1):17–28.
128. Borron SW, Stonerook M, Reid F. Efficacy of hydroxocobalamin for the treatment of acute cyanide poisoning in adult beagle dogs. Clin Toxicol 2006; 44(Suppl 1):5–15.
129. Bebarta VS, Tanen DA, Lairet J, et al. Hydroxocobalamin and sodium thiosulfate versus sodium nitrite and sodium thiosulfate in the treatment of acute cyanide toxicity in a swine (Sus scrofa) model. Ann Emerg Med 2010;55(4):345–51.
130. Bebarta VS, Pitotti RL, Dixon PS, et al. Hydroxocobalamin and epinephrine both improve survival in a swine model of cyanide-induced cardiac arrest. Ann Emerg Med 2012;60(4):415–22.
131. Fujita Y, Fujino Y, Onodera M, et al. A fatal case of acute hydrogen sulfide poisoning caused by hydrogen sulfide: hydroxocobalamin therapy for acute hydrogen sulfide poisoning. J Anal Toxicol 2011;35(2):119–23.
132. Haouzi P, Sonobe T, Torsell-Tubbs N, et al. In vivo interactions between cobalt or ferric compounds and the pools of sulphide in the blood during and after H2S poisoning. Toxicol Sci 2014;141:493–504.
133. Bebarta VS, Pitotti R, Boudreau S, et al. Intraosseous versus intravenous infusion of hydroxocobalamin for the treatment of acute severe cyanide toxicity in a swine model. Academic emergency medicine, in press.
134. Stellpflug SJ, Gardner RL, Leroy JM, et al. Hydroxocobalamin hinders hemodialysis. Am J Kidney Dis 2013;62(2):395.
135. Sutter M, Tereshchenko N, Rafii R, et al. Hemodialysis complications of hydroxocobalamin: a case report. J Med Toxicol 2010;6(2):165–7.

136. Avila J, Prasad D, Weisberg LS, et al. Pseudo-blood leak? A hemodialysis mystery. Clin Nephrol 2013;79(4):323–5.
137. Hall AH, Rumack BH. Hydrogen sulfide poisoning: an antidotal role for sodium nitrite? Vet Hum Toxicol 1997;39(3):152–4.
138. Pearce LL, Bominaar EL, Hill BC, et al. Reversal of cyanide inhibition of cytochrome c oxidase by the auxiliary substrate nitric oxide: an endogenous antidote to cyanide poisoning? J Biol Chem 2003;278(52):52139–45.
139. US Food and Drug Administration. Drug approval package: Nithiodote. Washington, DC: US Food and Drug Administration; 2011. Available at: http://www.accessdata.fda.gov/drugsatfda_docs/nda/2011/201444_nithiodote_toc.cfm. Accessed August 1, 2014.
140. Hall AH, Kulig KW, Rumack BH. Suspected cyanide poisoning in smoke inhalation: complications of sodium nitrite therapy. J Toxicol Clin Exp 1989;9(1):3–9.
141. Matteucci MJ, Reed WJ, Tanen DA. Sodium thiosulfate fails to reduce nitrite-induced methemoglobinemia in vitro. Acad Emerg Med 2003;10(4):299–302.
142. Baud F, Steffens W, Borron S, et al. Efficacy and safety of antidotes for acute poisoning by cyanides. Brussels (Belgium): European Centre for Ecotoxicology and Toxicology of Chemicals; 2013. Technical Report No. 121.
143. Hall AH, Dart R, Bogdan G. Sodium thiosulfate or hydroxocobalamin for the empiric treatment of cyanide poisoning? Ann Emerg Med 2007;49(6):806–13.
144. Kerns W 2nd, Beuhler M, Tomaszewski C. Hydroxocobalamin versus thiosulfate for cyanide poisoning. Ann Emerg Med 2008;51(3):338–9.
145. Renard C, Borron SW, Renaudeau C, et al. Sodium thiosulfate for acute cyanide poisoning: study in a rat model. Ann Pharm Fr 2005;63(2):154–61 [in French].
146. Bebarta VS. Antidotes for cyanide poisoning. Eur J Emerg Med 2013;20(1): 65–6.
147. Gourlain H, Buneaux F, Borron SW, et al. Interference of methylene blue with CO-oximetry of hemoglobin derivatives. Clin Chem 1997;43(6 Pt 1):1078–80.
148. Green D, Barry P, Green HD. Central cyanosis on a psychiatric unit treated at the Salford Royal Hospital. Thorax 2014. [Epub ahead of print].
149. Mostafazadeh B, Pajoumand A, Farzaneh E, et al. Blood levels of methemoglobin in patients with aluminum phosphide poisoning and its correlation with patient's outcome. J Med Toxicol 2011;7(1):40–3.
150. Bumbrah GS, Krishan K, Kanchan T, et al. Phosphide poisoning: a review of literature. Forensic Sci Int 2012;214(1–3):1–6.
151. Proudfoot AT. Aluminium and zinc phosphide poisoning. Clin Toxicol 2009;47(2): 89–100.
152. Lin CH, Fang CC, Lee CC, et al. Near-fatal methemoglobinemia after recreational inhalation of amyl nitrite aerosolized with a compressed gas blower. J Formos Med Assoc 2005;104(11):856–9.
153. Modarai B, Kapadia YK, Kerins M, et al. Methylene blue: a treatment for severe methaemoglobinaemia secondary to misuse of amyl nitrite. Emerg Med J 2002; 19(3):270–1.
154. Romanelli F, Smith KM, Thornton AC, et al. Poppers: epidemiology and clinical management of inhaled nitrite abuse. Pharmacotherapy 2004;24(1):69–78.
155. Bazylewicz A, Klopotowski T, Kicka M, et al. Acute poisoning due to chemical substances inducing methemoglobinemia–two cases report. Przegl Lek 2010; 67(8):636–9 [in Polish].
156. Prosser JM, Majlesi N, Chan GM, et al. Adverse effects associated with arginine alpha-ketoglutarate containing supplements. Hum Exp Toxicol 2009;28(5): 259–62.

157. Vevelstad M, Morild I. Lethal methemoglobinemia and automobile exhaust inhalation. Forensic Sci Int 2009;187(1–3):e1–5.
158. Suyama H, Morikawa S, Noma-Tanaka S, et al. Methemoglobinemia induced by automobile exhaust fumes. J Anesth 2005;19(4):333–5.
159. Aryal MR, Gupta S, Giri S, et al. Benzocaine-induced methaemoglobinaemia: a life-threatening complication after a transoesophageal echocardiogram (TEE). BMJ Case Rep 2013;2013. pii:bcr2013009398.
160. Khan R, Kuppaswamy BS. Cetacaine induced methemoglobinemia: overview of analysis and treatment strategies. W V Med J 2013;109(3):24–6.
161. Ash-Bernal R, Wise R, Wright SM. Acquired methemoglobinemia: a retrospective series of 138 cases at 2 teaching hospitals. Medicine 2004;83(5):265–73.
162. Lee E, Phua DH, Lim BL, et al. Severe chlorate poisoning successfully treated with methylene blue. J Emerg Med 2013;44(2):381–4.
163. Steffen C, Seitz R. Severe chlorate poisoning: report of a case. Arch Toxicol 1981;48(4):281–8.
164. Hunter L, Gordge L, Dargan PI, et al. Methaemoglobinaemia associated with the use of cocaine and volatile nitrites as recreational drugs: a review. Br J Clin Pharmacol 2011;72(1):18–26.
165. Naha K, Saravu K, Shastry BA. Blue vitriol poisoning: a 10-year experience in a tertiary care hospital. Clin Toxicol 2012;50(3):197–201.
166. Singh S, Sethi N, Pandith S, et al. Dapsone-induced methemoglobinemia: "Saturation gap"-The key to diagnosis. J Anaesthesiol Clin Pharmacol 2014;30(1):86–8.
167. Chang YJ, Ali H, Draper A, et al. An unusual cause of cyanosis in a patient with COPD. BMJ Case Rep 2013;2013. pii:bcr2012008092.
168. Canning J, Levine M. Case files of the medical toxicology fellowship at Banner Good Samaritan Medical Center in Phoenix, AZ: methemoglobinemia following dapsone exposure. J Med Toxicol 2011;7(2):139–46.
169. Park KH, Kim H, Lee CC, et al. Dapsone intoxication: clinical course and characteristics. Clin Toxicol 2010;48(6):516–21.
170. Sankar J, Devangare S, Dubey NK. Survival with 98% methemoglobin levels in a school-aged child during the "festival of colors." Pediatr Emerg Care 2013;29(10):1102–3.
171. Singh J, Gathwala G, Khanna A, et al. Acquired methemoglobinemia due to contaminated Holi colors - a rare but preventable complication. Indian J Pediatr 2013;80(4):351–2.
172. Zaki SA, Jadhav A, Chandane P. Methaemoglobinaemia during Holi festival. Ann Trop Paediatr 2009;29(3):221–3.
173. Wu YJ, Lin YL, Huang HY, et al. Methemoglobinemia induced by indoxacarb intoxication. Clin Toxicol 2010;48(7):766–7.
174. Park JS, Kim H, Lee SW, et al. Successful treatment of methemoglobinemia and acute renal failure after indoxacarb poisoning. Clin Toxicol 2011;49(8):744–6.
175. Bayat A, Kosinski RW. Methemoglobinemia in a newborn: a case report. Pediatr Dent 2011;33(3):252–4.
176. Oh JS, Choi KH. Methemoglobinemia associated with metaflumizone poisoning. Clin Toxicol 2014;52(4):288–90.
177. McRobb CM, Holt DW. Methylene blue-induced methemoglobinemia during cardiopulmonary bypass? A case report and literature review. J Extra Corpor Technol 2008;40(3):206–14.

178. Allegaert K, Miserez M, Lerut T, et al. Methemoglobinemia and hemolysis after enteral administration of methylene blue in a preterm infant: relevance for pediatric surgeons. J Pediatr Surg 2004;39(1):E35–7.
179. Merieau E, Suc AL, Beau-Salinas F, et al. Metoclopramide and neonatal methaemoglobinemia. Arch Pediatr 2005;12(4):438–41.
180. Mary AM, Bhupalam L. Metoclopramide-induced methemoglobinemia in an adult. J Ky Med Assoc 2000;98(6):245–7.
181. Hovenga S, Koenders ME, van der Werf TS, et al. Methaemoglobinaemia after inhalation of nitric oxide for treatment of hydrochlorothiazide-induced pulmonary oedema. Lancet 1996;348(9033):1035–6.
182. Gupta A, Jain N, Agrawal A, et al. A fatal case of severe methaemoglobinemia due to nitrobenzene poisoning. BMJ Case Rep 2011;2011. pii:bcr0720114431.
183. Shahani L, Sattovia S. Acquired methaemoglobinaemia related to phenazopyridine ingestion. BMJ Case Rep 2012;2012. pii:bcr2012006756.
184. Akbayram S, Akgun C, Dogan M, et al. Acquired methemoglobinemia due to application of prilocaine during circumcision. J Emerg Med 2012;43(1):120–1.
185. Trapp L, Will J. Acquired methemoglobinemia revisited. Dent Clin North Am 2010;54(4):665–75.
186. Kizer N, Martinez E, Powell M. Report of two cases of rasburicase-induced methemoglobinemia. Leuk Lymphoma 2006;47(12):2648–50.
187. Sohn CH, Seo DW, Ryoo SM, et al. Life-threatening methemoglobinemia after unintentional ingestion of antifreeze admixtures containing sodium nitrite in the construction sites. Clin Toxicol 2014;52(1):44–7.
188. Centers for Disease Control. Methemoglobinemia following unintentional ingestion of sodium nitrite–New York, 2002. MMWR Morb Mortal Wkly Rep 2002; 51(29):639–42.
189. Maric P, Ali SS, Heron LG, et al. Methaemoglobinaemia following ingestion of a commonly available food additive. Med J Aust 2008;188(3):156–8.
190. Kawasumi H, Tanaka E, Hoshi D, et al. Methemoglobinemia induced by trimethoprim-sulfamethoxazole in a patient with systemic lupus erythematosus. Intern Med 2013;52(15):1741–3.
191. Kohl BA, Domski A, Pavan K, et al. Use of telemedicine for the identification and treatment of sulfamethoxazole-induced methaemoglobinemia. J Telemed Telecare 2012;18(6):362–4.
192. Lavergne S, Darmon M, Levy V, et al. Methemoglobinemia and acute hemolysis after tetracaine lozenge use. J Crit Care 2006;21(1):112–4.
193. Burney RE, Wu SC, Nemiroff MJ. Mass carbon monoxide poisoning: clinical effects and results of treatment in 184 victims. Ann Emerg Med 1982;11(8): 394–9.
194. Borron S, Baud F. Acute cyanide poisoning: clinical spectrum, diagnosis, and treatment. Arh Hig Rada Toksikol 1996;47(3):307–22.
195. Burnett WW, King EG, Grace M, et al. Hydrogen sulfide poisoning: review of 5 years' experience. Can Med Assoc J 1977;117(11):1277–80.
196. Milby TH, Baselt RC. Hydrogen sulfide poisoning: clarification of some controversial issues. Am J Ind Med 1999;35(2):192–5.

Irritants and Corrosives

Richard Tovar, MD[a],*, Jerrold B. Leikin, MD[b]

KEYWORDS

- Corrosives • Irritants • Hazardous materials • Triage systems
- Communication of hazards • Contact dermatitis • Coagulative necrosis
- Liquefactive necrosis

KEY POINTS

- Irritant gas exposures predominantly affect the airways, causing tracheitis, bronchitis, and bronchiolitis.
- Complications of acute exposure may include adult respiratory distress syndrome, bacterial infections, and bronchiolitis obliterans (sometimes leading to pulmonary fibrosis).
- Diagnosis of acute exposure is usually obvious by history, but pulse oximetry and chest radiograph should be obtained. Follow-up evaluation should include spirometry and lung volume assessment.
- Treat acute irritant exposures supportively, and observe symptomatic patients and those at risk of delayed pulmonary injury for 24 hours.
- Corrosive compounds can cause significant immediate tissue destruction via direct contact.
- Skin decontamination involves a copious amount of water irrigation.
- Management of gastrointestinal exposure is mostly supportive, and includes endoscopy for significant ingestions.

INTRODUCTION

The US Occupational Safety and Health Administration (OSHA) defines an irritant toxic chemical as one whereby the skin or other organ system experiences reversible damage following the application of a test substance for up to 4 hours. OSHA defines a corrosive agent as one that produces irreversible damage to the skin or other organ systems; namely, visible necrosis into the organ system integumentary layers, following the application of a test substance for up to 4 hours. Corrosive reactions can cause coagulation or liquefaction necrosis. The damaged areas are typified by ulcers, bleeding, bloody scabs, and, by the end of observation at 14 days, discoloration caused by blanching of the skin, complete areas of alopecia, and scars.

Disclosures: None.

[a] Medical Toxicology, Clinical Forensic Medicine, TacticalTox, 3215 Golf Road #130, Delafield, WI 53018, USA; [b] Medical Toxicology, NorthShore University HealthSystems-OMEGA, University of Chicago Pritzker School of Medicine, 2150 Pfingsten Road, Suite 3000, Glenview, IL 60026, USA
* Corresponding author.
E-mail addresses: rttox@me.com; rttox@yahoo.com

Emerg Med Clin N Am 33 (2015) 117–131
http://dx.doi.org/10.1016/j.emc.2014.09.009
0733-8627/15/$ – see front matter © 2015 Elsevier Inc. All rights reserved.

emed.theclinics.com

Histopathology should be considered to evaluate questionable lesions. An example of the serious degree that chemical irritants and toxins can cause severe population toxicity is the release of chlorine gas from a train derailment on January 6, 2006, in Graniteville, South Carolina (**Fig. 1**). One rail tank car was estimated to have released approximately 60 tons of chlorine gas. The release resulted in at least 1 death and 250 exposures to residents of the surrounding area. More than 5000 residents were required to evacuate the scene, and the estimated cost of the cleanup, according to the National Transportation Safety Board, was more than $30 million.

IRRITANTS

Irritants are materials that can cause inflammation of the body surface with which they come into contact. The inflammation results from concentrations far below those needed to cause corrosion.[1] Corrosives are discussed in a separate section. Hazardous material irritants can be divided into those that cause irritation along with contact dermatitis and those that cause upper respiratory symptoms. Examples of irritant gas placards are shown in **Fig. 2**.

Dermatitis is a localized inflammation of the skin. Signs of skin inflammation include some or all of the following: redness, heat, swelling, and pain. More significant signs can include blisters, scales, or eschars. Skin becomes inflamed with exposure to hazardous materials, resulting in a nonallergic, irritant dermatitis. Other contributory factors to the extent of an irritant contact dermatitis are as follows.

- Substance chemical properties (eg, acid, alkali)
- Concentration of substance
- Duration and frequency of exposure
- Body surface area of the skin that is affected
- Preexisting skin condition (eg, abrasions, perspiration)

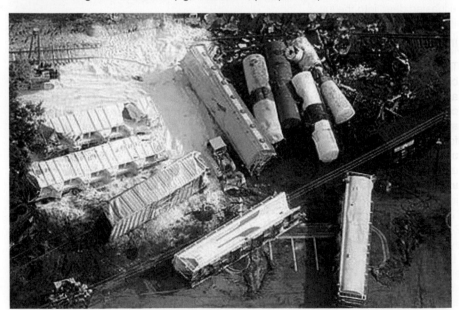

Fig. 1. Aerial picture of Graniteville crash site. (*From* United States Environmental Protection Agency. On-scene coordinator: Norfolk Southern Graniteville Derailment. Available at: http://www.epaosc.org/site/image_list.aspx?site_id=A4GY.)

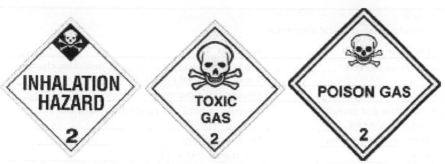

Fig. 2. Irritant gas placards.

Treatment usually consists of good skin decontamination, wound care, and steroid topical creams or ointments. Topical antibiotics are used for partial and full-thickness chemical burns to prevent secondary bacterial infections. Examples of hazardous substances in the workplace causing irritant dermatitis are listed in **Table 1**.

Irritant gases are those which, when inhaled, dissolve in the water of the respiratory tract mucosa and cause an inflammatory response, usually resulting from the release of acidic or alkaline radicals. Irritant gas exposures predominantly affect the airways, causing tracheitis, bronchitis, and bronchiolitis.

Table 2 lists common respiratory irritants found in hazardous material situations.

Irritant gases cause either immediate or delayed respiratory toxicity. The greater the water solubility of the gas, the more rapid is the reaction with water and the more likely it is to cause immediate toxicity and irritation of the upper respiratory tract (eg, chlorine or chloramine gas). Gases with low water solubility react with water at a slower rate, are inhaled deep into the lungs, and cause delayed toxicity and lower respiratory tract irritation (eg, phosgene). The inhalation of a large amount of highly water-soluble gas will overwhelm the respiratory system and cause upper and lower respiratory tract irritation.

Therefore, gases that are water soluble, such as hydrochloric acid (HCl), ammonia (NH$_3$), sulfur dioxide (SO$_2$), formaldehyde (CH$_2$O), chlorine gas (Cl$_2$), and acid vapors, cause immediate toxicity to the upper airway mucous membranes. Clinical symptoms consist of upper airway irritation, including a burning sensation of the eyes, throat, and upper airway.[2] Severe secondary upper airway edema and hypoxia may result from this type of exposure. Lack of immediate symptoms, combined with a brief observation period, can usually rule out significant toxicity.

Low water-soluble irritant gases, such as ozone, phosgene, and nitrogen oxides, can cause lower respiratory toxicity. The most severe form of lower tract respiratory injury is acute respiratory distress syndrome (ARDS). There is classically no evidence of immediate upper airway toxicity, and delayed lower respiratory symptoms for up to 12 hours can be observed. Phosgene has been reported to smell like freshly mown hay.

Besides causing immediate upper airway toxicity, chlorine gas can also act in a delayed fashion, causing lower tract injury. Hydrogen sulfide is another hazardous material (gas) that acts both as an irritant (upper airway edema) and an asphyxiant. In the case of hydrogen sulfide, the proposed mechanism of action is inhibition of oxygen utilization by the inhibition of cytochrome oxidase (asphyxia).[3] Finally, hydrogen sulfide has low water solubility and can also cause direct pulmonary injury, with symptoms ranging from cough and dyspnea to ARDS.[4]

Table 1
Irritants causing chemical dermatitis

Condition	Irritant
Agriculture workers	Artificial fertilizers, disinfectants, pesticides, cleaners, gasoline, diesel oil, plants and grains
Artists	Solvents, clay, plaster
Automobile and aircraft industry workers	Solvents, cutting oils, paints, hand cleansers
Bakers and confectioners	Flour, detergents
Bartenders	Detergents, wet work
Bookbinders	Solvents, glues
Butchers	Detergents, meat, waste
Cabinet makers and carpenters	Glues, detergents, thinners, solvents, wood preservatives
Cleaners	Detergents, solvents, wet work
Coal miners	Dust (coal, stone), wet conditions
Construction workers	Cement
Cooks and caterers	Detergents, vegetable juices, wet work
Dentists and dental technicians	Detergents, hand cleansers, wet work
Dry cleaners	Solvents
Electricians	Soldering fluxes
Electroplaters	Acids, alkalis
Floor layers	Solvents
Florists and gardeners	Manure, artificial fertilizers, pesticides, wet work
Hairdressers	Permanent wave solutions, shampoos, bleaching agents, wet work
Hospital workers	Detergents, disinfectants, foods, wet work
Homemakers	Detergents, cleansers, foods, wet work
Jewelers	Detergents, solvents
Mechanics	Oils, greases, gasoline, diesel fuel, cleaners, solvents
Metal workers	Cutting oils, solvents, hand cleansers
Nurses	Disinfectants, detergents, wet work
Office workers	Solvents, (photocopiers, adhesives)
Painters	Solvents, thinners, wallpaper adhesives, hand cleansers
Photography industry workers	Solvents, wet work
Plastics workers	Solvents, acids, styrene, oxidizing agents
Printers	Solvents
Rubber workers	Solvents, talc, zinc stearate, uncured rubber
Shoemakers	Solvents
Tannery workers	Acids, alkalis, reducing and oxidizing agents, wet work
Textile workers	Fibers, bleaching agents, solvents
Veterinarians and slaughterhouse workers	Disinfectants, wet work, animal entrails and secretions

Data from Canadian Center for Occupational Health and Safety (CCOHS). Irritant contact dermatitis, Available at: http://www.ccohs.ca/oshanswers/diseases/dermatitis.html. Accessed July 1, 2014. OSH Answers, 2008.

Table 2
Common respiratory irritants

Chemical	Sources of Exposure	Important Properties	Injury Produced	Dangerous Exposure Level Under 15 min (PPM Unless Otherwise Specified)
Acetaldehyde	Plastics, synthetic rubber industry, combustion products	High vapor pressure; high water solubility	Upper airway injury; rarely causes delayed pulmonary edema	
Acetic acid, organic acids	Chemical industry, electronics, combustion products	Water soluble	Ocular and upper airway injury	
Acid anhydrides	Chemicals, paints, and plastics industries; components of epoxy resins	Water soluble, highly reactive, may cause allergic sensitization	Ocular, upper airway injury, bronchospasm; pulmonary hemorrhage after massive exposure	
Acrolein	Plastics, textiles, pharmaceutical manufacturing, combustion products	High vapor pressure, intermediate water solubility, extremely irritating	Diffuse airway and parenchymal injury	
Ammonia	Fertilizers, animal feeds, chemicals, pharmaceuticals manufacturing	Alkaline gas, very high water solubility	Primarily ocular and upper airway burn; massive exposure may cause bronchiectasis	500
Antimony trichloride, antimony pentachloride	Alloys, organic catalysts	Poorly soluble, injury likely due to halide ion	Pneumonitis, noncardiogenic pulmonary edema	
Beryllium	Alloys (with copper), ceramics; electronics, aerospace and nuclear reactor equipment	Irritant metal, also acts as an antigen to promote a long-term granulomatous response	Acute upper airway injury, tracheobronchitis, chemical pneumonitis	25 $\mu g/m^3$
Boranes (diborane)	Aircraft fuel, fungicide manufacturing	Water-soluble gas	Upper airway injury, pneumonitis with massive exposure	
Hydrogen bromide	Petroleum refining		Upper airway injury, pneumonitis with massive exposure	

(continued on next page)

Table 2
(continued)

Chemical	Sources of Exposure	Important Properties	Injury Produced	Dangerous Exposure Level Under 15 min (PPM Unless Otherwise Specified)
Methyl bromide	Refrigeration, produce fumigation	Moderately soluble gas	Upper and lower airway injury, pneumonitis, central nervous system (CNS) depression and seizures	
Cadmium	Alloys with Zn and Pb, electroplating, batteries, insecticides	Acute and chronic respiratory effects	Tracheobronchitis, pulmonary edema (often delayed onset over 24–48 h); chronic low-level exposure leads to inflammatory changes and emphysema	100
Calcium oxide, calcium hydroxide	Lime, photography, tanning, insecticides	Moderately caustic, very high doses required for toxicity	Upper and lower airway inflammation, pneumonitis	
Chlorine	Bleaching, formation of chlorinated compounds, household cleaners	Intermediate water solubility	Upper and lower airway inflammation, pneumonitis and noncardiogenic pulmonary edema	5–10
Chloroacetophenone	Crowd-control agent, "tear gas"	Irritant qualities are used to incapacitate; alkylating agent	Ocular and upper airway inflammation, lower airway and parenchymal injury with massive exposure	1–10
o-Chlorobenzomalonitrile	Crowd-control agent, "tear gas"	Irritant qualities are used to incapacitate	Ocular and upper airway inflammation, lower airway injury with massive exposure	
Chloromethyl ethers	Solvents, used in manufacture of other organic compounds		Upper and lower airway irritation, also a respiratory tract carcinogen	
Chloropicrin	Chemical manufacturing, fumigant component	Former First World War gas	Upper and lower airway inflammation	15

Chromic acid (Cr(IV))	Welding, plating	Water soluble irritant, allergic sensitizer	Nasal inflammation and ulceration, rhinitis, pneumonitis with massive exposure	
Cobalt	High-temperature alloys, permanent magnets, hard metal tools (with tungsten carbide)	Nonspecific irritant, also allergic sensitizer	Acute bronchospasm and/or pneumonitis; chronic exposure can cause lung fibrosis	
Formaldehyde	Manufacture of foam insulation, plywood, textiles, paper, fertilizers, resins; embalming agents; combustion products	Highly water soluble, rapidly metabolized; primarily acts via sensory nerve stimulation; sensitization reported	Ocular and upper airway irritation; bronchospasm in severe exposure; contact dermatitis in sensitized persons	3
Hydrochloric acid	Metal refining, rubber manufacturing, organic compound manufacture, photographic materials	Highly water soluble	Ocular and upper airway inflammation, lower airway inflammation only with massive exposure	100
Hydrofluoric acid	Chemical catalyst, pesticides, bleaching, welding, etching	Highly water soluble, powerful and rapid oxidant, lowers serum calcium in massive exposure	Ocular and upper airway inflammation, tracheobronchitis and pneumonitis with massive exposure	20
Isocyanates	Polyurethane production; paints; herbicide and insecticide products; laminating, furniture, enameling, resin work	Low molecular weight organic compounds, cause irritants, sensitization in susceptible persons	Ocular, upper and lower inflammation; asthma, hypersensitivity pneumonitis in sensitized persons	0.1
Lithium hydride	Alloys, ceramics, electronics, chemical catalysts	Low solubility, highly reactive	Pneumonitis, noncardiogenic pulmonary edema	
Mercury	Electrolysis, ore and amalgam extraction, electronics manufacture	No respiratory symptoms with low level, chronic exposure	Ocular and respiratory tract inflammation, pneumonitis, CNS, kidney and systemic effects	1.1 mg/m^3

(continued on next page)

Table 2
(continued)

Chemical	Sources of Exposure	Important Properties	Injury Produced	Dangerous Exposure Level Under 15 min (PPM Unless Otherwise Specified)
Nickel carbonyl	Nickel refining, electroplating, chemical reagents	Potent toxin	Lower respiratory irritation, pneumonitis, delayed systemic toxic effects	$8\ \mu g/m^3$
Nitrogen dioxide	Silos after new grain storage, fertilizer making, arc welding, combustion products	Low water solubility, brown gas at high concentration	Ocular and upper airway inflammation, noncardiogenic pulmonary edema, delayed-onset bronchiolitis	50
Nitrogen mustards; sulfur mustards	Military gases	Causes severe injury, vesicant properties	Ocular, upper and lower airway inflammation, pneumonitis	$20\ mg/m^3$ (N), $1\ mg/m^3$ (S)
Osmium tetroxide	Copper refining, alloy with iridium, catalyst for steroid synthesis and ammonia formation	Metallic osmium is inert, tetroxide forms when heated in air	Severe ocular and upper airway irritation; transient renal damage	$1\ mg/m^3$
Ozone	Arc welding, copy machines, paper bleaching	Sweet-smelling gas, moderate water solubility	Upper and lower airway inflammation; asthmatics more susceptible	1
Phosgene	Pesticide and other chemical manufacture, arc welding, paint removal	Poorly water soluble, does not irritate airways in low doses	Upper airway inflammation and pneumonitis; delayed pulmonary edema in low doses	2
Phosphoric sulfides	Production of insecticides, ignition compounds, matches		Ocular and upper airway inflammation	
Phosphoric chlorides	Manufacture of chlorinated organic compounds, dyes, gasoline additives	Form phosphoric acid and hydrochloric acid on contact with mucosal surfaces	Ocular and upper airway inflammation	$10\ mg/m^3$

Selenium dioxide	Copper or nickel smelting, heating of selenium alloys	Strong vesicant, forms selenious acid (H_2SeO_3) on mucosal surfaces	Ocular and upper airway inflammation, pulmonary edema in massive exposure	
Hydrogen selenide	Copper refining, sulfuric acid production	Water soluble; exposure to selenium compounds gives rise to garlic odor breath	Ocular and upper airway inflammation, delayed pulmonary edema	
Styrene	Manufacture of polystyrene and resins, polymers	Highly irritating	Ocular, upper and lower airway inflammation, neurologic impairments	600
Sulfur dioxide	Petroleum refining, pulp mills, refrigeration plants, manufacturing of sodium sulfite	Highly water-soluble gas	Upper airway inflammation, bronchoconstriction, pneumonitis on massive exposure	100
Titanium tetrachloride	Dyes, pigments, sky writing	Chloride ions form HCl on mucosa	Upper airway injury	
Uranium hexafluoride	Metal coat removers, floor sealants, spray paints	Toxicity likely from chloride ions	Upper and lower airway injury, bronchospasm, pneumonitis	
Vanadium pentoxide	Cleaning oil tanks, metallurgy		Ocular, upper and lower airway symptoms	70
Zinc chloride	Smoke grenades, artillery	More severe than zinc oxide exposure	Upper and lower airway irritation, fever, delayed onset pneumonitis	200
Zirconium tetrachloride	Pigments, catalysts	Chloride ion toxicity	Upper and lower airway irritation, pneumonitis	

Reproduced from Pedersen LK, Johansen JD, Held E, et al. Augmentation of skin response by exposure to a combination of allergens and irritants - a review. Contact Dermatitis 2004;50(5):265–73.

Emergent medical evaluation of irritant gas exposures includes pulse oximetry and chest radiography. Clues to significant respiratory toxicity are hypoxemia and evidence of patchy consolidation on chest radiograph. Persistent respiratory symptoms are evaluated by computed tomography of the chest to look for bronchiolitis obliterans.

CORROSIVE CHEMICALS

Corrosive materials are liquid or solid substances that have the capability to cause full-thickness dermal injury on contact within a specified time period.[5] This class includes both acids and bases, and may include mixtures along with anhydrous compounds. An example of a hazardous material warning placard for corrosives is shown in **Fig. 3**.

Dermal contact with acid liquids results in protein desiccation, producing coagulative necrosis, whereas alkali substances can penetrate deeper, producing liquefactive necrosis and causing tissue saponification.[5] There are 6 mechanisms of action for chemical agents in biological systems.[6]

1. Oxidation: The protein denaturation is caused by inserting an oxygen, sulfur, or halogen atom to viable body proteins (sodium hypochlorite, potassium permanganate, and chromic acid).
2. Reduction: Reducing agents act by binding free electrons in tissue proteins. Heat may also be a product of a chemical reaction, thereby causing a mixed picture. The agents more likely to be encountered are hydrochloric acid, nitric acid, and alkyl mercuric compounds.
3. Corrosion: Corrosion causes protein denaturation on contact. Corrosive agents tend to produce a soft eschar, which may progress to shallow ulceration. Examples of corrosive agents are phenols, sodium hypochlorite, and white phosphorous.
4. Protoplasmic poisons: These poisons produce their effects by causing the formation of esters with proteins, or by binding or inhibiting calcium or other organic ions

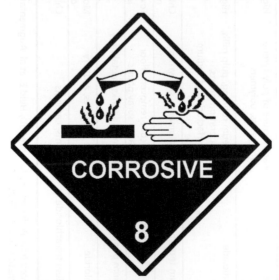

Fig. 3. Corrosive placard. (*From* Centers for Disease Control, The National Institute for Occupational Safety and Health (NIOSH). Available at http://www.cdc.gov/niosh/. Accessed July 1, 2014.)

necessary for tissue viability and function. Examples of ester formers are formic and acetic acids, while inhibitors include oxalic and hydrofluoric acids.

5. Vesicants: Vesicants produce ischemia with anoxic necrosis at the site of contact. These agents, characterized by producing cutaneous blisters, include mustard gas, dimethyl sulfoxide (DMSO), and Lewisite.

6. Desiccants: These substances cause damage by dehydration of tissues. The damage is often exacerbated by heat production, as these reactions are usually exothermic. This group contains find sulfuric acid and muriatic acid (concentrated hydrochloric acids).

A list of some of the common corrosive chemicals found in the academic laboratory is given in **Table 3**.

In general, treatment involves copious tepid water irrigation at the site of contact after removal of all clothing and jewelry. Chemical blisters should be broken to remove any blister fluid that may contain the offending corrosive.[7,8]

Chemical eye burns are classified into mild, moderate, and severe (**Fig. 4**). Corneal epithelial defects can range from superficial punctate keratopathy to sloughing of the entire epithelium. Mild to moderate burns do not demonstrate areas of perilimbal ischemia. By contrast, ischemic injury presents as blanching of conjunctival or episcleral vessels. Mild to moderate burns show areas of conjunctival epithelial defect, chemosis (conjunctival edema), hyperemia, hemorrhages, eyelid edema, mild anterior chamber reaction, and first-degree and second-degree burns of periocular skin. Severe ocular burns present with chemosis, conjunctival blanching, corneal edema, corneal opacification, moderate to severe anterior chamber reaction, increased intraocular pressure, and second-degree and third-degree burns of surrounding skin.

In addition, if the compound penetrates through the sclera, it can potentially cause local necrotic retinopathy.[9] Ocular exposures are treated similarly with copious water

Table 3
Common corrosive chemicals

Inorganic Acids	Inorganic Bases	Oxidizing Agents
Chromic acid	Ammonia, ammonium hydroxide	Bromine
Hydrochloric acid	Calcium hydroxide	Chlorine
Hydrofluoric acid	Calcium oxide	Chromic acid
Nitric acid	Potassium hydroxide	Fluorine
Perchloric acid	Sodium hydroxide	Nitric acid
Phosphoric acid		Perchloric acid
Sulfuric acid		
Organic Acids	**Dehydrating Agents**	**Other Compounds**
Butyric acid	Calcium oxide	Tin chloride
Formic acid	Glacial acetic acid	Potassium chromate
Glacial acetic acid	Phosphorous pentoxide	Phosphorous pentoxide
Oxalic acid	Sodium hydroxide	Phosphorous trichloride
Phenol	Sulfuric acid	
Salicylic acid		

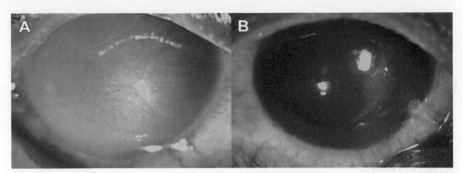

Fig. 4. Examples of severe corneal chemical burns. (*A*) Dua grade VI or Roper-Hall grade VI ocular chemical injury. (*B*) Dua and Roper-Hall grade II ocular chemical injury. (*From* Logothetis HD, Leikin SM, Patrianakos T. Management of anterior segment trauma. Dis Mon 2014;60(6):247–53; with permission.)

or saline irrigation to an end point of conjunctival sac runoff to a pH of 7. Two examples of the classification of chemical ocular injuries are shown in **Tables 4** and **5**.[10]

It should be noted that white phosphorus (which can be highly flammable) can cause hypocalcemia, resulting in a prolonged QT interval on electrocardiogram; intravenous calcium may be required.[11] Because it will react with ambient oxygen, tissue debridement to remove the solid particles and irrigation with water is important. Similarly, hydrofluoric acid (HF) can result in refractory hypocalcemia along with hypomagnesemia and hyperkalemia. The pain from HF burns may be severe and seem to be out of proportion to the physical signs at the site of exposure. Treatment of skin exposure includes copious irrigation, blister breakage, and calcium administration. Topical calcium gluconate gel (2.5%–10%) can be applied to the area of dermal exposure; subcutaneous (up to 0.5 mL per cm^3 skin surface area) or intra-arterial treatment via radial or brachial artery of affected limb (10 mL of 10% calcium gluconate diluted to 100 mL and infused over 4 hours titrated to pain relief) may be required. Calcium chloride or calcium gluconate can be given intravenously through a secure, preferably central venous access in cases of systemic hypocalcemia.[12]

Another special area of hazardous material exposure is that of ingested corrosives. Again, the basic tenets of airway stabilization and treatment of circulatory compromise hold sway. Caustic ingestions may cause widespread injury to the oral areas and upper airway. Usually, acids with pH less than 3 or bases with pH greater than 11 are of the greatest concern for caustic injury.[13] Among the most concerning injuries are

Table 4			
Roper Hall classification of chemical ocular injuries			
Grade	**Prognosis**	**Cornea**	**Conjunctival Limbus**
I	Good	Corneal epithelial damage	No ischemia
II	Good	Corneal haze, iris details visible	<1/3 limbal ischemia
III	Guarded	Total epithelial loss, stromal haze, iris details obscured	1/3–1/2 limbal ischemia
IV	Poor	Cornea opaque, iris and pupil obscured	>1/2 limbal ischemia

From Kuckelkorn R, Schrage N, Keller G, et al. Emergency treatment of chemical and thermal eye burns. Acta Ophthalmol Scand 2002;80(1):4–10; with permission.

Table 5
Dua classification of chemical ocular injuries

Grade	Prognosis	Clinical Findings	Conjunctival Involvement
I	Very good	0 Clock hours of limbal involvement	0%
II	Good	<3 Clock hours of limbal involvement	<30%
III	Good	Between 3–6 h of limbal involvement	30%–50%
IV	Good to guarded	Between 6–9 h of limbal involvement	50%–75%
V	Guarded to poor	Between 9–12 h of limbal involvement	75%–100%
VI	Very poor	Total limbus involved	Total conjunctival involvement

From Kuckelkorn R, Schrage N, Keller G, et al. Emergency treatment of chemical and thermal eye burns. Acta Ophthalmol Scand 2002;80(1):4–10; with permission.

those of esophageal and gastric injuries. Short-term complications include perforation and death. Long-term complications include stricture and increased lifetime risk of esophageal carcinoma. **Table 6** lists some of the most commonly ingested corrosive agents.[14]

The timing of endoscopy and the circumstances for its use, as recommended in the literature, are controversial. In the past there was a tendency to wait at least 24 hours to allow time for the injury to mature. Some investigators are now recommending earlier endoscopy and suggesting a wait of only 12 hours.[13] The recommendation not to perform endoscopy past 48 hours still stands, owing to a higher probability of perforation caused by ongoing weakening of the esophageal wall. **Table 7** is an example of endoscopic evaluation of the severity of a corrosive/caustic esophageal burn.

Most medical toxicologists and gastrointestinal specialists agree that strong alkali ingestions require endoscopy, while asymptomatic or questionable ingestions may be observed. The use of intravenous and oral steroids has been controversial. A randomized trial by Anderson and colleagues[15] found no difference in the incidence of stricture formation with the use of steroids. This study was underpowered, as the volume of patients in the study was relatively low.

Table 6
Commonly ingested caustic/corrosive agents

Type	Example
Alkali	Sodium hydroxide, potassium hydroxide, (oven cleaners, liquid agents, liquid drain cleaners, disk batteries), calcium and lithium hydroxide (hair relaxers), ammonia (household cleaners), dishwater detergents
Acid	Sulfuric acid, hydrochloric acid, nitric acid (toilet bowl cleaners, swimming pool cleaners, rust removers)
Bleaches and other caustics	Hypochlorous acid (bleach—generally neutral pH commercially), peroxide (mildew remover)

From Lupa M, Magne J, Guarisco JL, et al. Update on the diagnosis and treatment of caustic ingestion. Ochsner J 2009;9(2):54–9; with permission.

Table 7
Injury staging in corrosive esophageal burns

Injury	Findings
Grade 0	Normal mucosa
Grade 1 (mucosal)	Edema, hyperemia of mucosa
Grade 2a (transmucosal)	Blisters, hemorrhages, erosions, whitish membranes, exudates
Grade 2b	Grade 2a findings plus deep or circumferential ulceration
Grade 3a (transmural)	Small scattered area of ulceration and areas of necrosis
Grade 3b	Extensive necrosis

From Lupa M, Magne J, Guarisco JL, et al. Update on the diagnosis and treatment of caustic ingestion. Ochsner J 2009;9(2):54–9; with permission.

SUMMARY

This article constitutes a review of the toxic effects of hazardous substances known as irritants and corrosives. The treatment of both toxic hazardous materials is outlined, and mostly consists of conservative treatment. Further research is continuing to provide more aggressive reversal of some of the tissue destruction seen by irritant and corrosive tissue injury.

REFERENCES

1. U. S. Department of Labor, Occupational Safety & Health Administration, Marine terminals. 29 CFR 191728 App A. Washington, DC: U.S. Government Printing Office: 2014.
2. Rom WN, Ryon DL. Diseases caused by respiratory irritants and toxic chemicals. In: Stellman J, David A, Wagner G, editors. Encyclopedia of occupational health and safety. Geneva (Switzerland): International Labor Organization; 2011. p. 200–36.
3. Beauchamp RO Jr, Bus JS, Popp JA, et al. A critical review of the literature on hydrogen sulfide toxicity. Crit Rev Toxicol 1984;13(1):25–97.
4. Guidotti TL. Hydrogen sulphide. Occup Med 1996;46(5):367–71.
5. U. S. Department of Transportation. 49 CFR 173.136 class 8—definitions. Washington, DC: U.S. Government Printing Office; 2014.
6. Palao R, Monge I, Ruiz M, et al. Chemical burns: pathophysiology and treatment. Burns 2010;36(3):295–304.
7. Bruze M, Fregert S, Gruvberger B. Chemical skin burns. In: Kanerva L, Elsner P, Wahlberg JE, et al, editors. Handbook of occupational dermatology. Berlin: Springer; 2000. p. 325–32.
8. Hall AH, Maibach HI. Water decontamination of chemical skin/eye splashes: a critical review. Cutan Ocul Toxicol 2006;25(2):67–83.
9. Baker RS, Wilson RM, Flowers CW Jr, et al. A population-based survey of hospitalized work-related ocular injury: diagnoses, cause of injury, resource utilization, and hospitalization outcome. Ophthalmic Epidemiol 1999;6(3):159–69.
10. Kuckelkorn R, Schrage N, Keller G, et al. Emergency treatment of chemical and thermal eye burns. Acta Ophthalmol Scand 2002;80(1):4–10.
11. Bowen TE, Whelan TJ Jr, Nelson TG. Sudden death after phosphorus burns: experimental observations of hypocalcemia, hyperphosphatemia and electrocardiographic abnormalities following production of a standard white phosphorus burn. Ann Surg 1971;174(5):779–84.

12. Schauben JL, Wood A. Hydrofluoric acid. In: Walter FG, editor. Advanced Hazmat life support provider manual. Tucson (AZ): Arizona Board of Regents; 2014. p. 323–33.
13. Arevalo-Silva C, Eliashar R, Wohlgelernter J, et al. Ingestion of caustic substances: a 15-year experience. Laryngoscope 2006;116(8):1422–6.
14. Lupa M, Magne J, Guarisco JL, et al. Update on the diagnosis and treatment of caustic ingestion. Ochsner J 2009;9(2):54–9.
15. Anderson KD, Rouse TM, Randolph JG. A controlled trial of corticosteroids in children with corrosive injury of the esophagus. N Engl J Med 1990;323(10): 637–40.

Organophosphate and Carbamate Poisoning

Andrew M. King, MD*, Cynthia K. Aaron, MD

KEYWORDS

- Organophosphate • Carbamate • Pesticides • Insecticides • Nerve agents
- Chemical warfare • Atropine • Oxime

KEY POINTS

- Organophosphates (OPs) and carbamates have a variety of applications, but are primarily used agriculturally as pesticides.
- OPs and carbamates are responsible for the deaths of hundreds of thousands of people every year.
- Acute toxicity results from acetylcholinesterase (AChE) enzyme inhibition and subsequent excessive nicotinic and muscarinic stimulation in the central and autonomic nervous systems and the neuromuscular junction.
- Good supportive care, decontamination, aggressive antimuscarinic therapy, early seizure control, and early antidotal oxime therapy are the keys to good outcomes.

INTRODUCTION
Epidemiology

Experts believe that acute poisoning from acetylcholinesterase (AChE)-inhibiting insecticides is responsible for more deaths than any other class of drug or chemical.[1] They are a particular problem in the developing world, where highly toxic pesticides are readily available and are used in the suicides of hundreds of thousands of people every year.[2] With an estimated case fatality rate of 10% to 20%, the subsequent health care burden of those who do not die after a suicidal ingestion is an order of magnitude higher.[3,4] The disease burden of OP and carbamate toxicity is much less in developed countries. In contrast with the 25,288 people who committed suicide with pesticides in India in 2010,[5] the American Association of Poison Control Centers in 2012 received a combined 4150 calls for OP and carbamate exposures, resulting in a total of 3 deaths.[6] Although unintentional agricultural poisonings do occur, they are generally less severe.[7,8]

Disclosure Statement: The authors of this paper have no disclosures.
Department of Emergency Medicine, Children's Hospital of Michigan Regional Poison Control Center, Detroit Medical Center, Wayne State University School of Medicine, 4707 Street Antoine, Suite 302, Detroit, MI 48201, USA
* Corresponding author.
E-mail address: aking@dmc.org

Emerg Med Clin N Am 33 (2015) 133–151
http://dx.doi.org/10.1016/j.emc.2014.09.010
0733-8627/15/$ – see front matter © 2015 Elsevier Inc. All rights reserved.

Uses

Commercially, organophosphorus chemicals have a number of applications, but are mostly employed as pesticides in a variety of settings (**Box 1** from[9]). They protect commercial and food crops from damaging insect vectors. They also control insect infestations in commercial and residential settings. It should be noted that the Environmental Protection Agency has banned or plans to remove many OPs from the United States and thus OP use for many of these applications has been sharply curtailed. Some medical indications for organophosphates (OPs) include the eradication of corporeal insect infestations in humans and animals. One organic phosphorus chemical is used for glaucoma (diisopropyl phosphorofluorodate).

Militarized OPs (also known as nerve agents) are classified as chemical weapons and weapons of mass destruction. Despite the manufacture of hundreds of thousands of tons of these chemicals by various countries during the 20th century, only small amounts have been deployed in a number of clandestine situations, including the Iran–Iraq war, the Iranian attack on the Kurds, and more recently in the Syrian Civil war in August 2013, resulting in more than 1400 deaths.[10] Before this, the most notable use of nerve agents was the 1995 terrorist attack in Tokyo, Japan, which left 11 dead and more than 5000 victims seeking medical attention.[11] These recent episodes are tragic reminders of the persistent threat posed by nerve agents.

By volume, carbamates are used most frequently as pesticides. However, they do have number of interesting medical indications (**Table 1**).

History

OPs are of particular historical interest given their development and use as chemical weapons. The early part of the 20th century saw the development of the G-series of nerve agents (tabun, sarin, and soman) by the Germans, the V-series (VE, VG, VM,

---

Box 1
Sources of organophosphorus pesticides

Domestic

- Garden sheds—in particular insecticidal preparations but also other products that are marketed as fertilizers but contain some organophosphorus pesticides, available as solid or liquid formulations

- Surface and room sprays

- Baits for cockroaches and other insects (eg, chlorpyrifos)

- Shampoos against head lice (eg, malathion)

- Pet preparations (eg, pet washes, collars)

Industrial or occupational

- Crop protection and livestock dipping

- Large scale internal control, including fumigation

Terrorism or warfare (nerve agents)

- Sarin, for example, was used in the Tokyo subway attack, and both tabun and sarin were used during the Iraq–Iran conflict; although nerve agents share a similar mechanism of toxicity with organophosphorus pesticides, their treatment is a specialized topic and not dealt with in this review

From Roberts DM, Aaron CK. Management of acute organophosphorus pesticide poisoning. BMJ 2007;334(7594):629-34; with permission.

Table 1 Human disease treated with carbamates	
Indication	**Carbamate**
Myasthenia gravis	Edrophonium, pyridostigmine
Antimuscarinic poisoning	Physostigmine
Alzheimer's disease	Rivastigmine, donepezil, galantamine, tacrine
Glaucoma	Physostigmine, ecthiopate
Neuromuscular blockade reversal	Pyridostigmine, neostigmine
Elapid envenomation	Neostigmine
Adynamic ileus	Neostigmine

and VX) by the allies, and, more recently, the ultratoxic group of agents called the Novichok or newcomer agents by the Russians.[12] Many tens of thousands of tons of nerve agents were produced and stockpiled by various countries during World War II. Since then, most countries, in compliance with the Chemical Weapons Convention of 1997, have destroyed or scuttled more than 80% of their declared stockpiles.[13] However, as the incidents in Tokyo and Syria have reminded us, nerve agents continue to be a threat in the hands of terrorists and other militant groups.

The delayed peripheral neuropathy caused by certain OPs (also known as OP-induced delayed peripheral neuropathy [OPIDN]) has led to many well-known, toxin-induced epidemics throughout the world. The Ginger Jake paralysis that affected thousands of Americans during prohibition was caused by an organic phosphorus adulterant (triorthocresyl phosphate, added to Jamaican Ginger ["jake"] extract) to pass US Department of Agriculture inspections. Consumption of this adulterated extract resulted in lower extremity weakness, paraparesis, paralysis, and impotence.[14,15] Similar outbreaks of OPIDN have subsequently been reported in Sri Lanka, Vietnam, and other developing countries.[16,17]

Physostigmine and its carbamate derivates have an interesting and tragic past as well. Physostigmine is the ordeal bean of Old Calabar (*Physostigma venenosum Balfour*), and was the first carbamate isolated by Westerners.[18] Since then, a number of carbamates have been synthesized and employed as fungicides and insecticides. Unfortunately, it was this synthesis that led to the largest industrial accident in history[19] in 1984 during production of the carbamate carbaryl at The Union Carbide Corporation's factory in Bhopal, India. Methyl isocyanate accidentally leaked, immediately killing more than 3800 people and leaving thousands more suffering health effects and premature death.

AGENTS OF TOXICITY
Biochemistry

The general structures of carbamates and OPs are shown below (**Fig. 1**). *N*-Methyl carbamate compounds are the only carbamate derivatives that inhibit AChE. Other derivatives, such as thiocarbamates, do not inhibit AChE and are be discussed in this article. The major carbamates and their relative toxicities are found in **Table 2**.[20] A number of these are not available commercially in the United States.

The structure–function relationship of organic phosphorus compounds is clinically relevant in that each derivative's chemical properties relates to its toxic potential. The general structure includes a phosphoryl group (O = P) or a thiophosphoryl group (P = S), 2 lipophilic R groups, and the leaving group (X; see **Fig. 1**). The X group or leaving group serves as a means of classifying the various OPs.[1] These groups tend to

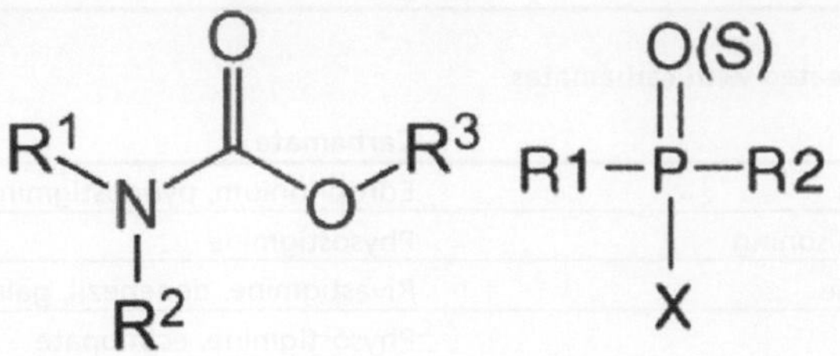

Fig. 1. N-Methyl carbamates contain a common NCOO structure with various side chains R1-R3 (*left*). The basic structure of an organophosphate (OP) is shown on the *right*. Each OP contains a phosphoryl or thiophosphoryl group, 2 side chains, and a leaving group (X).

share certain physical and pharmacodynamic characteristics, but generally do not affect acute management.

Pharmacokinetics

A number of pharmacokinetic properties are important with respect to onset and duration of toxicity. These include route of exposure, lipophilicity, and volume of distribution, whether the agent requires metabolism before it can exert its toxic effects, serum paraoxonase activity (an intrinsic enzyme capable of hydrolyzing certain OPs), and elimination. Important pharmacodynamic properties include potency, rate of AChE inhibition, and rate of aging.

Route

- OPs and carbamates are absorbed through all routes
- Ingestion and inhalation lead to immediate onset of symptoms if vaporized or misted.
- Dermal exposure may have immediate local effects (local diaphoresis and fasciculations) and delayed systemic effects.[21]

Table 2
The main carbamate insecticides in use and their relative toxic potency (estimated human values)

High Toxicity (LD_{50} <50 mg/kg)	Moderate Toxicity (LD_{50} = 50–200 mg/kg)	Low Toxicity (LD_{50} >200 mg/kg)
Aldicarb (Temik)	Bufencarb (Bux)	BPMC (Fenocarb)
Aldoxycarb (Standak)	Carbosulfan	Carbaryl (Sevin)
Aminocarb (Metacil)	Pirimicarb (Pirimor)	Isoprocarb (Etrofolan)
Bendiocarb (Ficam)	Promecarb	MPMC (Meobal)
Carbofuran (Furadan)	Thiodicarb (Larvin)	MTMC (Metacrate, Tsumacide)
Dimetan (Dimetan)	Trimethacarb (Broot)	XMC (Cosban)
Dimetilan (Snip)		
Dioxacarb (Eleocron, Famid)		
Formetanate (Carzol)		
Methiocarb (Mesurol)		
Methomyl (Lannate, Nudrin)		
Oxamyl (Vydate)		
Propoxur (Baygon)		

Data from National Crime Records Bureau. Accidental Deaths and Suicides in India - 2010. Available at: http://ncrb.nic.in/ADSI2010/home.htm. Accessed June 4, 2014.

Pharmacokinetic Properties

- OPs are lipophilic compounds with some sequestering in fat stores.
- Highly lipophilic agents may have a delay in symptoms development.[22,23]
- Highly lipophilic agents cause protracted toxicity.[24,25]
- Redistribution of lipid soluble OPs from fat stores can "repoison" a patient.
- Carbamates are inactivated more quickly and generally do not cause prolonged toxicity.

Metabolism and Subsequent Activation

- OPs are either "oxons" (which can directly inhibit AChE) or "thions" (which require desulfuration to the oxon form to become maximally active).
- Once "thions" (P = S) are oxidized to "oxons"(P = O), they have enhanced toxicity.
- Carbamates do not require metabolism to become active.

Toxicodynamics

OPs and carbamates both inhibit synaptic AChE. Synaptic AChE normally prevents further downstream neurotransmission by hydrolyzing acetylcholine to acetic acid and choline. Acetic acid feeds into the Krebs cycle, whereas choline is taken back up by the neuron and resynthesized to new acetylcholine. Subsequently, acetylcholine accumulates in the nerve or myoneuronal synapse, which leads to characteristic toxic manifestations (cholinergic toxidrome). True AChE is found not only in nervous tissue, but also on the surface of erythrocytes (erythrocyte or red blood cell cholinesterase). Butyrylcholinesterase (also known as pseudocholinesterase or plasma cholinesterase) is found primarily in the liver and is responsible for xenobiotic metabolism (eg, cocaine, succinylcholine). It is important to note that erythrocyte AChE activity more closely mirrors neuronal AChE activity than does butyrylcholinesterase, and is a better marker for neuronal physiologic status.[26–28]

Toxicodynamic Differences Between Organophosphates and Carbamates

The unique pharmacodynamics of organosphosphates and carbamates and their differences in interaction with AChE play a role in the clinical toxicity differences as well as implications for antidotal therapy.

Within the anticholinesterase protein catalytic site lays a serine hydroxyl group (–OH). The serine group becomes phosphorylated once the leaving group (X) is released. At this point, the OP–serine bond can spontaneously hydrolyze and the enzyme regains its function, or, an R group leaves (ages), it becomes irreversibly phosphorylated, and the enzyme is permanently inhibited (**Fig. 2**). The relative speeds of these processes have major implications with respect to administration of the antidotal oximes.

Antidotal oximes increase the rate of hydrolysis and reactivation and prevent irreversible aging. Although those OPs with shorter R-group side chains age more quickly, they also reactivate more quickly and are theoretically more responsive to oxime therapy, provided it is administered early. In contrast, although there is more time to administer oximes to patients poisoned with long-R chain OPs, a greater amount of oxime administered over a longer period of time is required.[21] The reverse can be argued as well; administration of oximes to dimethyl phosphoryl–poisoned patients is less likely to benefit precisely because of those OPs propensity to age quickly.[29] In other words, by the time the oxime is available to facilitate hydrolysis and reactivate AChE, the OP has already aged. Unfortunately, once aged, oximes

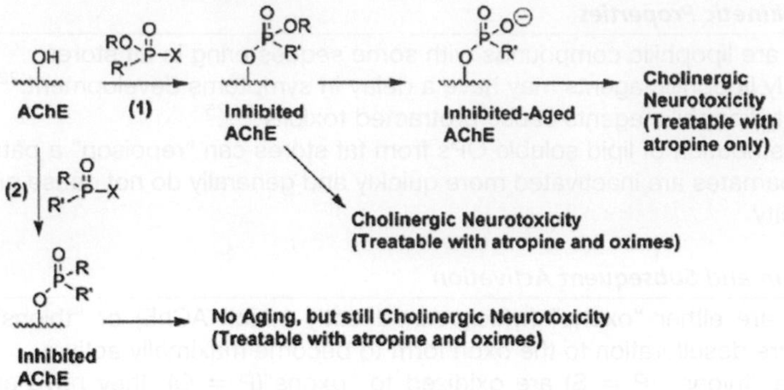

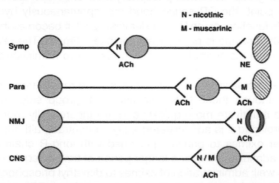

Fig. 2. Phosphonyl (1) and phosphinyl (2) organophosphate molecules bind to the acetyl-cholinesterase enzyme with resultant loss of the leaving group (X). The acetylcholinesterase (AChE) enzyme is now inhibited in both cases and cholinergic toxicity ensues. Before the loss of the R group in (1), both complexes are treatable with atropine and oximes. However, after the loss of the R group (1), the OP has "aged" and the AChE enzyme is irreversibly inhibited.

cannot reactivate the enzyme and any further AChE activity requires the de novo synthesis of additional AChE enzyme[30]

Carbamates also inhibit AChE enzyme in an identical fashion; however, the carbamate–AChE bond is weaker than that formed by OPs. Thus, carbamate–AChE bonds spontaneously hydrolyze more rapidly and AChE function returns typically within 24 to 48 hours. In contrast with OPs, carbamates cannot age and prolonged toxicity is uncommon.

Pathophysiology

The 2 acetylcholine receptor subtypes found in humans and animals are the muscarinic and nicotinic receptors. These receptors are further subclassified according to their locations in the body and what occurs after acetylcholine binds to the receptor. In general, muscarinic receptors are found in the central nervous system (CNS), exocrine glands, and the hollow end-organs innervated by the parasympathetic system, and nicotinic receptors are located in the postganglionic neurons of both the parasympathetic and sympathetic chains, the adrenal medulla, and the neuromuscular junction (**Fig. 3**).[31] Both are found in the brain.

Fig. 3. Graphic representation of the acetylcholine-relevant physiology and anatomy. (*From* Cannard K. The acute treatment of nerve agent exposure. J Neurol Sci 2006;249(1):86–94; with permission.)

Excess acetylcholine at the 2 receptor subtypes results in different end-organ effects. When poisoned by OP and carbamate xenobiotics, toxicity varies and may manifest with primarily nicotinic effects (hypertension, tachycardia, fasciculations, weakness, mydriasis), muscarinic effects (miosis, bradycardia, bronchospasm, bronchorrhea), or a combination of the two. Acetylcholine excess at the neuromuscular junction results in a type II paralysis in the same way succinylcholine depolarizes and paralyzes skeletal muscle. Additionally, cholinergic neurons interact with other neurotransmitter systems ultimately leading to γ-aminobutyric acid (GABA) inhibition and N-methyl-ᴅ-aspartate activation, which may in part be responsible for CNS-mediated respiratory depression and seizure activity.[32–35] **Table 3** summarizes the clinical effects of cholinergic toxicity.

CLINICAL MANIFESTATIONS

Onset and severity of toxicity depend on a variety of factors, including agent, route, formulation, amount, and duration of exposure. For example, death may occur within minutes of inhalational exposure to nerve agents, whereas symptoms from dermal exposures of highly lipophilic agents requiring activation may be delayed by up to 48 hours.[36] Time to onset of symptoms after ingestion tends to be slightly delayed compared with inhalation, with clinical effects expected to begin within 30 to 90 minutes.

Similarly, initial and presenting symptoms depend on the route of exposure. Ingestion often presents with vomiting and other gastrointestinal symptoms, whereas aerosol exposure causes ocular and respiratory symptoms. Dermal exposure may present with localized sweating and fasciculations. Both dermal and inhalational exposures are recognized occupational hazards and exposure can occur during formulation

Table 3
Clinical effects of organophosphate poisoning (acetylcholine excess)

Anatomic Site of Action	Signs and Symptoms
Muscarinic effects	
Sweat glands	Sweating
Pupils	Constricted pupils
Lacrimal glands	Lacrimation
Salivary glands	Excessive salivation
Bronchial tree	Wheezing
Gastrointestinal	Cramps, vomiting, diarrhea, tenesmus
Cardiovascular	Bradycardia, decrease in blood pressure
Ciliary body	Blurred vision
Bladder	Urinary incontinence
Nicotinic effects	
Striated muscle	Fasciculations, cramps, weakness, twitching, paralysis, respiratory embarrassment, cyanosis, arrest
Sympathetic ganglia	Tachycardia, elevated blood pressure
Central nervous system effects	Anxiety, restlessness, ataxia, convulsions, insomnia, coma, absent reflexes, Cheyne-Stokes respirations, respiratory and circulatory depression

From Bradberry SM, Vale J. Organophosphorus and carbamate insecticides. In: Wallece K, Brent J, Burkhart KK, editors. Critical care toxicology: diagnosis and management of the critically poisoned patient. Philadelphia: Elsevier Mosby; 2005. p. 940; with permission.

manufacture, mixing, or spraying. Nonsuicidal ingestion can occur when workers do not adhere to appropriate industrial hygiene.

Clinical effects are owing to stimulation of the muscarinic and nicotinic receptors (see **Table 3**). Muscarinic stimulation causes defecation, urination, miosis, bradycardia, bronchorrhea, bronchospasm, emesis, lacrimation, and salivation (remembered by the mnemonic DUMBBBELS). Stimulation of the nicotinic receptors in the sympathetic ganglia and neuromuscular junction will cause *m*ydriasis, *t*achycardia, *w*eakness, *h*ypertension, and *f*asciculations (*M*onday–*T*uesday–*W*ednesday–*T*hursday–*F*riday).[37] The "mixed" nicotinic and muscarinic clinical effects can be confusing and lead to misdiagnosis.[38] Clinical effects owing to nicotinic receptor stimulation tend to occur first in more severe poisonings.[39]

CNS effects are varied and can be both nonspecific and severe. These effects include headache, dizziness, restless, anxiety, insomnia, confusion, tremor, dysarthria, ataxia, seizures, coma, and central respiratory depression.[40] Finally, given the balance needed between the dopamine and cholinergic systems, it is not surprising that both acute and delayed extrapyramidal symptoms occur.[41–43]

Muscle weakness and paralysis is of particular importance, which contributes to respiratory arrest and death. Severe OP poisoning results in depolarizing paralysis, preceded by muscle twitching and fasciculations. Mechanical ventilation is often necessary because striated intercostal and diaphragmatic muscles become paralyzed.

Additionally troubling is the "intermediate syndrome," which develops after acute exposure to certain highly lipophilic OPs.[44] This syndrome, which occurs a few days after a well-defined cholinergic phase, is defined by the development of diffuse weakness, often leading to respiratory failure requiring ventilatory assistance.[45] It is so named because it typically occurs after the initial cholinergic phase and before the delayed-neuropathic phase (see Intermediate syndrome, elsewhere in this article).

Inhibition of neuropathy target esterase by certain OPs leads to a syndrome known as OPIDN. OPIDN typically develops weeks after an acute exposure. A characteristic progression of symptoms occurs, starting with paresthesias in the hands and feet leading to sensory loss, weakness, ataxia, and distal muscle flaccidity. Those who develop OPIDN may recover after a few months; however, in some cases, the effects are permanent (see Organic Phosphorus-Induced Delayed Neuropathy, elsewhere in this article). OPs and carbamates affect a number of additional organ systems. The various cardiac effects are shown in **Box 2**.

Ventricular dysrhythmias occur a few days after admission and may be related to direct myocardial damage from interstitial inflammation, myocarditis, or patchy pericarditis, which has been described in post mortem histopathology.[46–49] The prognostic utility of the QTc interval with respect to respiratory failure and mortality has been described in at least 3 studies,[50–52] but this is not a consistent finding.[53,54] QT prolongation and Torsades de pointes is reported with relative frequency.[49,55] Pancreatitis and hyperamylasemia have been reported[56] and has a reported incidence of 12% of OP-poisoned patients in 1 case series.[57] Hyperglycemia and hypokalemia are the most common metabolic abnormalities.[58]

Hypotension can occur in up to 17% of OP-poisoned patients based on 1 case series and may have a variety of etiologies.[59] OP- and carbamate-poisoned patients are invariably volume depleted (emesis, diaphoresis, urination, etc), which indicates a need for fluid resuscitation during atropinization. Additionally, OPs may cause additional hypotension by a generalized decrease in the sympathetic outflow from the medulla ("sympatholysis").[60–62] This has been a particular issue with dimethoate. Hypotension refractory to fluid resuscitation should be managed with direct-acting vasopressors, the choice of agent depending on the physiologic parameters of the

Box 2
Cardiac manifestations of organophosphorus insecticide poisoning
Bradycardia, tachycardia
Ventricular arrhythmias
Torsades de pointes
Ventricular fibrillation
Asystole
ECG changes
ST-segment changes
Peaked T waves
AV block
QT interval prolongation
Histopathologic changes
Lysis of myofibrils
Z-band abnormalities
Abbreviations: AV, atrioventricular; ECG, electrocardiogram.
Adapted from Bradberry SM, Vale J. Organophosphorus and carbamate insecticides. In: Wallece K, Brent J, Burkhart KK, editors. Critical care toxicology: diagnosis and management of the critically poisoned patient. Philadelphia: Elsevier Mosby; 2005. p. 940. Table 91–2; with permission.

individual patient. Other medications or therapies that can be considered for refractory shock include methylene blue or lipid emulsion therapy.[63] Neither of these treatments has been evaluated in the setting of OP or carbamate poisoning and should be considered off-label indications.

MANAGEMENT
Diagnostics

The diagnosis of OP or carbamate poisoning is typically a clinical diagnosis based on history and physical examination. In the United States, an exposure is usually known and reported by the patient, bystanders, coworkers, or emergency medical services. The simultaneous presence of both muscarinic and nicotinic effects should strongly suggest OP exposure and empiric, immediate treatment is warranted. Similarly, any multicasualty incident where multiple victims have seizures, became comatose, or suffer cardiac arrest should raise suspicion for nerve agent release. Nevertheless, the diagnosis can be elusive, especially in the case of mild toxicity or atypical presentations; laboratory evaluation and consultation with a medical toxicologist or poison center may help.

Exposure is typically confirmed in 1 of 2 ways. The first method involves detection of organophosphorus metabolites (para-nitrophenol or dialkyl phosphate) in the urine. The second approach involves the assay of AChE and is most useful when the diagnosis is not evident or when mild or chronic toxicity is present. Cholinesterase activity levels are often not readily available within a practical time window for emergency clinicians.[64–66] However, laboratory testing can provide useful parameters to follow while managing an intoxicated patient and can give insight into the disease course and response to therapy.[22,27,67–69] In general, erythrocyte cholinesterase activity corre- lates best with neuronal AChE activity at the neuromuscular junction and is the preferred test to evaluate oxime effectiveness.[70] Plasma cholinesterase activity can also be useful, but there are a number of mitigating factors and differences with plasma cholinesterase assays that affect their utility.[22,26,27,67–69]

Clinical Management

Removal from the source and patient decontamination is often performed before health care facility arrival and ideally should be performed by health care providers in appropriate personal protective equipment. Although secondary contamination from exposed individuals is likely minimal, level C personal protective equipment used by properly trained, hospital-based health care providers is recommended.[71] See the article by Holland for further information on personal protective equipment and decontamination.

Further decontamination should be addressed only after initial stabilization and injury assessment. Removal of all clothing and equipment may substantially reduce re- sidual exposure directly to the patient and prevent off-gassing of fumes.[72] The patient should then be washed down with soap and water. Alternative methods of decontam- ination include dilute alkaline soap, military reactive skin decontamination lotion tow- elettes, sponges, or lotion. Dry decontamination can be performed with talcum powder, flour, or Fuller's earth ([73]available online at http://www.bt.cdc.gov/agent/ agentlistchem.asp).[74] Any agent used for decontamination is hazardous waste and should be disposed of appropriately.

Most patients who succumb to OP or carbamate exposure die from loss of airway and respiratory drive or from seizures. Threats to airway patency include salivation, emesis and aspiration, bronchorrhea, bronchospasm, pulmonary edema, seizures, CNS depression, muscular weakness, and overt paralysis. In severely poisoned pa- tients, early control of airway and breathing is often required and may need to be per- formed concurrently with decontamination. Rapid atropinization should be initiated even before oxygen administration because oxygenation may be impossible until se- cretions are controlled.[75,76] The need for rapid sequence intubation depends on the clinical situation and response to aggressive and early atropinization. If succinylcho- line is used for rapid sequence intubation, there will be prolonged paralysis because succinylcholine is metabolized by plasma cholinesterases.[77,78] Although not contrain- dicated, the use of succinylcholine for rapid sequence intubation is discouraged and short-acting, nondepolarizing agents are preferred.

Because seizures can be lethal in cholinesterase-inhibiting agent intoxication, aggressive seizure control with benzodiazepines is paramount and may increase sur- vival, prevent CNS injury, and avoid cardiac dysrhythmias.[74] Although any GABAergic agent is likely to be effective, an initial dose of 10 mg of intravenous diazepam is sug- gested given its rapid onset and ease of titration, although any parenteral benzodiaz- epine may be used. If intravenous access is not immediately available, intramuscular lorazepam or midazolam can be substituted. Other often-employed anticonvulsants are unlikely to be effective.[79] Specific therapeutic recommendations are discussed elsewhere in this article.

Gastrointestinal decontamination after OP or carbamate ingestion is of unknown benefit; however, emesis is common and further removal via gastric aspiration or lavage is unlikely to have added benefit. OPs are often dissolved in various hydrocar- bons and attempted mechanical decontamination may lead to pulmonary aspiration and pneumonitis. It may however, be reasonable to attempt gastric aspiration under appropriate conditions if the patient's airway is intact or protected. Further decontamination with activated charcoal may be reasonable to limit agent absorption. However, a large, prospective, randomized, clinical trial for all self-poisonings in rural Asia utilizing therapy with multidose activated charcoal did not find improved outcomes with multidose activated charcoal administration.[80] Furthermore, the use of activated charcoal should be balanced against atropine-induced ileus and subsequent risk of aspiration and charcoal pneumonitis.[81]

PHARMACOLOGY AND TREATMENT OPTIONS

The pharmacologic section is divided into 3 main sections based on their therapeutic mechanisms: Antimuscarinic agents, oxime therapy, and seizure control with benzodiazepines. The options available to most health care facilities include antimuscarinics, oximes, and benzodiazepines.

Antimuscarinics

Atropine
Atropine is a competitive inhibitor of muscarinic receptors both in the CNS and peripheral nervous systems. Atropine has no effect at nicotinic receptors and cannot ameliorate symptoms caused by nicotinic stimulation. It is readily available in most hospitals and easily titrated, given its quick onset of action. Atropine is indicated to reverse any clinical evidence of muscarinic toxicity, especially respiratory embarrassment from bronchorrhea, bronchospasm, and pulmonary edema. Atropine has the added advantage of helping to control seizures as well as cardiac toxicity.[82–84]

Rapid administration of atropine in rapidly escalating doses is recommended. Patient should receive 1 to 2 mg of atropine initially, and the dose should be doubled every 5 minutes until pulmonary secretions are dried and the patient has an adequate heart rate and blood pressure.[76] Once control is achieved with bolus dosing, an atropine infusion should be initiated at 10% to 20% of the total dose required to stabilize the patient per hour.[85] Very large doses may be required and the clinician may quickly exhaust the hospital's supply of atropine. Early discussion with pharmacy regarding the mobilization of hospital and regional stores is suggested. See the article by elsewhere in this issue on resources for information on mobilizing Chempacks.

Glycopyrrolate
Because atropine is able to cross the blood–brain barrier, CNS anticholinergic toxicity may occur before adequate control of peripheral cholinergic symptoms. Atropine treatment can be replaced with glycopyrrolate, a peripheral antimuscarinic agent without CNS muscarinic receptor activity. Despite limited evidence, glycopyrrolate is not inferior to atropine, and should be considered an appropriate alternative to atropine if atropine supply is limited.[86] Finally, if bronchorrhea and bronchoconstriction are the primary forms of toxicity, ipratropium can be administered by inhalation with direct effects on the target end organ.[87,88] Indications for antimuscarinic pharmacologic therapy are provided in **Table 4**.

Oxime Therapy

Early initiation of oxime therapy prevents OP aging by reactivating enzymes and improving outcomes. The main goal of oxime therapy is reversal of nicotinic effects and muscular weakness/paralysis. In vitro experiments demonstrate effective reactivation of OP-poisoned AChE.

Table 4
Recommended symptom based treatment for cholinergic poisoning

Sign/Symptom	Agent
Salivation, lacrimation, nausea, vomiting, diarrhea	Atropine, glycopyrrolate
Bronchorrhea, bronchospasm	Atropine, ipratropium, glycopyrrolate
Hypotension	Fluids, atropine, vasopressors, inotropes
Bradycardia	Atropine, glycopyrrolate
Eye pain	Ophthalmic preparations that are mydriatics and cycloplegics
Muscle weakness	Oxime therapy
Respiratory failure	Intubation and ventilation, oxime therapy (muscle weakness)
Seizures	Benzodiazepines (diazepam, midazolam, lorazepam)

Unfortunately, robust demonstration of clinical efficacy remains elusive.[89,90] The most recent Cochrane review evaluated the existing randomized, controlled trials and concluded that the "current evidence was insufficient to indicate whether oximes are harmful or beneficial"; however, study heterogeneity limited the ability to group results.[89] Lower quality evidence suggests efficacy[91–95] and oxime therapy continues to be recommended by many authorities until better evidence emerges that demonstrates a lack of benefit or harm. A recent, retrospective analysis from India found that mortality, in combination with poisoning severity and duration of ventilation, was dependent on delay in oxime administration.[96]

The most commonly utilized oximes include pralidoxime (2-PAM, Protopam), obidoxime (Toxigonin), P2S, and TMB-4. The various oximes are dosed differently and optimal dosing regiments are debated. The suggested US textbook dosing of pralidoxime (1–2 g IV, then 1 g every 6–12 hours or 500 mg/h) may be inadequate.[92,97–99] The World Health Organization recommends a higher dosing regiment (30 mg/kg bolus, then 8 mg/kg/h or 30 mg/kg every 4 hours). The recommended obidoxime dosing regimen is 4 mg/kg, then 0.5 mg/kg/h or 2 mg/kg every 4 hours.[74] In all situations, the dosing should be individualized, depending on patient response.

Administration of oximes to carbamate-poisoned patient is likewise controversial. However, the preponderance of the data suggests that oxime therapy in the setting of carbamate toxicity improves morbidity and mortality[28,67,100]; empiric oxime therapy should be employed in any patient presenting with cholinergic symptoms.[20]

Adverse reactions reported with oxime administration include hypertension, vomiting, and short-lived augmentation of neuromuscular block and may be dosing rate related.[91,101,102]

Benzodiazepines

In animal models, duration of seizure activity has been correlated with the extent of neuronal damage. Benzodiazepines should be utilized as early as possible to halt seizure activity. There are no head-to-head studies in humans that suggest 1 agent is superior to another. Once an intravenous line is established, a benzodiazepine can be easily titrated. A reasonable initial dose of diazepam is 5 to 10 mg IV repeated every 5 minutes until seizure control is obtained. If an IV is not established, diazepam has erratic intramuscular bioavailability and alternative agents such as midazolam or lorazepam should be considered. Intranasal and buccal formulations of midazolam are viable alternatives if no intravenous access is available. Midazolam has a relatively short elimination half-life when compared with other benzodiazepines owing to its relatively high water solubility and may require redosing.

NONPHARMACOLOGIC TREATMENT OPTIONS

Good supportive care is the cornerstone of management of any poisoned patient. Patients poisoned with OPs and carbamates often develop respiratory failure and require intubation and ventilation. Respiratory failure suggests a poor prognosis.[103] The usual care of a ventilated patient should be maintained such as elevation of the head of the bed deep venous thrombosis prophylaxis, and lung-protective ventilatory settings. There is no strong evidence to suggest that hemodialysis or hemoperfusion improve outcomes in the setting of OP and carbamate toxicity.[104]

SPECIAL CONSIDERATIONS
The Intermediate Syndrome

Upon resolution of the acute cholinergic phase and before the development of delayed neuropathy, the intermediate syndrome may occur. A few days after poisoning and during resolution of the cholinergic crises, some OP-poisoned patients develop severe weakness leading to respiratory failure with the need for (re-)intubation and mechanical ventilation in otherwise seemingly improved, conscious patients.[44] The amount of weakness is variable[23] and demonstrates a spectrum of findings. The first clinical signs of intermediate syndrome are bulbar muscle insufficiency and a simple bedside test is the inability to lift one's head off of the bed. The intermediate syndrome may persist for several weeks. The pathophysiology of the intermediate syndrome remains unclear, but seems to be multifactorial[74] and care remains supportive.

Organic Phosphorus-Induced Delayed Neuropathy

Delayed peripheral neurologic dysfunction, occurring weeks after an acute poisoning, is well-documented after acute exposures (ie, OPIDN). OPIDN is a separate entity from the intermediate syndrome with a different pathophysiologic process. OPIDN results from phosphorylation and inhibition of neuropathy target esterase, leading to a "dying back" neuronopathy with preservation of the cell body.[105] Exposure to certain OPs, such as triorthocresyl phosphate, can cause OPIDN in the absence of a cholinergic toxidrome. Historically, contaminated food products and beverages have led to a number of epidemics in the United States, Vietnam, and Sri Lanka. Onset of OPIDN is variable, often within weeks and months of exposure. Recovery is similarly variable and may take months or years.[14,106] Interestingly, delayed neuropathy owing to the carbamates carbaryl, carbofuran, and m-tolyl methyl carbamate has also been described.[107–110]

SUMMARY

The outcomes of victims of carbamate and OP poisoning are multifactorial. In general, outcome depends on the severity of poisoning (amount, duration, and agent), certain individual factors including one's intrinsic ability to metabolize certain OPs, preexisting disease, time to receipt of medical therapy, access to specialists, and hospital capabilities. Despite good supportive and antidotal care, mortality remains high, especially in the case of OP poisoning. Therapy includes supportive care and aggressive and early administration of antimuscarinic agents and oximes. Patients poisoned by OPs should be observed closely after the resolution of acute cholinergic toxicity for development of the intermediate syndrome and OPIDN. In general, although acute carbamate toxicity should resolve within 24 to 48 hours, clinicians should be aware of the potential for these patients to develop delayed neuropathy as well.

REFERENCES

1. Eddleston M, Clark R. Insecticides: organophosphorus compounds and carbamates. In: Nelson LS, editor. Goldfrank's toxicologic emergencies. New York: McGraw Hill Medical; 2011. p. 1450–66.
2. Gunnell D, Eddleston M, Phillips MR, et al. The global distribution of fatal pesticide self-poisoning: systematic review. BMC Public Health 2007;7:357.
3. Gunnell D, Eddleston M. Suicide by intentional ingestion of pesticides: a continuing tragedy in developing countries. Int J Epidemiol 2003;32(6):902–9.
4. Eddleston M. Patterns and problems of deliberate self-poisoning in the developing world. QJM 2000;93(11):715–31.
5. National Crime Records Bureau. Accidental deaths and suicides in India - 2010. Available at: http://ncrb.nic.in/ADSI2010/home.htm. Accessed June 4, 2014.
6. Mowry JB, Spyker DA, Cantilena LR Jr, et al. 2012 Annual Report of the American Association of Poison Control Centers' National Poison Data System (NPDS): 30th Annual Report. Clin Toxicol (Phila) 2013;51(10):949–1229.
7. Maddy KT, Edmiston S, Richmond D. Illness, injuries, and deaths from pesticide exposures in California 1949–1988. Rev Environ Contam Toxicol 1990;114: 57–123.
8. Wesseling C, McConnell R, Partanen T, et al. Agricultural pesticide use in developing countries: health effects and research needs. Int J Health Serv 1997; 27(2):273–308.
9. Roberts DM, Aaron CK. Management of acute organophosphorus pesticide poisoning. BMJ 2007;334(7594):629–34.
10. Government Assessment of the Syrian Government's Use of Chemical Weapons on August 21, 2013. 2013. Available at: http://www.whitehouse.gov/the-press-office/2013/08/30/government-assessment-syrian-government-s-use-chemical-weapons-august-21. Accessed June 5, 2014.
11. Okumura T, Takasu N, Ishimatsu S, et al. Report on 640 victims of the Tokyo subway sarin attack. Ann Emerg Med 1996;28(2):129–35.
12. Mirzayanov VS. State secrets: an insider's chronicle of the Russian Chemical Weapons Program. Denver (CO): Outskirts Press, Inc; 2009. p. 142–5, 179–80.
13. Organisation for the Prohibition of Chemical Weapons. Demilitarisation. Available at: http://www.opcw.org/our-work/demilitarisation/. Accessed June 5, 2014.
14. Morgan JP, Penovich P. Jamaica ginger paralysis. Forty-seven-year follow-up. Arch Neurol 1978;35(8):530–2.
15. Morgan JP, Tulloss TC. The jake walk blues. A toxicologic tragedy mirrored in American popular music. Ann Intern Med 1976;85(6):804–8.
16. Senanayake N, Jeyaratnam J. Toxic polyneuropathy due to gingili oil contaminated with tri-cresyl phosphate affecting adolescent girls in Sri Lanka. Lancet 1981;1(8211):88–9.
17. Dennis DT. Jake walk in Vietnam. Ann Intern Med 1977;86(5):665–6.
18. Proudfoot A. The early toxicology of physostigmine: a tale of beans, great men and egos. Toxicol Rev 2006;25(2):99–138.
19. Broughton E. The Bhopal disaster and its aftermath: a review. Environ Health 2005;4(1):6.

20. Rosman Y, Makarovsky I, Bentur Y, et al. Carbamate poisoning: treatment recommendations in the setting of a mass casualties event. Am J Emerg Med 2009;27(9):1117–24.
21. Aaron CK. Organophosphates and carbamates. Chapter 76. In: Haddad Shannon MW, Borron SW, Burns MJ, editors. Haddad and Winchester's clinical management of poisoning and drug overdose. Philadelphia: Saunders Elsevier; 2007. p. 1171–84.
22. Eddleston M, Eyer P, Worek F, et al. Differences between organophosphorus insecticides in human self-poisoning: a prospective cohort study. Lancet 2005; 366(9495):1452–9.
23. Eddleston M, Mohamed F, Davies JO, et al. Respiratory failure in acute organophosphorus pesticide self-poisoning. QJM 2006;99(8):513–22.
24. Davies JE, Barquet A, Freed VH, et al. Human pesticide poisonings by a fat-soluble organophosphate insecticide. Arch Environ Health 1975;30(12):608–13.
25. Soummer A, Megarbane B, Boroli F, et al. Severe and prolonged neurologic toxicity following subcutaneous chlorpyrifos self-administration: a case report. Clin Toxicol (Phila) 2011;49(2):124–7.
26. Coye MJ, Barnett PG, Midtling JE, et al. Clinical confirmation of OP poisoning of agricultural workers. Am J Ind Med 1986;10(4):399–409.
27. Coye MJ, Barnett PG, Midtling JE, et al. Clinical confirmation of OP poisoning by serial cholinesterase analyses. Arch Intern Med 1987;147(3):438–42.
28. Lifshitz M, Rotenberg M, Sofer S, et al. Carbamate poisoning and oxime treatment in children a clinical and laboratory study. Pediatrics 1994;93(4):652–5.
29. Eyer P. The role of oximes in the management of organophosphorus pesticide poisoning. Toxicol Rev 2003;22(3):165–90.
30. Taylor P. Anticholinesterase agents. In: Brunton LL, Lazo JS, Parker KL, editors. Goodman and Gilman's the pharmacological basis of therapeutics. New York: McGraw-Hill; 2006. p. 201–16.
31. Katzung BG. Section II: autonomic drugs, introduction to autonomic pharmacology. In: Katzung BG, editor. Basic and clinical pharmacology. New York: Lange Medical Books/McGraw-Hill; 2004. p. 75–93.
32. Bird SB, Gaspari R, Dickson EW. Early death due to severe OP poisoning is a centrally mediated process. Acad Emerg Med 2003;10(4):295–8.
33. Dickson EW. Diazepam inhibits organophosphate-induced central respiratory depression. Acad Emerg Med 2003;10(12):1303–6.
34. Dekundy A, Kaminski RM, Zielinska E, et al. NMDA antagonists exert distinct effects in experimental organophosphate or carbamate poisoning in mice. Toxicol Appl Pharmacol 2007;219(2–3):114–21.
35. Kozhemyakin M, Rajasekaran K, Kapur J. Central cholinesterase inhibition enhances glutamatergic synaptic transmission. J Neurophysiol 2010;103(4):1748–57.
36. Sakamoto T, Sawada Y, Nishide K, et al. Delayed neurotoxicity produced by an organophosphorus compound (Sumithion). A case report. Arch Toxicol 1984; 56(2):136–8.
37. Advanced Hazmat Life support Provider Manual, 3rd edition. Walter FG, editor. Arizona Board of Regents for the University of AZ, Tucson. 2003.
38. Zwiener RJ, Ginsburg CM. Organophosphate and carbamate poisoning in infants and children. Pediatrics 1988;81(1):121–6.
39. Bradberry SM, Vale J. Organophosphorus and carbamate insecticides. In: Wallece K, Brent J, Burkhart KK, et al, editors. Critical care toxicology: diagnosis and management of the critically poisoned patient. Philadelphia: Elsevier Mosby; 2005. p. 937–45.

40. Asari Y, Kamijyo Y, Soma K. Changes in the hemodynamic state of patients with acute lethal organophosphate poisoning. Vet Hum Toxicol 2004;46(1):5–9.
41. Joubert J, Joubert PH, van der Spuy M, et al. Acute organophosphate poisoning presenting with choreo-athetosis. J Toxicol Clin Toxicol 1984;22(2):187–91.
42. Senanayake N, Sanmuganathan PS. Extrapyramidal manifestations complicating organophosphorus insecticide poisoning. Hum Exp Toxicol 1995;14(7): 600–4.
43. Shahar E, Andraws J. Extra-pyramidal parkinsonism complicating organophosphate insecticide poisoning. Eur J Paediatr Neurol 2001;5(6):261–4.
44. Senanayake N, Karalliedde L. Neurotoxic effects of organophosphorus insecticides. An intermediate syndrome. N Engl J Med 1987;316(13):761–3.
45. De Bleecker J, Van Den Neucker K, Willems J. The intermediate syndrome in organophosphate poisoning: presentation of a case and review of the literature. J Toxicol Clin Toxicol 1992;30(3):321–9 [discussion: 331–2].
46. Kiss Z, Fazekas T. Organophosphates and torsade de pointes ventricular tachycardia. J R Soc Med 1983;76(11):984–5.
47. Chacko J, Elangovan A. Late onset, prolonged asystole following organophosphate poisoning: a case report. J Med Toxicol 2010;6(3):311–4.
48. Anand S, Singh S, Nahar Saikia U, et al. Cardiac abnormalities in acute organophosphate poisoning. Clin Toxicol (Phila) 2009;47(3):230–5.
49. Wang MH, Tseng CD, Bair SY. Q-T interval prolongation and pleomorphic ventricular tachyarrhythmia ('Torsade de pointes') in organophosphate poisoning: report of a case. Hum Exp Toxicol 1998;17(10):587–90.
50. Chuang FR, Jang SW, Lin JL, et al. QTc prolongation indicates a poor prognosis in patients with organophosphate poisoning. Am J Emerg Med 1996;14(5):451–3.
51. Hrabetz H, Thiermann H, Felgenhauer N, et al. Organophosphate poisoning in the developed world - a single centre experience from here to the millennium. Chem Biol Interact 2013;206(3):561–8.
52. Shadnia S, Okazi A, Akhlaghi N, et al. Prognostic value of long QT interval in acute and severe organophosphate poisoning. J Med Toxicol 2009;5(4):196–9.
53. Akdur O, Durukan P, Ozkan S, et al. Poisoning severity score, Glasgow coma scale, corrected QT interval in acute organophosphate poisoning. Hum Exp Toxicol 2010;29(5):419–25.
54. Yurumez Y, Yavuz Y, Saglam H, et al. Electrocardiographic findings of acute organophosphate poisoning. J Emerg Med 2009;36(1):39–42.
55. Bar-Meir E, Schein O, Eisenkraft A, et al. Guidelines for treating cardiac manifestations of organophosphates poisoning with special emphasis on long QT and Torsades De Pointes. Crit Rev Toxicol 2007;37(3):279–85.
56. Moore PG, James OF. Acute pancreatitis by acute organophosphate poisoning. Postgrad Med J 1981;57(672):660–2.
57. Sahin I, Onbasi K, Sahin H, et al. The prevalence of pancreatitis in organophosphate poisonings. Hum Exp Toxicol 2002;21(4):175–7.
58. Saadeh AM. Metabolic complications of OP and carbamate poisoning. Trop Doct 2001;31(3):149–52.
59. Saadeh AM, Farsakh NA, al-Ali MK. Cardiac manifestations of acute carbamate and organophosphate poisoning. Heart 1997;77(5):461–4.
60. Chang AY, Chan JY, Kao FJ, et al. Engagement of inducible nitric oxide synthase at the rostral ventrolateral medulla during mevinphos intoxication in the rat. J Biomed Sci 2001;8(6):475–83.
61. Yen DH, Yen JC, Len WB, et al. Spectral changes in systemic arterial pressure signals during acute mevinphos intoxication in the rat. Shock 2001;15(1):35–41.

62. Yeo V, Young K, Tsuen CH. Anticholinesterase-induced hypotension treated with pulmonary artery catheterization-guided vasopressors. Vet Hum Toxicol 2002; 44(2):99–100.
63. Jang DH, Nelson LS, Hoffman RS. Methylene blue for distributive shock: a potential new use of an old antidote. J Med Toxicol 2013;9(3):242–9.
64. Rehiman S, Lohani SP, Bhattarai MC. Correlation of serum cholinesterase level, clinical score at presentation and severity of organophosphate poisoning. JNMA J Nepal Med Assoc 2008;47(170):47–52.
65. Aygun D, Doganay Z, Altintop L, et al. Serum acetylcholinesterase and prognosis of acute organophosphate poisoning. J Toxicol Clin Toxicol 2002;40(7):903–10.
66. Rajapakse BN, Thiermann H, Eyer P, et al. Evaluation of the test-mate ChE (cholinesterase) field kit in acute organophosphorus poisoning. Ann Emerg Med 2011;58(6):559–64.e6.
67. Lifshitz M, Shahak E, Sofer S. Carbamate and organophosphate poisoning in young children. Pediatr Emerg Care 1999;15(2):102–3.
68. Davies JO, Eddleston M, Buckley NA. Predicting outcome in acute organophosphorus poisoning with a poison severity score or the Glasgow coma scale. QJM 2008;101(5):371–9.
69. Yager J, McLean H, Hudes M, et al. Components of variability in blood cholinesterase assay results. J Occup Med 1976;18(4):242–4.
70. Thiermann H, Szinicz L, Eyer P, et al. Correlation between red blood cell acetylcholinesterase activity and neuromuscular transmission in organophosphate poisoning. Chem Biol Interact 2005;157-8:345–7.
71. Macintyre AG, Christopher G, Eitzen E Jr, et al. Weapons of mass destruction events with contaminated casualties: effective planning for health care facilities. JAMA 2000;283(2):242–9.
72. Kales SN, Christiani D. Acute chemical emergencies. N Engl J Med 2004; 350(8):800–8.
73. Sidell FR, Borak J. Chemical warfare agents II nerve agents. Ann Emerg Med 1992;21(7):865–71.
74. Koenig, KL, Boatright CJ, Hancock JA, et al. Health care facility-based decontamination of victims exposed to chemical, biological, and radiological materials. Am J Emerg Med 2008;26(1):71–80.
75. Konickx LA, Bingham K, Eddleston M. Is oxygen required before atropine administration in organophosphorus or carbamate pesticide poisoning? - a cohort study. Clin Toxicol (Phila) 2014;52(5):531–7.
76. Eddleston M, Buckley NA, Checketts H, et al. Speed of initial atropinisation in significant organophosphorus pesticide poisoning—a systematic comparison of recommended regimens. Clin Toxicol 2004;42(6):865–75.
77. Sener EB, Ustun E, Kocamanoglu S, et al. Prolonged succinylcholine-induced paralysis in OP insecticide poisoning. Acta Anaesthesiol Scand 2002;46(8):1046–8.
78. Selden BS, Curry SC. Prolonged succinylcholine-induced paralysis in organophosphate insecticide poisoning. Ann Emerg Med 1987;16(2):215–7.
79. Shih T, McDonough JH Jr, Koplovitz I. Anticonvulsants for soman-induced seizure activity. J Biomed Sci 1999;6(2):86–96.
80. Eddleston M, Juszczak E, Buckley NA, et al. Multiple-dose activated charcoal in acute self-poisoning: a randomised controlled trial. Lancet 2008;371(9612): 579–87.
81. Mizutani T, Naito H, Oohashi N. Rectal ulcer with massive haemorrhage due to activated charcoal treatment in oral organophosphate poisoning. Hum Exp Toxicol 1991;10(5):385–6.

82. Shih TM, Koviak TA, Capacio BR. Anticonvulsants for poisoning by the organo-phosphorus compound soman: pharmacological mechanisms. Neurosci Bio-behav Rev 1991;15(3):349–62.

83. Shih TM, Rowland TC, McDonough JH. Anticonvulsants for nerve agent-induced seizures: the influence of the therapeutic dose of atropine. J Pharmacol Exp Ther 2007;320(1):154–61.

84. McDonough JH Jr, Jaax NK, Crowley RA, et al. Atropine and/or diazepam therapy protects against soman-induced neural and cardiac pathology. Fundam Appl Toxicol 1989;13(2):256–76.

85. Eddleston M, Buckley NA, Eyer P, et al. Management of acute organophosphorus pesticide poisoning. Lancet 2008;371(9612):597–607.

86. Choi PT, Quinonez LG, Cook DJ, et al. The use of glycopyrrolate in a case of intermediate syndrome following acute organophosphate poisoning. Can J Anaesth 1998;45(4):337–40.

87. Perrone J, Henretig F, Sims M, et al. A role for ipratropium in chemical terrorism preparedness. Acad Emerg Med 2003;10(3):290.

88. Shemesh I, Bourvin A, Gold D, et al. Chlorpyrifos poisoning treated with ipratropium and dantrolene: a case report. J Toxicol Clin Toxicol 1988;26(7):495–8.

89. Buckley NA, Eddleston M, Li Y, et al. Oximes for acute organophosphate pesticide poisoning. Cochrane Database Syst Rev 2011;(2):CD005085.

90. Eddleston M, Eyer P, Worek F, et al. Pralidoxime in acute organophosphorus insecticide poisoning–a randomised controlled trial. PLoS Med 2009;6(6):e1000104.

91. Eddleston M, Szinicz L, Eyer P, et al. oximes in acute organophosphorus pesticide poisoning a systematic review of clinical trials. QJM 2002;95(5):275–83.

92. Worek F, Bäcker M, Thiermann H, et al. Reappraisal of indications and limitations of oxime therapy in organophosphate poisoning. Hum Exp Toxicol 1997;16(8):466–72.

93. Kurtz PH. Pralidoxime in the treatment of carbamate intoxication. Am J Emerg Med 1990;8(1):68–70.

94. Petroianu G, Ruefer R. Poisoning with organophosphorus compounds. Emerg Med (Fremantle) 2001;13(2):258–60.

95. Shih TM, Skovira JW, O'Donnell JC, et al. Treatment with tertiary oximes prevents seizures and improves survival following sarin intoxication. J Mol Neurosci 2010;40(1–2):63–9.

96. Ahmed SM, Das B, Nadeem A, et al. Survival pattern in patients with acute organophosphate poisoning on mechanical ventilation: a retrospective intensive care unit-based study in a tertiary care teaching hospital. Indian J Anaesth 2014;58(1):11–7.

97. Thiermann H, Szinicz L, Eyer F, et al. Modern strategies in therapy of OP poisoning. Toxicol Lett 1999;107(1–3):233–9.

98. Schexnayder S, James LP, Kearns GL, et al. The pharmacokinetics of continuous infusion pralidoxime in children with organophosphate poisoning. J Toxicol Clin Toxicol 1998;36(6):549–55.

99. Willems JL, De Bisschop HC, Verstraete AG, et al. Cholinesterase reactivation in organophosphorus poisoned patients depends on the plasma concentrations of the oxime pralidoxime methylsulphate and of the organophosphate. Arch Toxicol 1993;67(2):79–84.

100. Dawson RM, Poretski M. Carbamylated acetylcholinesterase: acceleration of decarbamylation by bispyridinium oximes. Biochem Pharmacol 1985;34(24):4337–40.

101. Medicis JJ, Stork CM, Howland MA, et al. Pharmacokinetics following a loading plus a continuous infusion of pralidoxime compared with the traditional short infusion regimen in human volunteers. J Toxicol Clin Toxicol 1996;34(3): 289–95.
102. Thompson DF, Thompson GD, Greenwood RB, et al. Therapeutic dosing of pralidoxime chloride. Drug Intell Clin Pharm 1987;21(7–8):590–3.
103. Noshad H, Ansarin K, Ardalan MR, et al. Respiratory failure in organophosphate insecticide poisoning. Saudi Med J 2007;28(3):405–7.
104. Altintop L, Aygun D, Sahin H, et al. In acute organophosphate poisoning, the efficacy of hemoperfusion on clinical status and mortality. J Intensive Care Med 2005;20(6):346–50.
105. Richardson RJ, Hein ND, Wijeyesakere SJ, et al. Neuropathy target esterase (NTE): overview and future. Chem Biol Interact 2013;203(1):238–44.
106. Senanayake N. Tri-cresyl phosphate neuropathy in Sri Lanka: a clinical and neurophysiological study with a three year follow up. J Neurol Neurosurg Psychiatry 1981;44(9):775–80.
107. Lotti M, Moretto A. Do carbamates cause polyneuropathy? Muscle Nerve 2006; 34(4):499–502.
108. Yang PY, Tsao TC, Lin JL, et al. Carbofuran-induced delayed neuropathy. J Toxicol Clin Toxicol 2000;38(1):43–6.
109. Umehara F, Izumo S, Arimura K, et al. Polyneuropathy induced by m-tolyl methyl carbamate intoxication. J Neurol 1991;238(1):47–8.
110. Dickoff DJ, Gerber O, Turovsky Z. Delayed neurotoxicity after ingestion of carbamate pesticide. Neurology 1987;37(7):1229–31.

Intentional and Inadvertent Chemical Contamination of Food, Water, and Medication

Charles McKay, MD[a],*, Elizabeth J. Scharman, PharmD, DABAT, BCPS[b]

KEYWORDS

- Chemical terrorism • Food contamination • Water contamination
- Medication contamination • Risk communication • Supply chain

KEY POINTS

- Food, water, and medication production, processing, and distribution involve multiple potential points of entry for chemical contamination.
- Developing a clinical case definition based on toxidrome recognition is the most important epidemiologic step early in a chemical contamination event.
- Laboratory investigation and identification of a chemical compound as the cause can be time and labor intensive, expensive, and frustrating, with attendant problems of confounding or associated noncausal substances.
- The number and location of affected individuals can facilitate identification of the likely point of entry of a chemical contaminant through the use of bow-tie modeling.
- Risk communication is an important aspect of the response to potential chemical contamination of food, water, or medication.
- The resources of a regional poison control center or medical toxicologist can be used as an entry to the public health system and considerations regarding tracking potential contamination of food, water, or medication.
- Following large-scale contamination events, the public health impact associated with an outbreak of mass epidemic illness must also be addressed, especially in the absence of an available biological marker to differentiate stress response from toxic injury.

Disclosures: None.
[a] Division of Medical Toxicology, Department of Emergency Medicine, CT Poison Control Center, American College of Medical Toxicology, Hartford Hospital, University of Connecticut School of Medicine, 263 Farmington Avenue, Farmington, CT 06030, USA; [b] Department Clinical Pharmacy, WVU School of Pharmacy, WV Poison Center, 3110 Maccorkle Ave SE, Charleston, WV 25304, USA
* Corresponding author.
E-mail address: cmckay@toxphysician.com

Emerg Med Clin N Am 33 (2015) 153–177
http://dx.doi.org/10.1016/j.emc.2014.09.011
emed.theclinics.com

INTRODUCTION

The delivery of toxins or contaminants via food supply, water, or medications has a long history, particularly as a means of altering political futures. In 585 BC, the city of Kirra in modern-day Greece was besieged by attacking clans in the First Sacred War. The attackers discovered a buried pipe bringing fresh water to Kirra and reportedly poisoned it with hellebore, weakening the city occupants by inducing vomiting and diarrhea.[1] Recordings of other targeted terroristic poisonings at feasts or other gatherings date back several millennia.[2,3] Technological, legislative, and regulatory efforts to forestall terrorist goals of targeted or widespread poisoning by contamination of food, water, or medication supplies continue. This article uses examples of contamination of these critical supply chains to highlight the production and distribution components that provide common points of vulnerability for attack, and the resources and measures to counter such attempts.

Production and Distribution Systems as a Framework

Most modern societies have developed highly specialized production and distribution methods to deliver large quantities of goods such as medications to populations that are both congregated in large cities and more widely dispersed, while maintaining standards of uniform composition and potency. The same is true for food and water. Separation of the many steps and multiple components required to produce, package, and widely distribute these critical entities affords numerous opportunities for inadvertent or intentional contamination; this complexity can also create barriers and delays in identification of, and notification about, contamination. Production and distribution systems can be depicted as a bow-tie model, as shown in **Fig. 1**. Many raw materials or tributaries combine to make a processed or finished product, which is then collected, stored, and distributed via a series of outlets until eventually reaching a large number of consumers. This simple unidirectional flow example of network theory has been used to model the impact of introduction of a small amount of the potent botulinum toxin into the milk supply.[4]

Using Bow-tie Analysis to Identify the Point of Introduction of Chemical Contaminant

From an epidemiologic point of view, the in-flow/out-flow concept is critically important in determining the need and location for investigations, recalls, testing, and communications. These same issues need to be addressed in individual patient encounters. For

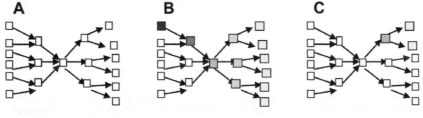

A   **B**   **C**

Raw   Finished Distrib- Consumers   Raw   Finished Distrib- Consumers   Raw   Finished Distrib- Consumers
Material Product utors   Material Product utors   Material Product utors

Fig. 1. (*A*) Bow-tie production and distribution. (*B*) Insertion of a large amount of a compound early in the production can have a widespread but diluted effect for many consumers. (*C*) Insertion of a smaller amount of a compound late in the distribution process requires less substance for effect, but affects fewer individuals. (*From* Centers for Disease Control. CDC estimates of foodborne illness in the United States: overview of attribution of foodborne illness. Available at: www.cdc.gov/foodborneburden/attribution/overview.html.)

example, symptoms of palpitations or light-headedness that are associated by the individual with eating at a restaurant may be coincidental, attributable to underlying medical illness, environmental heat, or emotional stress. However, they could also represent early symptoms of food toxicity or foodborne illness from a variety of preformed biological toxins or chemical contaminants, such as the sodium azide poisoning of iced tea drinkers at a Texas restaurant in 2010.[5] When several people rapidly became ill while still at the restaurant, it might reasonably be assumed that there was a shared exposure, but was it in the air, the food, or the water? Because not everyone in the restaurant at one time was affected, a shared airborne exposure (eg, carbon monoxide) was unlikely. In the same way, not all victims were present at exactly the same time, making the problem of line-of-sight transmission of psychogenic reactions unlikely. Investigation in this event quickly focused on the common iced tea urn, with analysis for cardiovascular toxins eventually identifying hydrazoic acid as a reaction product of sodium azide and water. However, although the clinical syndrome of rapid onset of hypotensive symptoms was quickly identified and appropriate supportive care initiated, the analysis and identification of the causative chemical agent took months. Interviews of other restaurant patrons and evaluation of contemporaneous emergency department visits identified only 1 additional victim, confirming the far right side (distribution) of the bow-tie model intrusion of a contaminant. Epidemiologic response tools, such as the Electronic Surveillance System for the Early Notification of Community-based Epidemics (ESSENSE),[6] which tracks emergency department visits or poison center calls, were also used to screen for other cases.

Early access to clinical partners such as regional poison control centers or medical toxicologists can assist in developing a clinical picture based on toxidrome recognition, determining which, if any, laboratory tests should be obtained and where to obtain this testing, and contacting public health entities for further investigation or intervention. The nature and extent of any needed public communication and involvement of law enforcement can also be better ascertained when properly applying the bow-tie tool.

TYPES OF FOODBORNE ILLNESS

The term foodborne illness is used to describe illness resulting from the consumption of food products. This term is preferred to the term food poisoning because it encompasses a broader range of food source contaminants and is technically more appropriate. Foodborne illness needs to be distinguished from coincidental onset of symptoms while a person is eating, or noncausal food-associated illness.

Foodborne illness may be the result of bacterial, viral, or parasitic contamination, or noninfectious toxins such as ciguatera. Illness can also be the result of toxins produced by bacterial contamination (eg, botulism). Although foodborne illness from infectious contamination is usually the result of improper food preparation or handling practices, bacterial contamination has also been the means of terrorist acts.[7] Foodborne illness may also be the result of foreign body contamination, insect infestation, or the introduction of nonfood substances. Foreign body contamination or other non–foreign body contaminants (eg, chemicals) can be introduced inadvertently or deliberately, based on a desire to substitute a less expensive compound, circumvent a regulatory restriction or standard, or to cause harm. State public health laboratories have increased capabilities and capacities to address these issues through the Food Emergency Response Network (FERN).[8]

FOOD CONTAMINATION

The US Centers for Disease Control and Prevention (CDC) tracks a variety of foodborne illnesses. More than 1 in every 6 Americans becomes ill from some food they eat every year. Because these under-report the scope of the problem, some investigators have explored using social media as a more robust means of monitoring foodborne illness outbreaks, at least those associated with dining out.[9] **Fig. 2** shows the broad categories of food commodities tracked by the CDC and the relative attribution of reported diseases. Although most people recover, 1 in 300 people with symptoms are treated in a hospital and more than 3000 people die.[10] Most of these cases reflect identified microorganism contamination; much of this biocontamination occurs during food handling or prepreparation of complex food items (containing multiple food items/commodity categories). In some instances, the food may have originated from outside the country, and therefore may not have been subjected to the preparation practices guiding food production in the United States.

Contaminant Identification

Of nearly 200 chemical contamination events involving US food in the last 30 years, as reported by one consumer advocacy group, with each event affecting 2 to 133 people, more than one-half were characterized as "suspected or unknown chemical,"

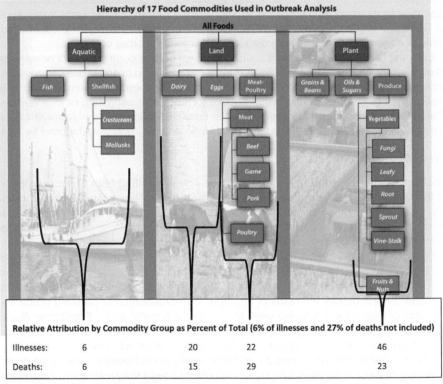

Fig. 2. Food categories and attribution of foodborne disease outbreaks in the United States. Commodity groups appear in orange cells; 17 commodities are italicized and appear in green cells. (*From* Centers for Disease Control. CDC estimates of foodborne illness in the United States: overview of attribution of foodborne illness. Available at: www.cdc.gov/foodborneburden/attribution/overview.html; and *From* Painter JA, Ayers T, Woodruff R, et al. Recipes for foodborne outbreaks: a scheme for categorizing and grouping implicated foods. Foodborne Pathog Dis 2009;6:1259–64, with permission.)

highlighting the analytical challenges noted earlier.[11] Although regulations focus on ensuring food safety and quality based on accidental contamination by biological organisms, these same principles apply to intentional chemical contamination. Chemical regulatory focus by the Center for Food Safety and Applied Nutrition (CFSAN) has been on pesticide residues, heavy metals, and natural toxins such as mycotoxins, although several other biopersistent chemicals are also monitored.[12] The US Food and Drug Administration (FDA) and the Department of Agriculture (USDA) have primary responsibility for regulating food quality and safety, although the number of agencies with some involvement is much larger. The USDA is responsible through the Food Safety Inspection Service (FSIS) for meat, poultry, and egg safety, whereas the FDA is responsible for all other food products. Recognizing the need for improved oversight and coordination, Congress passed the Food Safety Modernization Act in 2010 and FDA published its draft approach to designating high-risk foods in 2014.[13] Analytical capabilities have increased within many state departments of health and other cooperative laboratories following the 2001 terrorist attacks. This Laboratory Response Network (LRN)[14] may be able to assist when questions of chemical contamination arise.

Impact of Site of Contamination

As depicted in **Table 1**, chemical contamination or threat thereof on the food production/processing side of the bow tie have much greater impact than when they occur on the distribution side. Production of large batches with uniform mixing increases the extent of spread of an introduced contaminant. Multiple points of access exist from farm to storage to shipment to processing and manufacture, as well as throughout the distribution network. From a chemical terrorism point of view, products with short shelf lives are preferred vehicles, because they are less likely to be stored away unused and be available for removal or recall once a source of symptoms is recognized. The psychological impact of a contamination event can spread greatly beyond the physically affected individuals. As noted earlier, many complex food products are composed of raw materials from other countries. The extent of this outsourcing was highlighted in 2008 by the melamine scare (and the previous 2007 melamine-attributable animal deaths from contaminated pet food). Melamine is an industrial compound widely used to form plastics; another related and potentially contaminating compound (cyanuric acid) is used to stabilize pool water disinfectants (**Fig. 3**). Melamine is 66% nitrogen by weight; this characteristic was used by unscrupulous farmers and dairy companies in China to falsely increase the apparent protein content of milk and milk powder when measured by total nitrogen content.[15] During late 2008, as many as 300,000 Chinese children (most less than 3 years old) were evaluated for exposure and resulting crystalluria/hematuria. Thousands were hospitalized with acute kidney injury; at least 6 died.[16] Although there were no significant illnesses in the United States, the identification of melamine in several products with dairy ingredients sourced from China caused widespread public concern. The US problem was more of a risk communication issue, in that mere identification of melamine did not indicate risk.[17,18]

WATER CONTAMINATION

Safe and plentiful water, available at the turn of a handle, has been the assumed status quo for almost all Americans for decades. More than 84% of the US population is served by public water systems, defined by the Environmental Protection Agency

Table 1
Examples of chemical contamination of the food supply

Bow-Tie Site of Introduction	Chemical Exposure (Intentional or Inadvertent)	Site/Date	Number of People Affected	Health Effects	Acute vs Chronic Health Effects
Raw material: harvested fruit in Chili	Cyanide-tainted fruit[19] (intentional)	US imports/1989	All US Chilean fruit imports for 3 wk; $300,000,000 loss to Chile	None; hoax with telephone alert; 3 μg of cyanide identified in 2 punctured grapes	Acute (economic)
Production: substitution of 225–450 kg (500–1000 pounds) of PBB flame retardant for magnesium oxide cattle feed	PBB[20,21] (inadvertent)	Michigan/1973 (secondary contamination via cattle excrement in pastures recreated event in 1977)	Potentially 9 million Michigan residents; quarantine >500 farms; ~ 30,000 cattle, 4500 swine, 1500 sheep, and 1.5 million chickens and food products destroyed	Emotional impact of biopersistent contamination; constitutional and depressive symptoms; abnormal immunologic studies of uncertain significance	Chronic
Production: inappropriate use of carbamate insecticide on melons	Aldicarb-contaminated watermelons (inadvertent)	California and 10 other states, provinces/1985	1350 cases (California) with 483 cases elsewhere; 17 hospitalized; clusters of 1–13 people affected	Cholinergic symptoms including seizures, coma, hypotension	Acute
Processing: addition of nonbioavailable high-nitrogen-content chemical to milk and/or animal feed	Melamine-adulterated milk/powdered milk[16,22] (inadvertent)	Multiple provinces, China/2008 (repeat events continue)	~ 300,000 infants and children with urinary stones of 22,384,000 examined; >50,000 hospitalized; 6 known deaths (impact on United States considered minimal)	Crystalluria with hematuria and obstruction; renal tubular injury	Subacute to chronic

Processing: refined aniline denaturant in rapeseed oil (illicit use as cooking oil)	TOS[23] (inadvertent)	Madrid, Spain/1981	19,904 people; ~400 of 1224 deaths attributed to TOS	Systemic nonnecrotizing vasculitis usually presenting as noncardiogenic pulmonary edema, eosinophilia, myalgia, and rash	Acute and chronic
Processing: undercooked chili sauce at plant in Georgia	Botulinum-contaminated chili sauce[24] (inadvertent)	Three US states (Indiana, Texas, Ohio)/2007	At least 8 people in 3 states	Bulbar dysfunction with motor paralysis	Acute to subacute
Distribution: nicotine insecticide added to 115 kg (250 pounds) of ground beef in single store	Nicotine-contaminated ground beef[25] (intentional)	Detroit, MI/2003	At least 92 people	Nausea and vomiting, other cholinergic symptoms	Acute
Distribution: preserved bamboo shoots served at local festival	Botulism-contaminated bamboo shoots[26] (inadvertent)	Thailand/2006	209 people; 42 with respiratory failure requiring mechanical ventilation for as long as 1 mo	Bulbar dysfunction with motor paralysis and autonomic instability	Acute
Local distribution: arsenic placed in church coffee pot by member	Arsenate-contaminated water[27] (intentional)	New Sweden, ME/2003	15 people sickened; 1 death	Vomiting/diarrhea; hemodynamic shock; persistent neuropathy	Acute and chronic
Consumer: single container	Cyanide-contaminated yogurt[28] (intentional)	New Jersey/1989	One death	Rapid collapse	Acute

Note that the number of people affected generally decreases as the site of contaminant introduction moves from the production to the distribution side.

Abbreviations: PBB, polybrominated biphenyls; TOS, toxic oil syndrome.

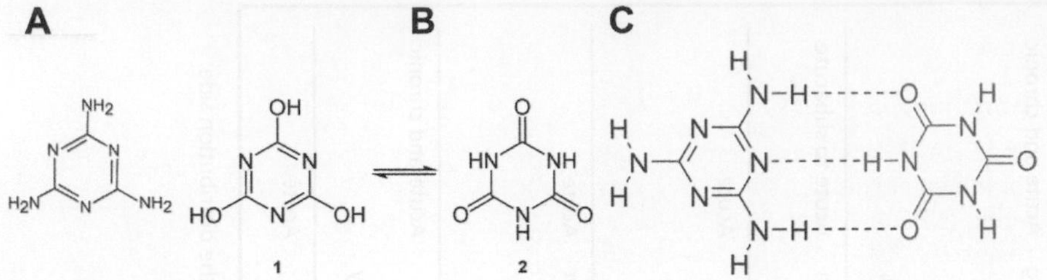

A   **B**   **C**

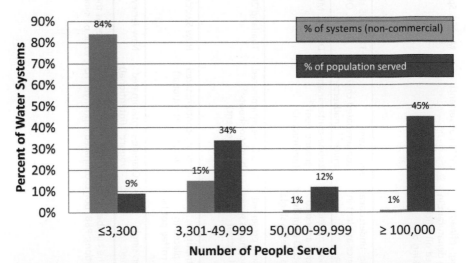

Fig. 3. Chemical structures of (*A*) melamine, (*B*) cyanuric acid, and (*C*) melamine–cyanuric acid complex.

(EPA) as those systems that regularly (60 or more days per year) supply drinking water to at least 25 persons or 15 separate connections. Two-thirds of the approximately 160,000 public drinking water systems use surface water (rivers, lakes, and reservoirs), whereas one-third have a groundwater source (wells and aquifers). For those relying on private water systems, most water comes from small wells.[29] Using the bow-tie model, rain, runoff, and groundwater flow can be considered the raw materials, potentially picking up chemical solutes as the water is collected together at 1 point. The distribution network for water is both extensive and vulnerable. Although most public water systems serve fewer than 3300 people each, some large systems service more than 100,000 people (**Fig. 4**). Most of the millions of miles of distribution system pipes have been in place for more than 30 to 100 years and are vulnerable to leaking and accidental contamination. The EPA has estimated that there is an average of 1 line break per year for every 1000-person system, leading to a high likelihood of cross-connections in water flow.[30] The greatest vulnerability for intentional introduction of a chemical contaminant to the water system is

Fig. 4. Comparison of community water systems: number of systems versus number of people served by those systems. (*Data from* Kongsaengdao S, Samintarapanya K, Rusmeechan S, et al. An outbreak of botulism in Thailand: clinical manifestations and management of severe respiratory failure. Clin Infect Dis 2006;43(10):1247–56.)

by creating backflow and overcoming the low pressure at the end of a water distribution network.

Contamination Identification

The EPA, in most cases via state environmental agencies, has regulatory responsibility for the safety of public drinking water systems. National Primary Drinking Water Regulation (NPDWR) standards, first codified in the Safe Drinking Water Act in 1974 (last revised in 1996) include maximum contaminant levels for more than 80 elements and chemical compounds, as well as several micro-organisms.[31] Municipal and private water companies are required to test and report on the status of their water product relative to these standards. However, the EPA does not regulate the testing methodology; most systems use intermittent rather than continuous monitoring for chemical contaminants. In addition, testing requirements are limited to those identified contaminants listed in the Safe Drinking Water Act. This potential vulnerability is being addressed as a portion of the critical infrastructure assessment pursuant to Executive Order 13636; several routine and innovative techniques are being considered.[32,33] Note that systems that do not qualify as public water systems are not under EPA regulations, and homeowners are usually responsible for their own testing. In areas of the country with significant groundwater contribution from mountain ranges, arsenic and radon contamination of private water sources is a matter of concern. Several regions and states provide information for homeowners.[34]

Millions of people in the United States drink bottled water, many as their sole source of drinking water. As opposed to tap water, bottled water is considered a food product and is regulated by the FDA under the Food, Drug, and Cosmetic Act; Title 21 of the Code of Federal Regulations part 129 covers the regulations relating to the Processing and Bottling of Bottled Drinking Water. The plastic containers are regulated as a food contact substance; they are governed by food additive regulations. Contaminant standards set by NPDWR may apply to bottled water or the standard may be different if the contaminant is not found in water used for bottled water (eg, allowed lead levels are lower in bottled water because there is no likely contribution by lead in public water system pipes). Recalls of bottled water products are common and testing of bottled water for some contaminants, like coliform bacteria, differs from that for public water systems.[35]

The CDC tracks reported water-borne illness outbreaks. In 2009 to 2010, there were 33 outbreaks affecting 1040 people reported. Almost all of the serious cases and all of the deaths were attributable to legionella infection. Contamination is not only from biological sources. One chemical exposure affecting 3 people was attributed to sodium hydroxide–contaminated water.[36] Over an 18-year period, 459 events with more than 12,000 associated illnesses have been reported. Fifteen of these outbreaks (679 associated illnesses) were caused by chemical contaminants.[30] Many water-associated events are not reported and ascertaining the cause is often difficult. As listed in **Table 2**, obvious odor or visible changes to water can be quickly recognized, but analytical analysis for compounds other than the chemical compound H_2O can be complicated by natural minerals and introduced disinfectants, as well as the increasing sophistication of laboratory equipment, resulting in the problem of the so-called receding zero: it has become technologically possible to detect extremely small concentrations of chemicals (parts per trillion), whereas the corresponding knowledge on the public health implications of these (very) low-level exposures, if there are any, is lacking.[37] It further complicates investigations that the mere identification of a compound does not indicate that it is responsible for observed symptoms and signs.

Table 2
Examples of chemical contamination of the water supply

Bow-Tie Site of Introduction	Chemical Exposure	Site/Date	Number of People Affected	Health Effects	Acute vs Chronic Health Effects
Raw material: Yippie political theater threat to introduce LSD into drinking water supply at 1968 Democratic National Convention	LSD[43] (and other intentional threats[44])	Lake Michigan, Chicago, IL/1968	None directly; large security presence at convention with riots	None; threat only	None
Raw material: Elk River contamination from above-ground storage tank	4-Methylcyclohexane methanol[45] (inadvertent)	Charleston, WV/2014	300,000 no-use water warning	Odor, skin rashes, nonspecific complaints	Acute
Raw material: 4.1 million cubic meters of wet ash released into Tennessee River tributaries	Coal ash[46] (inadvertent)	Harriman, TN/2008 (and other sites: North Carolina[47])	22 residents evacuated; 165 properties sold to TVA	None; concern about heavy metal contamination and particulate-related respiratory irritation	—
Production: waste off site: dry cleaning plant. On site: industrial spills, leaking underground storage tanks, waste disposal sites	Trichloroethylene, perchloroethylene, vinyl chloride, benzene, multiple other chemicals (VOCs)[48] (inadvertent)	Camp Lejeune Marine Corps Base, North Carolina/1953–1987 (investigation started in 2009)	Up to 750,000 (service members and families) exposed to contaminated tap water	Concerns for higher cancer rates, birth defects (neural tube defects), amyotrophic lateral sclerosis	Chronic with delayed identification of contamination

Description	Contaminant	Location/Date	Number affected	Clinical effects	Severity
Processing: security fence cut at 12 million gallon reservoir	Unknown[49] (intentional)	Seattle, OR/2002	None; cost of emptying reservoir; increased water security	None identified	NA
Distribution: 60 gallons of foam accidentally pumped into hydrant	Fire retardant foam[50] (inadvertent)	Charlotte, NC/1997	40,000 households; no water use for 1.5 d	None	NA
Distribution: (cross-connection): water for soup contaminated by boiler additive	Nitrites[51] (inadvertent)	New Jersey/1992	49 children; 14 with MetHb >20%	Cyanosis, nausea, abdominal pain, vomiting, dizziness	Acute
Distribution: possible plot to introduce 4 kg (9 pounds) of a cyanide compound into US embassy water supply	Potassium ferrocyanide[52] (intentional)	Rome, Italy/2002	None	None; plot disrupted	NA

Note that the number of people affected generally decreases as the site of contaminant introduction moves from the production to the distribution side.
Abbreviations: LSD, lysergic acid diethylamide; MetHb, methemoglobinemia; NA, not applicable; TVA, Tennessee valley authority; VOC, volatile organic compounds; Yippie, Youth International Party.

Impact of Site of Contamination

From a terrorist viewpoint, characteristics of the ideal water contaminant include an agent that causes illness and is:

- Odorless and tasteless
- Colorless
- Resistant to water treatment procedures
- Water stable (not subject to hydrolysis)
- Water soluble
- Low LD_{50} (median lethal dose; ie, high toxicity)

Several compounds have been assessed and ranked for relative water toxicity, using the ratio of solubility in water to lethal dose.[38] As with the milk vehicle model mentioned earlier, botulinum toxin leads the list of theoretic water toxins. Many other chemical compounds that are of significant acute toxicity would be diluted beyond effect if introduced into a large water supply, or potentially removed or inactivated by water treatment procedures. Most water systems (particularly those that use surface water, which is most of them) process water by flocculation and sedimentation to remove large particulates, then filtration through sand, gravel, or charcoal (removing micrometer-sized particles), then disinfection (using a halide such as chlorine) as depicted in **Fig. 5**. Only after this is the water distributed to end users, usually with free residual chlorine content of considerably more than 0.2 mg/L.[39]

The January 2014 Elk River chemical spill just upstream from Charleston, West Virginia, provides an example of the impact of water contamination on a large scale.

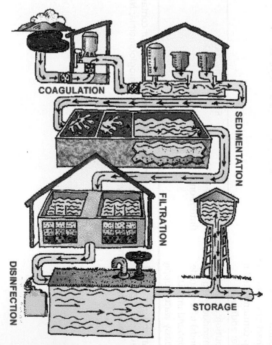

Fig. 5. Community water treatment steps. (*From* United States Environmental Protection Agency. Water treatment process. Available at: http://water.epa.gov/learn/kids/drinkingwater/watertreatmentplant_index.cfm.)

An above-ground storage tank containing approximately 37,855 L (10,000 gallons) of a coal flotation product containing a mixture of 88.5% 4-methylcyclohexane methanol (MCHM), 7.3% propylene glycol phenyl ether (PPH), and water leaked into the Elk River at a point 2.5 km (2.4 km) above the sole intake valve for a public water system serving 300,000 people in 9 counties. A do-not-use order was announced the evening of the spill; water was to be used for firefighting and toilet flushing only. The water was cleared for use in zones beginning 4 days later, with all sections cleared 8 days after the spill. During the 2 weeks after the spill, hospitals recorded 369 water contamination–related hospital visits, the WV Poison Center recorded 2000 human exposures, and (according to the CDC Community Assessment for Public Health Emergency Response survey), 21.7% of households reported someone having symptoms they thought were related to water contamination.[40,41] No hospital admissions were determined to be related to water contamination. Although the environmental health screening value was set by the CDC at 1 ppm for MCHM and 1.2 ppm for PPH (below which water was cleared for use), it was determined after the water crisis ended that the odor threshold was even lower. The noxious licorice smell of MCHM was detectible down to 0.022 ppm (22 parts per billion). The lingering water odor and the ability to taste MCHM led to persisting distrust of water safety long after water zones had reopened; the state of emergency was not lifted until 42 days after the last zone was opened for use. During the water crisis, more than 19.5 million bottles of water, 8.7 million liter containers of water, and 3 million gallons of bulk water were distributed by the National Guard; more than 3000 water samples were tested (Elizabeth Scharman, PharmD 2014). Public schools in the area were closed for weeks and businesses lost thousands of dollars. It caused outrage in the community that a company was allowed to store such large quantities of a chemical with no human health exposure information, and no previously established test to detect its presence in water, in such proximity to the intake valve of a public water system. The lack of extensive human health effect information for MCHM, the inability of the water company to shut off water coming into the intake valve following the spill, the lack of regulations applying to the chemicals involved, and the distrust of state public health partners fueled fear in the community. Multiple instances of social media postings of untrue or misleading information helped to spread the fear quickly. This incident brings to light several potential vulnerabilities in the public water drinking system:

- Available filtration systems may be overwhelmed by a large volume of contaminant
- Backup storage capacity in a water system is an important safety redundancy
- Consideration of the odor and taste of a contaminant can be a serious public health issue (even in the absence of clinically significant toxicity of that contaminant at the levels present)
- Unregulated above-ground storage tanks near public water supplies are a vulnerability for a large number of communities (eg, 800,000 people in Charlotte, NC, are downstream of coal ash waste located just 3 miles from the public water source intake)

Because of the critically important role played by water in daily life, and its often limited access, many organizations and governmental authorities have provided public health educational and response tools to address concerns about water quality. One of these, the physician online reference guide to water-borne disease and health effects of water pollution developed by the American College of Preventive Medicine, provides continuing medical education and a tool kit for clinicians.[42]

MEDICATION CONTAMINATION

The FDA is responsible for ensuring that prescription and over-the-counter medications in the United States are safe and effective. To that end, the FDA regulates all steps in the process of manufacture under the concept of current good manufacturing practice regulations.[53] This authority came in a series of acts precipitated by the substitution of diethylene glycol for the more expensive glycerin solvent in the liquid formulation of an early antibiotic, sulfanilamide, in 1937. This substitution resulted in the deaths of 105 people of the known 353 people exposed. The Food, Drug, and Cosmetic Act of 1938 increased regulatory authority of the FDA for medication safety. However, substitution of diethylene glycol in several medications and consumer products continues to result in poisoning outbreaks in different parts of the world.[54] The ongoing problem of intermittent medication shortages is partially caused by production halts by the FDA because of identified lack of pharmaceutical manufacturers' compliance with regulatory standards for documenting purity or sterility or other good manufacturing processes.[55] Additional problems with compounding pharmacies, which traditionally have been regulated by the state in which the entity is sited, have become apparent when these entities have done large-scale production and distribution. The multistate outbreak of fungal meningitis and other closed-space infection from methylprednisolone acetate contaminated at the site of processing in 2013 highlighted a problem with use and regulation of these entities.[56]

Given the frequency with which all of these problems occur, the potential for intentional and inadvertent contamination is even greater with products marketed outside the FDA's usual regulatory oversight. These products include dietary supplements,[57] which occupy a legislated limbo by the 1994 Dietary Supplement Health and Education Act.[58] They are regulated as food, but routinely illegally promoted as active medications; foreign products brought into the United States, such as Chinese patent medicines, Ayurvedic medication, or other culturally based medical practices that frequently make use of heavy metals[59]; and counterfeit medications, a market considered larger than the illicit drug of abuse market.[60]

Contamination Identification

Identification of chemically adulterated medication can be difficult. In contrast with the situations described for food and water, in which small or large segments of the general population may be affected, medications are often given to individuals who are already ill. Thus, additional clinical symptoms or death could be attributed to the underlying medical condition, intercurrent medical illness, or drug-drug interactions, resulting in a missed or delayed identification of drug adulteration. The major postmarketing mechanism for identification of adverse medication reactions, FDA's MedWatch program, is a voluntary reporting system, and causality may be difficult to determine.[61] Voluntary reporting via regional poison control centers to the National Poison Data System has similarly been used to identify illicit drug supply adulteration because of the increased number of emergency department visits,[62,63] but incoming calls depend on the clinician recognizing the potential for drug-related adverse events. Other surveillance mechanisms, such as health insurance–based monitoring, the standards-setting organization, US Pharmacopeia,[64] or organ-specific programs such as the Drug-Induced Liver Injury Network[65] can play an important role, but are not well coordinated centrally and may have significant time lags in identifying signals. Analytical testing by chromatographic techniques is an excellent mechanism to identify contaminants, but has been largely applied only to confiscated and black market drug analysis.[66] For solid medication preparations, comparison of potential counterfeit tablets with infrared spectra of a known branded product has been used as an accurate screening method.[67]

Impact of Site of Contamination

The frequent occurrence of manufacturing errors provides a window into the multinational sourcing of medication components, with active pharmaceutical ingredients being manufactured in one place and shipped with other ingredients to another site for batch processing and addition of excipients for medication delivery or aesthetics, labeling, and distribution to third parties for delivery to pharmacies and other retail outlets. As examples, star anise, in addition to its use as a flavoring agent, was the major source of shikimic acid, itself the major precursor of the anti-influenza medication, oseltamivir. Until a process for *Escherichia coli*–mediated synthesis of shikimic acid was developed, China was the major source of star anise.[68] Such international dependence for a raw material is not only strategically unwise, it also provides opportunity for product adulteration. This opportunity was seen recently with a large number of allergic reactions reported with use of one brand of heparin. The ultimate cause was identified as the substitution of a cheaper, but less active and allergenic, raw material (active pharmaceutical ingredient [API]) from multiple Chinese suppliers.[69,70]

At the other end of the production-distribution chain, the batching process used by most pharmaceutical manufacturers allows errors at switchover transition from one product to another, resulting in one API being packaged and labeled as another. Still further down the chain, individual pharmacies can mislabel product, affecting a single or small number of individuals. The most famous example of end-distribution medication tampering was the so-called Chicago Tylenol murders in 1982.[71] Substitution of several capsules in multiple drug stores resulted in 7 deaths from cyanide poisoning. The response to this included legislation making drug tampering a federal offense and an industry response that resulted in the standard of triple-sealed tamper-evident packaging for over-the-counter medications (now amended to 2 tamper-evident seals).[72] **Table 3** lists some examples of medication adulteration along this supply chain.

RECOGNIZING CLINICAL MANIFESTATIONS

As outlined in **Tables 1–3** listing examples of past food, water, and medication contamination, identification of the causative agent or even the existence of a contamination event is not always easy or rapid. Clinicians face competing challenges: identify toxic symptoms and reassure those with unrelated symptoms while all are facing a stressful situation. Local and national experts, as appropriate, can assist by providing alerts to emergency and primary care providers, and by formulating clinical case definitions. However, these definitions often undergo revisions as more information becomes available and may take some time to develop; clinicians must depend on obtaining a good history of associated events and timing, while being aware of symptom clusters that may identify toxidromes. The importance of a system-wide approach, making use of all available resources, has been emphasized previously both here and elsewhere.[79] The CDC has provided a symptom-based approach to some agents, as listed in **Table 4**.[80] The American College of Emergency Physicians and other organizations have prepared graphic material to display in emergency departments to assist in toxidrome recognition in the mass casualty situation. Although these resources can be outdated, the National Library of Medicine has incorporated several resources and expert input into an online interactive Chemical Hazards Emergency Medical Management (CHEMM).[81] This resource is valuable because it allows a clinical picture to be built of a potentially poisoned patient using the CHEMM Intelligent

Table 3
Examples of chemical contamination of the medication supply

Bow-Tie Site of Introduction	Chemical Exposure	Site/Date	Number of People Affected	Health Effects	Acute vs Chronic Health Effects
Raw ingredient (API): Chinese suppliers substituted animal cartilage–based oversulfated chondroitin sulfate for pig intestine–based product	Baxter Healthcare brand heparin[70] (intentional)	United States and at least 10 other countries/2008	Thousands; >100 reported deaths in United States	Allergic reactions (angioedema, hypotension, dyspnea, gastrointestinal symptoms)	Acute
Production: substitution of DEG for glycerin or propylene glycol in an acetaminophen elixir	DEG[73] (intentional)	Haiti/1995–1996 (and multiple other events[46])	106 children with renal failure, 93 of whom died	Vomiting, mental status changes, renal failure	Acute
Production: aegeline substituted for illegal stimulant (DMAA) in OxyElite Pro dietary supplement	Aegeline[74–76] (intentional)	Hawaii/2013	Approximately 30 cases; 1 death	Loss of appetite, jaundice consequent to hepatic injury	Acute to subacute
Production: 200 times indicated selenium and 17 times indicated chromium content added to dietary supplements Total Body Formula and Total Body Mega Formula	Selenium (and chromium)[77] (inadvertent)	9 US states/2008	At least 43 people	Muscle cramps, diarrhea, joint pain, fatigue, hair loss, and nail changes days to weeks while using product	Subacute
End distribution: tampering of Tylenol brand acetaminophen capsules on pharmacy shelves	Cyanide[71] (intentional)	Chicago, IL 1982 (and numerous copycat events[78])	7 people died	Sudden cardiovascular collapse	Acute

Note that the number of people affected generally decreases as the site of contaminant introduction moves from the production to the distribution side.
Abbreviations: DEG, diethylene glycol; DMAA, 1,3-dimethylamylamine.

Table 4
Selected clinical syndromes and potential chemical causes

Category[a]	Clinical Syndrome	Potential Chemical Cause
Cholinergic crisis	• Salivation, diarrhea, lacrimation, bronchorrhea, diaphoresis, and/or urination • Miosis, fasciculations, weakness, bradycardia or tachycardia, hypotension or hypertension, altered mental status, and/or seizures	• Nicotine[b] • Organophosphate insecticides[b] 　○ Decreased acetylcholinesterase activity • Carbamate insecticides • Medicinal carbamates (eg, physostigmine)
Generalized muscle rigidity	• Seizurelike, generalized muscle contractions or painful spasms (neck and limbs) and usually tachycardia and hypertension	• Strychnine 　○ Intact sensorium
Oropharyngeal pain and ulcerations	• Lip, mouth, and pharyngeal ulcerations and burning pain	• Paraquat[b] 　○ Dyspnea and hemoptysis secondary to pulmonary edema or hemorrhage; can progress to pulmonary fibrosis over days to weeks • Diquat • Caustics (ie, acids and alkalis) • Inorganic mercuric salts • Mustards (eg, sulfur)
Cellular hypoxia	• Mild: nausea, vomiting, and headache • Severe: altered mental status, dyspnea, hypotension, seizures, and metabolic acidosis	• Cyanide[b] (eg, hydrogen cyanide gas or sodium cyanide) 　○ Bitter almond odor[c] • Sodium monofluoroacetate[b] 　○ Hypocalcemia or hypokalemia • Carbon monoxide • Hydrogen sulfide • Sodium azide • Methemoglobin-causing agents
Peripheral neuropathy and/or neurocognitive effects	• Peripheral neuropathy signs and symptoms: muscle weakness and atrophy, glove-and-stocking sensory loss, and depressed or absent deep tendon reflexes • Neurocognitive effects: memory loss, delirium, ataxia, and/or encephalopathy	• Mercury (organic)[b] 　○ Visual disturbances, paresthesias, and/or ataxia • Arsenic (inorganic)[b] 　○ Delirium and/or peripheral neuropathy • Thallium 　○ Delirium and/or peripheral neuropathy • Lead 　○ Encephalopathy • Acrylamide 　○ Encephalopathy and/or peripheral neuropathy

(continued on next page)

Table 4 (continued)		
Category[a]	Clinical Syndrome	Potential Chemical Cause

Severe gastrointestinal illness, dehydration	• Abdominal pain, vomiting, profuse diarrhea (possibly bloody), and hypotension, possibly followed by multisystem organ failure	• Arsenic[b]
		• Ricin[b]
		  ○ Inhalation an additional route of exposure; severe respiratory illness possible
		• Colchicine
		• Barium
		  ○ Hypokalemia common

[a] Not intended as a complete differential diagnosis for each syndrome or a list of all chemicals that might be used in a covert chemical release.

[b] Potential agents for a covert chemical release based on historical use (ie, intentional or inadvertent use), high toxicity, and/or ease of availability.

[c] Unreliable sign.

From Patel M, Schier J, Belson M, et al. Recognition of illness associated with exposure to chemical agents–United States, 2003. MMWR Morb Mortal Wkly Rep 2003; 52(39):938–40.

Syndromes Tool (CHEMM-IST).[82] Differentiating fear response from toxic exposure can be particularly difficult. Even for suspected substances that are often considered all or none in their clinical presentation, such as cyanide salts, patient and provider fear or lack of understanding can interfere with good medical care.[76] Recognizing that people respond to the unknown with uncertainty can be the first step toward formulating a reasonable approach that involves them in the solution.[83,84]

MANAGEMENT

The axiom that supportive care forms the basis of emergency medical care is also true in settings of mass exposure events. One of the issues that arise during mass casualty events is the problem of limited resources, which can include difficulty in determining a diagnosis and initiating treatment, as well as mobilizing adequate numbers of personnel, supplies, and treatment modalities. A recently published systematic review of the disaster medicine literature evaluated response strategies in mass casualty events; it identified little evidence for effective, proven strategies to manage or allocate scarce resources, particularly for chemical exposure events.[85] Hospital-based antidote supplies have long been recognized as deficient; a consensus panel recently reviewed the rationale for immediate availability of several antidotes.[86] However, maintaining stocks of infrequently used, and sometimes expensive, medications encounters the problem of the often arbitrary out-date for these agents. Although the Medical Letter and professional organizations such as the American College of Medical Toxicology and the American Academy of Clinical Toxicology have called for a resolution to this largely bureaucratic problem,[87] there has only been limited success, as exemplified by the Department of Defense's Shelf Life Extension Program[88] regulating the ongoing extensions of the out-dates for nerve agent antidotes regionally located in the Chem-Pack program.[89] Regional poison control centers maintain lists of antidote availability at regional hospitals and can be accessed through their toll-free number of 1-800-222-1222. In contrast with most other acute emergencies, individual cases of potential contamination of food, water, or medication require immediate notification of relevant regulatory agencies and careful crafting of messages to the public. The local or state health department is the point of first contact; this too can sometimes be facilitated by the regional poison control center and its toxicology directors. **Box 1** summarizes

> **Box 1**
> **Assistance in identification of a potential food, water, or medication contamination event**
>
> - Obtain a history of onset of symptoms and any association with new medication refills or purchases, or eating/drinking.
> - Identify any concerns regarding food, water, or medication appearance or taste.
> - Query as to others who shared these items and their condition.
> - Identify any prominent organ effects or laboratory findings of concern.
> - If possible, obtain sample of potentially contaminated material.
> - If assessment raises concern regarding contamination, contact the regional poison control center (PCC) at 1-800-222-1222 and report concerns.
> - If a toxidrome with a specific antidote is being considered, the PCC can assist in identifying and/or locating these medical countermeasures. The PCC can also identify additional resources, such as medical toxicologists, if the hospital does not have a medical toxicologist on staff.
> - If other reports from regional caregivers, or consistent with notices on American Association of Poison Control Centers (AAPCC) listserv, Epi-X, or other reporting sources, the PCC directors may draft a press release for dissemination to hospitals in conjunction with state department of public health notification to assist in defining the clinical picture, possible diagnostic studies, and treatment.
> - Incorporate additional public health, laboratory, and investigative resources as appropriate.

some commonsense management points that may assist in the early recognition and response to potentially contaminated food, water, or medication supplies.

SPECIAL CONSIDERATIONS

As noted earlier in this article, children were at particular risk in the modeling of poisoning of the milk supply by botulinum toxin because of their larger intake of milk compared with adults and their smaller mass and increased respiratory rate.[4] In general, this same principle can apply to other toxins and toxicants delivered via food or water in terms of at-risk populations. As noted earlier, medication tampering has the potential for asymmetric impact on those with underlying health issues for which the medications were indicated in the first place.

SUMMARY

Food, water, and medication production, processing, and distribution involve multiple potential points of entry for chemical contamination. These points of entry can be inadvertent or intentional. Past experience indicates that these issues will continue to present challenges in prevention, rapid identification, and response. Several regulatory agencies have ultimate responsibility for each of these areas, but early recognition of introduced contamination will continue to be based on clinical suspicion. Given that analytical testing can be delayed, a complete history of travel and medication use (including specific questioning about supplements, over-the-counter products, and ethnic products), timing of onset and nature of symptoms, inquiries about others with symptoms, and recognition of potential toxidromes forms the foundation for subsequent investigation. Regional poison control centers are a valuable resource for assistance and potential case finding, and they can serve as an entry point to additional medical toxicology and public health resources. State public health laboratories participate in a national LRN, with specific capabilities to deal with potential food issues via the FERN.

The number and location of affected individuals can facilitate identification of the likely point of entry of a chemical contaminant through the use of bow-tie modeling. In general, the earlier in the production-distribution chain the contamination occurred, the more widely dispersed and greater in number will be the impact. This epidemiologic tool can be important when crafting a public response, which may include recalls or no-use warnings. Appropriate and ongoing risk communication is an important aspect of the overall response to potential chemical contamination of food, water, or medication, in order to avoid inappropriate responses based on fear or inaccurate information.

REFERENCES

1. Mayor A. Greek fire, poison arrows, and scorpion bombs: Biological and chemical warfare in the ancient world. New York: The Overlook Press, Peter Mayer Publishers; 2003.
2. Thompson CJ. Poisons and poisoners. New York: Barnes & Noble Books; 1993.
3. Appian of Alexandria. Appian's history of Rome: the Mithridatic Wars; XVI: paragraph 111. c 120 AD [translated by Horace White, 1899]. Proc Natl Acad Sci USA.
4. Wein LM, Liu Y. Analyzing a bioterror attack on the food supply: the case of botulinum toxin in milk. Proc Natl Acad Sci U S A 2005;102(28):9984–9. Available at: http://www.pnas.org/content/102/28/9984.full. Accessed July 13, 2014.
5. Schwarz ES, Wax PM, Kleinschmidt KC, et al. Sodium azide poisoning at a restaurant – Dallas County, Texas, 2010. MMWR Morb Mortal Wkly Rep 2012; 61(25):457–60.
6. Lombardo JS, Burkom H, Pavlin J. ESSENCE II and the framework for evaluating syndromic surveillance systems. MMWR Morb Mortal Wkly Rep 2004;53(Suppl): 159–65.
7. Torok TJ, Tauxe RV, Wise RP, et al. A large community outbreak of salmonellosis caused by intentional contamination of restaurant salad bars. JAMA 1997;278: 389–95.
8. Food Emergency Response Network. USDA audit report 24601-6-At; March 2011. Available at: http://www.usda.gov/oig/webdocs/24601-6-AT.pdf. Accessed July 13, 2014.
9. Kuehn BM. Agencies use social media to track foodborne illness. JAMA 2014. http://dx.doi.org/10.1001/jama.2014.7731. Available at: http://jama.jamanetwork.com/article.aspx?articleID=1885471&utm_source=Silverchair Information Systems&utm_medium=email&utm_campaign=JAMA%3AOnline First06%2F25%2F2014. Accessed July 13, 2014.
10. Estimates of foodborne illness in the United States. CDC; 2014 (2011 data). Available at: http://www.cdc.gov/foodborneburden/. Accessed July 13, 2014.
11. Food Safety Network: Outbreak alert! Database. Center for Science in the Public Interest. Available at: http://www.cspinet.org/foodsafety/outbreak/outbreaks.php?column=pathogenGroup&colval=Other Chemicals/Toxins. Accessed July 13, 2014.
12. Food: chemical contaminants. FDA, 2014. Available at: http://www.fda.gov/Food/FoodborneIllnessContaminants/ChemicalContaminants/default.htm. Accessed July 13, 2014.
13. Food and Drug Administration. FDA's draft approach for designating high-risk foods as required by section 204 of FSMA. Available at: http://www.fda.gov/

downloads/Food/GuidanceRegulation/FSMA/UCM380212.pdf. Accessed July 13, 2014.

14. The Laboratory Response Network partners in preparedness. Emergency preparedness and response. CDC; 2013. Available at: http://www.bt.cdc.gov/lrn/. Accessed July 13, 2014.

15. Hau AK, Kwan TH, Li PK. Melamine toxicity and the kidney. J Am Soc Nephrol 2009;20:245–50. Available at: http://jasn.asnjournals.org/content/20/2/245.full.pdf+html. Accessed July 13, 2014.

16. Timeline: China milk scandal. BBC News; January 25, 2010. Available at: http://news.bbc.co.uk/2/hi/7720404.stm. Accessed July 13, 2014.

17. Melamine contamination in China. News & Events. US FDA January 5, 2009. Available at: http://www.fda.gov/NewsEvents/PublicHealthFocus/ucm179005.htm. Accessed July 13, 2014.

18. Melamine and cyanuric acid: toxicity, preliminary risk assessment and guidance on levels in food. World Health Organization; 2008. Available at: http://www.who.int/foodsafety/fs_management/Melamine.pdf. Accessed July 13, 2014.

19. No new traces of poisoned Chilean fruit. Philly.com; March 15, 1989. Available at: http://articles.philly.com/1989-03-15/news/26129183_1_chilean-fruit-cyanide-laced-grapes-almeria-star. Accessed July 13, 2014.

20. Reich MR. Environmental politics and science: the case of PBB contamination in Michigan. Am J Public Health 1983;73:302–13. Available at: http://www.ncbi.nlm.nih.gov/pmc/articles/PMC1650578/pdf/amjph00638-0078.pdf. Accessed July 13, 2014.

21. Decades later, PBB contamination suspected in illnesses and deaths. Detroit, MI: Detroit Free Press; 2012. Available at: http://www.freep.com/article/20120923/NEWS06/309230153/Toxic-aftermath. Accessed July 13, 2014.

22. Tu WW, Yang H, Luo H, et al. One-year followup of melamine-associated renal stones in Sichuan and Hong Kong. Hong Kong J Paediatr 2012;17:12–23. Available at: http://www.hkjpaed.org/pdf/2012;17;12-23.pdf. Accessed July 13, 2014.

23. Terracino B, editor. Toxic oil syndrome: ten years of progress. World Health Organization; 2004. ISBN 9289010630. Available at: http://www.euro.who.int/__data/assets/pdf_file/0005/98447/E84423.pdf. Accessed July 13, 2014.

24. Botulism associated with canned chili sauce, July-August 2007. CDC; August 24, 2007. Available at: http://www.cdc.gov/botulism/botulism.htm. Accessed July 13, 2014.

25. Boulton M, Stanbury M, Wade D, et al. Nicotine poisoning after ingestion of contaminated ground beef—Michigan, 2003. MMWR Morb Mortal Wkly Rep 2003;52(18):413–6. Available at: http://www.cdc.gov/mmwr/preview/mmwrhtml/mm5218a3.htm. Accessed July 13, 2014.

26. Kongsaengdao S, Samintarapanya K, Rusmeechan S, et al. An outbreak of botulism in Thailand: clinical manifestations and management of severe respiratory failure. Clin Infect Dis 2006;43(10):1247–56. Available at: http://cid.oxfordjournals.org/content/43/10/1247.full.pdf+html. Accessed July 13, 2014.

27. AG, state police close investigation of 2003 New Sweden poisonings; conclude Bondeson acted alone. Office of the Maine Attorney General; April 18, 2006. Available at: http://www.maine.gov/ag/news/article.shtml?id=48446. Accessed July 13, 2014.

28. FBI finds no yogurt tampering. Philly.com; January 13, 1989. Available at: http://articles.philly.com/1989-01-13/news/26123322_1_potassium-cyanide-breyers-black-cherry-yogurt-county-prosecutor-samuel-asbell. Accessed July 13, 2014.

29. Basic information about water security. Water: water security. EPA; 2011. Available at: http://water.epa.gov/infrastructure/watersecurity/basicinformation.cfm. Accessed July 13, 2014.

30. EPA. Potential contamination due to cross-connections and backflow and associated health risks. Issue Paper US EPA Office of Ground Water and Drinking Water (OGWDW); 2001. Available at: http://www.epa.gov/safewater/disinfection/tcr/pdfs/issuepaper_tcr_crossconnection-backflow.pdf. Accessed July 13, 2014.

31. Drinking water contaminants. Water. EPA; 2013. Available at: http://water.epa.gov/drink/contaminants/index.cfm#List. Accessed July 13, 2014.

32. US EPA response to Executive Order 13636, improving critical infrastructure and cybersecurity. Available at: http://water.epa.gov/infrastructure/watersecurity/upload/EO_13696_10-b-_EPA_response.pdf. Accessed July 13, 2014.

33. van der Gaag B, Volz J. Real-time on-line monitoring of contaminants in water: developing a research strategy from utility experiences and needs. Kiwa Water Research BTO 2008.028; 2008. Available at: http://www.waterrf.org/PublicReportLibrary/4025.pdf. Accessed July 13, 2014.

34. Private drinking water wells. Water. EPA; 2012. Available at: http://water.epa.gov/drink/info/well/index.cfm. Accessed July 13, 2014.

35. Bottled water code of practice. International Bottled Water Association; 2012. Available at: http://www.bottledwater.org/files/IBWA_MODEL_CODE_2012_1212_FINAL_0.pdf. Accessed July 13, 2014.

36. Hilborn ED, Wade TJ, Hicks L, et al. Surveillance for waterborne disease outbreaks associated with drinking water and other nonrecreational water – United States, 2009-2010. MMWR Morb Mortal Wkly Rep 2013;62(35):714–20. Available at: http://www.cdc.gov/mmwr/preview/mmwrhtml/mm6235a3.htm?s_cid=mm6235a3_w#tab1. Accessed July 13, 2014.

37. Fairley CK, Sinclair MI, Rizak S. Monitoring drinking water: the receding zero. Med J Aust 1999;171(8):397–8.

38. Clark RM, Deininger RA. Protecting the nation's critical infrastructure: the vulnerability of U.S. water supply system. JCCM 2000;8(2):73–80.

39. CDC. Chlorine residual testing fact sheet, SWS project. Available at: http://www.cdc.gov/safewater/publications_pages/chlorineresidual.pdf. Accessed July 13, 2014.

40. Disaster response and recovery needs of communities affected by the Elk River chemical spill, West Virginia; April 2014. CDC/National Center for Environmental Health, Division of Environmental Hazards and Health Effects/Health Studies Branch. Available at: http://www.bt.cdc.gov/chemical/MCHM/westvirginia2014/. Accessed July 13, 2014.

41. Elk River chemical spill health effects: findings of emergency department record review; April 2014. Collaborative investigation by the West Virginia Bureau for Public Health (WVBPH) and the Agency for Toxic Substances Disease Registry (ATSDR). Available at: http://www.bt.cdc.gov/chemical/MCHM/westvirginia2014/. Accessed July 13, 2014.

42. Meinhardt PL. Recognizing waterborne disease and the health effects of water pollution: a physician online reference guide. And physician preparedness for acts of water terrorism: a physician online readiness guide. Available at: http://www.waterhealthconnection.org/. Accessed July 13, 2014.

43. Boehm LK. Popular culture and the enduring myth of Chicago, 1871–1968. London: Routledge; 2004.

44. Davies L. French transport workers threaten to pollute river Seine. The Guardian; 20 August 2009. Available at: http://www.theguardian.com/environment/2009/aug/20/france-transport-river-seine-pollution. Accessed July 13, 2014.

45. West Virginia chemical spill causes huge disruption for residents. The Guardian, January 12, 2014. Available at: http://www.theguardian.com/world/2014/jan/12/west-virginia-chemical-spill-disruption. Accessed July 13, 2014.
46. Tennessee Department of Health. Public Health Assessment: Tennessee Valley Authority Kingston Fossil Plant: Coal ash release. Available at: http://www.atsdr.cdc.gov/HAC/pha/TVAKingstonFossilPlant/TVAKingstonFossilPlantFinalPHA09072010.pdf. Accessed July 13, 2014.
47. Shoichet CE. Spill spews tons of coal ash into North Carolina river. CNN US; 9 February 2014. Available at: http://www.cnn.com/2014/02/09/us/north-carolina-coal-ash-spill/. Accessed July 13, 2014.
48. ATSDR. Camp Lejeune, North Carolina. Agency for Toxic Substances & Disease Registry; 2014. Available at: http://www.atsdr.cdc.gov/sites/lejeune/. Accessed July 13, 2014.
49. Boykin M. EPA R10 water contamination incident response protocols and preparedness; 2008. Presentation. Available at: http://www.ttemidev.com/oscadmin2008/conference/materials/203/8_Boykin_Water.pdf. Accessed July 13, 2014.
50. Krouse M. Backflow incident sparks improvements. Opflow 2001;27(2):1, 4–5,7,14.
51. Shih RD, Marcus SM, Genese CA, et al. Methemoglobinemia attributable to nitrite contamination of potable water through boiler fluid additives—New Jersey, 1992 and 1996. MMWR Morb Mortal Wkly Rep 1997;46(9):202–4. Available at: http://www.cdc.gov/mmwr/preview/mmwrhtml/00046656.htm. Accessed July 13, 2014.
52. Croddy E, Osborne M, McCloud K. Chemical terrorist plot in Rome? James Martin Center for Nonproliferation Studies; Monterey Institute of International Studies. 2002. Available at: http://cns.miis.edu/stories/020311.htm. Accessed July 13, 2014.
53. Facts about current good manufacturing practices (cGMPs). Drugs. FDA; 2013. Available at: http://www.fda.gov/Drugs/DevelopmentApprovalProcess/Manufacturing/ucm169105.htm. Accessed July 13, 2014.
54. Diethylene glycol. Health Council of the Netherlands; 2007. Available at: www.gezondheidsraad.nl/pdf/php?ID=1606&;p=1. Accessed July 13, 2014.
55. FDA. Strategic plan for preventing and mitigating drug shortages. October 2013. Available at: http://www.fda.gov/downloads/drugs/drugsafety/drugshortages/ucm372566.pdf. Accessed July 13, 2014.
56. Wookcock J. Examining drug compounding. Statement before the Subcommittee on Health, Committee on Energy and Commerce, US House of Representatives; May 23, 2013. Available at: http://www.fda.gov/NewsEvents/Testimony/ucm353654.htm. Accessed July 13, 2014.
57. Ching CK, Lam YH, Chan AY, et al. Adulteration of herbal antidiabetic products with undeclared pharmaceuticals: a case series in Hong Kong. Br J Clin Pharmacol 2011;73(5):795–800. Available at: http://www.ncbi.nlm.nih.gov/pmc/articles/PMC3403207/pdf/bcp0073-0795.pdf. Accessed July 13, 2014.
58. Dietary supplements. FDA; 2014. Available at: http://www.fda.gov/Food/Dietarysupplements/default.htm. Accessed July 13, 2014.
59. Byard RW. A review of the potential forensic significance of traditional herbal medicines. J Forensic Sci 2010;55(1):89–92.
60. Mackey TK, Liang BA. The global counterfeit drug trade: patient safety and public health risks. J Pharm Sci 2011;100(11):4571–9. Available at: file:///C:/Users/CN/Downloads/d912f50a49024c2a16.pdf. Accessed July 13, 2014.

61. MedWatch: the FDA safety information and adverse event reporting program. Available at: http://www.fda.gov/Safety/MedWatch/. Accessed July 13, 2014.

62. Hamilton RJ, Perrone J, Hoffman R, et al. A descriptive study of an epidemic of poisoning caused by heroin adulterated with scopolamine. J Toxicol Clin Toxicol 2000;38(6):597–608.

63. Hoffman RS, Kirrane BM, Marcus SM. Clenbuterol Study Investigators. A descriptive study of an outbreak of clenbuterol-containing heroin. Ann Emerg Med 2008; 52(5):548–53.

64. Mahady GB, Dog TL, Barrett ML, et al. United States Pharmacopeia review of black cohosh case reports of hepatotoxicity. Menopause 2008;15(4):628–38. Available at: http://www.drlowdog.com/Assets/pdf_files/BlackCohoshReview_USP.pdf. Accessed July 13, 2014.

65. Fontana RJ, Seeff LB, Andrade RJ, et al. Standardization of nomenclature and causality assessment in drug-induced liver injury: summary of a clinical research workshop. Hepatology 2010;52(2):730–42. Available at: http://www.ncbi.nlm.nih.gov/pmc/articles/PMC3616501/pdf/nihms445212.pdf. Accessed July 13, 2014.

66. Thevis M, Schrader Y, Thomas A, et al. Analysis of confiscated black market drugs using chromatographic and mass spectrometric approaches. J Anal Toxicol 2008;32:232–40. Available at: http://www.muscle-core.com/files/Analysis_AAS.pdf. Accessed July 13, 2014.

67. Storme-Paris I, Rebiere H, Matoga M, et al. Challenging near infrared spectroscopy discriminating ability for counterfeit pharmaceuticals detection. Anal Chim Acta 2010;658(2):163–74.

68. Ghosh S, Chisti Y, Banerjee UC. Production of shikimic acid. Biotechnol Adv 2012;30(6):1425–31.

69. FDA media briefing on heparin; March 19, 2008. Available at: http://www.fda.gov/downloads/NewsEvents/Newsroom/MediaTranscripts/UCM169335.pdf. Accessed July 13, 2014.

70. Kishimoto TK, Viswanathan K, Ganguly T, et al. Contaminated heparin associated with adverse clinical events and activation of the contact system. N Engl J Med 2008;358(23):2457–67.

71. Manning J. "The Tylenol murders", material things (The Eighties Club); 2000. Available at: eightiesclub.tripod.com/id298.htm. Accessed July 13, 2014.

72. Tamper-evident packaging requirements for over-the-counter human drug products. Final Rule; 21 CFR Part 211; 1998. Available at: http://www.fda.gov/ohrms/dockets/98fr/110498a.txt. Accessed July 13, 2014.

73. Malebranche R, Hecdivert C, Lassegue A, et al. Fatalities associated with ingestion of diethylene glycol-contaminated glycerin used to manufacture acetaminophen syrup—Haiti, November 1995-June 1996. MMWR Morb Mortal Wkly Rep 1996;45(30):649–50. Available at: http://www.cdc.gov/mmwr/preview/mmwrhtml/00043194.htm. Accessed July 13, 2014.

74. Park SY, Johnston D, Taylor E, et al. Notes from the field: acute hepatitis and liver failure following the use of a dietary supplement intended for weight loss or muscle building – May-October 2013. MMWR Morb Mortal Wkly Rep 2013;62(40): 817–9. Available at: http://www.cdc.gov/mmwr/preview/mmwrhtml/mm6240a1.htm. Accessed July 13, 2014.

75. Fabricant D. FDA uses new authorities to get OxyElite Pro off the market. FDA-Voice; November 18, 2013. Available at: http://blogs.fda.gov/fdavoice/index.php/tag/aegeline/. Accessed July 13, 2014.

76. Cohen PA. Hazards of hindsight–monitoring the safety of nutritional supplements. N Engl J Med 2014;370:1277–80. Available at: http://www.nejm.org/doi/full/10.1056/NEJMp1315559. Accessed July 13, 2014.

77. Total Body Formula, Total Body Mega Formula. Safety. FDA; Update 5/1/2008. Available at: http://www.fda.gov/Safety/MedWatch/SafetyInformation/SafetyAlertsfor HumanMedicalProducts/ucm070027.htm. Accessed July 13, 2014.

78. Bell R. The Tylenol terrorist: copycat criminals. Crimelibrary. Available at: http://www.crimelibrary.com/terrorists_spies/terrorists/tylenol_murders/4.html. Accessed July 13, 2014.

79. Kirk MA, Deaton ML. Bringing order out of chaos: effective strategies for medical response to mass chemical exposure. Emerg Med Clin North Am 2007;25(2):527–48.

80. Patel M, Schier J, Belson M, et al. Recognition of illness associated with exposure to chemical agents–United States, 2003. MMWR Morb Mortal Wkly Rep 2003;52(39):938–40. Available at: http://www.cdc.gov/mmwr/preview/mmwrhtml/mm5239a3.htm#tab. Accessed July 13, 2014.

81. CHEMM: Chemical Hazards Emergency Medical Management. US Department of Health and Human Services, Office of the Assistant Secretary for Preparedness and Response, Office of Planning and Emergency Operations/National Library of Medicine, Division of Specialized Information Services. Available at: http://chemm.nlm.nih.gov/. Accessed July 13, 2014.

82. CHEMM Intelligent Syndromes Tool (CHEMM-IST). US Department of Health and Human Services, Office of the Assistant Secretary for Preparedness and Response, Office of Planning and Emergency Operations/National Library of Medicine, Division of Specialized Information Services. Available at: http://chemm.nlm.nih.gov/chemmist.htm. Accessed July 13, 2014.

83. McKay CA. Risk assessment and risk communication. In: Nelson L, Lewin N, Howland MA, et al, editors. Goldfrank's toxicologic emergencies. 9th edition. New York (NY): McGraw-Hill; 2010. Chapter 129.

84. Covello VT. The EPA's seven cardinal rules of risk communication. Available at: http://www.wvdhhr.org/bphtraining/courses/cdcynergy/content/activeinformation/resources/epa_seven_cardinal_rules.pdf. Accessed July 13, 2014.

85. Timble JW, Ringel JS, Fox S, et al. Systematic review of strategies to manage and allocate scarce resources during mass casualty events. Ann Emerg Med 2013;61(6):677–89.

86. Dart RC, Borron SW, Caravati EM, et al. Expert consensus guidelines for stocking of antidotes in hospitals that provide emergency care. Ann Emerg Med 2009;54(3):386–94. Available at: http://www.supplements.annemergmed.com/PDF/Guidelines.pdf. Accessed July 13, 2014.

87. Antidote shortages: impact and response. American College of Medical Toxicology and American Academy of Clinical Toxicology position statement. Available at: http://acmt.net/_Library/docs/AntidoteShortages111512.pdf. Accessed July 13, 2014.

88. Department of Defense. Shelf life management manual. DOD 4140.27-M/DLA J-373; 2003. Available at: https://www.shelflife.hq.dla.mil/policy_DoD4140_27.aspx. Accessed July 13, 2014.

89. Chempack. US Department of Health and Human Services, Office of the Assistant Secretary for Preparedness and Response, Office of Planning and Emergency Operations/National Library of Medicine, Division of Specialized Information Services. Available at: http://chemm.nlm.nih.gov/chempack.htm. Accessed July 13, 2014.

Emergency Department Management of Patients Internally Contaminated with Radioactive Material

Ziad Kazzi, MD[a,b,*], Jennifer Buzzell, MS[a], Luiz Bertelli, PhD[c],
Doran Christensen, DO[d]

KEYWORDS

- Radioactive terrorism • Contamination • Radioactive elements • Radiation dosage
- Chelation therapy

KEY POINTS

- Patients can become contaminated with radioactive material after the detonation of an improvised nuclear device, a nuclear power plant accident, or a radioactive dispersal device incident.
- Depending on the scenario, radioactive material can enter the body through ingestion, inhalation or injection.
- Life-saving care of a patient contaminated with radioactive material should not be delayed to perform a radiation survey or decontamination.
- Once stabilized, a patient should be undressed, surveyed for contamination, and washed with soap and water.
- In addition to supportive care, chelators can remove certain radioactive materials, such as cesium-137, plutonium, americium, and curium.

INTRODUCTION
Definition

Emergency physicians care for a wide range of illnesses and injuries, including those that are sustained during a radiologic or nuclear emergency. There are several

Disclosure Statement: No financial support was provided to any author in relationship to this article. No author declares a conflict of financial interest in relationship to this article.

CDC disclosure statement: "The findings and conclusions in this report are those of the authors and do not necessarily represent the views of the Centers for Disease Control and Prevention/the Agency for Toxic Substances and Disease Registry."

[a] National Center for Environmental Health, Centers for Disease Control and Prevention, 4770 Buford Highway, Northeast, MS-F59, Atlanta, GA 30341-3717, USA; [b] Department of Emergency Medicine, Emory University, 531 Asbury Cir-Annex, Suite N-340, Atlanta, GA 30322, USA; [c] Los Alamos National Laboratory, Mailstop G761, Los Alamos, NM 87545, USA; [d] Radiation Emergency Assistance Center/Training Site, PO Box 117, Oak Ridge TN 37831, USA
* Corresponding author. 4770 Buford Highway, Northeast, MS-F59, Atlanta, GA 30341-3717.
E-mail address: ZKAZZI@emory.edu

Emerg Med Clin N Am 33 (2015) 179–196
http://dx.doi.org/10.1016/j.emc.2014.09.008
0733-8627/15/$ – see front matter © 2015 Elsevier Inc. All rights reserved.

emed.theclinics.com

possible scenarios that cause people to become exposed to ionizing radiation; the most common incidents reported to the Radiation Emergency Assistance and Training Site involve inadvertent exposure to radiation from a radioactive source used in a medical or industrial setting. The Radiation Emergency Assistance and Training Site offers 24–7 assistance to health care professionals or the public with questions about ionizing radiation. Occasionally, a transportation accident involving radioactive material can occur. Less frequently, a nuclear power plant malfunction leads to the release of radioactive material in the environment. This has occurred only a few times in history, yet they have had a large impact on the environment (Fukushima 2011) and public health (Chernobyl 1986). Additionally, the US Government recommends that states prepare for 15 National Planning Scenarios, two of which involve radiation. These are the detonation of an improvised nuclear device and a radiologic dispersal device.[1]

These radiologic or nuclear incidents occur infrequently and some occur rarely; however, they can be potentially devastating. When they do occur, they cause a disproportionate amount of fear and concern in the public and emergency responders, including emergency physicians.[2–4] This fact is combined with a suboptimal amount of health care provider knowledge about the evaluation and care of victims as supported by several previous studies.[5,6]

Radioactive material exists in a solid, liquid, or gaseous physical form. They can occur naturally in the environment (eg, uranium, thorium, and potassium)[7] or are manufactured in a reactor (eg, polonium and plutonium). Although some of these materials are stored in secured locations, like nuclear power plants or military facilities, the majority are available for use in broad range of industries and for a number of applications, including radiography, sterilization of products, materials testing, and medicine. In fact, the International Atomic Energy Agency and US Nuclear Regulatory Commission report the loss of a significant number of sources, some of which are never recovered.[8]

Patients can become contaminated with radioactive material when the substance in question deposits on their body surface or enters their body through the gastrointestinal tract, the respiratory tract, open wounds, or, less commonly, through intact skin. These routes of exposure need to be differentiated from scenarios in which the patient is exposed to an external source of ionizing radiation, that is, from a source that is external to the body and not contaminating skin or clothing.[9]

This article discusses the emergency department evaluation and management of a patient who is externally and or internally contaminated with radioactive material.

HISTORICAL BACKGROUND: GOIANIA BRAZIL AND MR LITVINENKO

To better illustrate the concept of contamination with radioactive material, a description of 2 important historical incidents follows.

The radiologic incident in Goiania, Brazil (1987)

On September 28, 1987, a woman visited the clinic at the local Goiania health department in Brazil.[10] She claimed that her family members and herself had fallen ill because of handling an unknown solid substance. This material was eventually identified as cesium-137 that originated from the theft of an abandoned teletherapy source on September 13, 1987. The material consisted of about 100 g of cesium-137 in the form of the chloride salt. During the 16 days that followed the theft of the source, several people came into contact with the material and fell ill. They were initially misdiagnosed with food poisoning or allergic reactions by local physicians. In total, 249 people were found to be contaminated with cesium-137 and 4 people died, including a 6-year-old girl who handled the material while eating food. The incident caused severe economic and social impacts. More than 125,000 people presented for monitoring for contamination with the radioactive material. To this day, the psychological consequences of this incident are still apparent in the exposed population.[11]

The poisoning of Mr Alexander Litvinenko with Polonium-210 (2006)

On November 1, 2006, Mr Alexander Litvinenko developed a gastrointestinal illness after a business meeting at a London restaurant.[12] On November 23, 2006, he died from acute radiation syndrome (ARS). On the preceding day, he was discovered to be internally contaminated with a minute yet lethal amount of polonium-210. The particular radioactive properties of this radionuclide facilitated its evasion of early detection tests that were performed and highlighted the hazardous nature of this radioactive element when internalized into the body. In the aftermath of his death, English public health authorities conducted screening of potentially contaminated areas and people. This process included identifying foreign nationals who could have been contaminated during travel and who had to be screened for polonium-210 in their home country.[13]

AGENTS OF TOXICITY
Mechanism of Injury

Basic definitions (intake, uptake and deposition–initial deposition, excretion)
Radioactive material can enter the body through inhalation, ingestion, or injection. The skin is usually an effective barrier, except when it is damaged (eg, burn) or open (eg, wound). Infrequently, certain radioactive elements may have chemical properties or can be formulated in a manner that makes them absorbable through intact skin. Tritium, which is present in nuclear power plants, is an example of an element that can be absorbed through intact skin. Other than tritium, most radioactive materials are metals or have metallike properties and are not easily absorbed through intact skin.[14]

An intake is defined as the result of a radioactive element entering the physical confines of the human body (eg, the nares or the mouth). This occurs before uptake (or absorption) of the element into the circulation (eg, into blood or lymph). Once the element enters the circulation, it is distributed in the body and is deposited in various organs or tissues on the basis of its chemical rather than its radioactive properties. For example, iodine-131 deposits primarily in the thyroid gland and cesium-137 behaves like potassium and distributes uniformly in muscle tissue.[15]

After deposition into various organs and tissues, the element undergoes elimination. The elimination biological half-life varies for different elements and in different patients. For example, the biological half-life for iodine is approximately 57 days and depends on individual factors like thyroid gland activity and iodine content.[16] Elimination occurs via different routes including urine, feces, sweat, lungs, and saliva. For example, cesium-137 is naturally primarily eliminated in urine rather than feces. However, when oral Prussian blue chelation therapy is administered, fecal elimination becomes the dominant route.[17] Additionally, some elements deposit in bone after being absorbed into the circulation and are less amenable to excretion. For example, strontium has a long biological half-life of approximately 50 years.[18]

Radiation physics basics (ionizing radiation, radiobiology)
Some atoms are radioactive because they contain too much energy and they emit radiation from the nucleus to reach a more favorable, stable energy state (this process is

called radioactive decay). The greater the number of decays per unit time the greater the activity of the material and the more radioactive it is. The unit of activity is the becquerel, where 1 becquerel is equivalent of 1 disintegration or decay per second. As time elapses, the activity of the material decreases because of physical (radioactive) decay. The rate of decay of a specific element is governed by the corresponding physical half-life. For example, the physical half-life of iodine-131 is about 8 days whereas the physical half-life of cesium-137 is about 30 years.[19,20] Therefore, radioactive elements that are internalized are subject to both the biological elimination and physical decay processes.[21]

The effective half-life reflects both processes and is shorter than either one. The effective half-life can be calculated as 1/effective half-life = (1/biological half-life + 1/physical half-life.) For example, iodine-131 has an approximate biological half-life of 57 days and a physical half-life of 8 days. The effective half-life is approximately 7 days (1/effective half-life = 1/8 + 1/57 = 0.1425).

Radioactive elements are potentially hazardous to people because of the radiation that they emit during decay. This radiation carries enough energy to ionize another atom and is appropriately called ionizing radiation. When this radiation energy deposits in a cell, it can damage genetic material or induce the production of free radicals from water molecules in a process called hydrolysis. These highly reactive species in turn damage genetic material or cellular constituents, which could cause cell damage and death. Gamma rays, alpha particles, beta particles, positrons, and neutrons are examples of ionizing radiation and originate from the nucleus of an atom. X-rays are also ionizing; however, they are not released from the nucleus of an atom. They can be generated by a machine or occur naturally when an electron drops from an orbital with higher energy down to a lower energy orbital shell. Typically, x-rays are lower in energy than gamma rays.[22,23] In comparison, ultraviolet, visible light, and radio waves do not have enough energy and are unable to ionize atoms. They belong to the category of nonionizing radiation. Every radioactive atom decays to a more stable state by emitting 1 or more types of ionizing radiation. For example, every 137-cesium atom decays by emitting a single gamma ray and a single beta particle and becomes stable barium-137 after going through a barium-137 m (metastable) state.[20] On the other hand, every polonium-210 atom decays by emitting an alpha particle and becomes the stable atom lead-206.[24]

The specific decay information for every radioactive element is available through a variety of sources and can be used to better characterize the health hazards from external or internal contamination with the corresponding element or material (eg, The Health Physics Society Webpage http://hps.org/publicinformation/radardecaydata.cfm). The amount of ionizing radiation energy that deposits in the body or in a specific organ is called absorbed dose and is expressed using the unit gray (Gy) that reflects the energy in joules deposited per kilogram of tissue. The gray is defined as 1 J/kg.[25] The biological health effect equivalent of an absorbed dose in gray is expressed using the unit sievert (Sv) and is called equivalent dose. It is calculated by multiplying the dose in gray by a dimensionless radiation weighting factor (previously termed quality factor- "Q").[26] **Table 1** below shows the radiation weighting factor for several radiation types.

Committed equivalent dose and committed effective dose
The committed equivalent dose is the dose that will be received by an organ after intake of radioactive material into the body over 50 years for adults and 70 years for children. To account for differences in sensitivity between tissues, the equivalent dose to each organ is multiplied by a tissue weighting factor, which is the factor by

Table 1
Radiation weighting factors in ICRP Publication 60

Type and Energy Range	Radiation Weighting Factor
Photons, all energies	1
Electrons and muons, all energies	1
Neutrons, energy	
<10 keV	5
>10 keV–100 keV	10
>100 keV–2 MeV	20
>2 MeV–20 MeV	10
>20 MeV	5
Protons, energy >2 MeV	5
Alpha particles, fission fragments, heavy nuclei	20

Data from ICRP. 1990 Recommendations of the International Commission on Radiological Protection. ICRP Publication 60; 1991. Ann. ICRP 21 (1–3).

which the equivalent dose in a tissue or organ is weighted to represent the relative contributions of that tissue or organ to the total detriment resulting from uniform irradiation of the body. The committed effective dose is the sum of the products of the committed organ equivalent doses and the appropriate organ weighting factors. Committed doses are evaluated over 50 years for adults, and from intake to age 70 years for children. The recommended values of the tissue weighting factors are given in **Table 2**.[27]

The United States has historically used a different set of units than those listed. This can lead to errors when interpreting measurements or other types of data during

Table 2
Tissue weighting factors in ICRP Publication 60

Organ or Tissue	Tissue Weighting Factor
Gonads	0.20
Bone marrow (red)	0.12
Colon	0.12
Lung	0.12
Stomach	0.12
Bladder	0.05
Breast	0.05
Liver	0.05
Esophagus	0.05
Thyroid	0.05
Skin	0.01
Bone surface	0.01
Remainder	0.05

The values have been developed from a reference population of equal numbers of both sexes and a wide range of ages. In the definition of effective dose they apply to workers, to the whole population, and to either sex.

Data from ICRP. 1990 Recommendations of the International Commission on Radiological Protection. ICRP Publication 60; 1991. Ann. ICRP 21 (1–3).

emergencies. The United States Health Physics Society has recommended using the international system of units (SI) for future activities.[28] The conversion between SI units and the ones traditionally used traditional in the United States is listed in **Table 3**.

CLINICAL MANIFESTATIONS
Stochastic and Deterministic

The primary goal of the evaluation and management of patients who are contaminated with a radioactive material is to prevent the occurrence of adverse deterministic and stochastic health effects. Deterministic clinical effects occur when the radiation dose to the body or organ is great enough to damage critical cells and lead to organ malfunction like bone marrow failure and neutropenia. The severity and rate of manifestation of these effects are dose dependent. An example of a deterministic effect is the sunburn; the longer one is in the sun, the greater the redness. By the same token, clinically relevant deterministic effects do not occur if the dose received by the organ or body is below a certain threshold (eg, 1 Gy of absorbed dose in general is considered to be the threshold for the development of ARS). Additional factors that determine the type and severity of clinical effects include dose rate, type of ionizing radiation, type and volume of tissue affected, individual patient susceptibilities, co-morbid conditions, and concomitant injuries.[23] On the other hand, stochastic effects occur in a random, probabilistic manner and do not require the dose received to be greater than a threshold. Stochastic effects include cancer and birth defects. The greater the dose of radiation deposited in an organ or in the body, the greater the chance of developing the effect, although there is no dose–response relationship between the radiation dose and these effects.[23] Last, although genetic hereditary effects have been observed in animals exposed to radiation, they have not been seen in human population studies.[29]

Chemical toxicity from uranium

The chemical toxicity of the element occasionally is more significant than the clinical effects caused by exposure to the emitted radiation. This is especially true for internal contamination with soluble compounds of natural uranium. This element is radioactive, but causes chemical nephrotoxicity at a lesser concentration in the body than what is required to deliver a radiation dose that is great enough to cause any stochastic clinical effects.[30] Therefore, when dealing with internal contamination with one of the isotopes of natural uranium, the main concern is for renal damage from the toxic uranyl ion.

MANAGEMENT
Staff Protection and Safety (Personal Protective Equipment and Concern About Hazards from Body Fluid like Urine, Blood Samples, Management of Waste)

Radiation protection principles

Every effort should be made to keep the dose received by the public and responders including health care providers as low as possible.[31] This is known as the ALARA

Table 3
Conversion between SI Units and units traditionally used in the United States

SI Units	Units Used in the United States	Conversion
Gray (Gy)	Rad	1 Gy = 100 Rad
Sievert (Sv)	Rem	1 Sv = 100 Rem
Becquerel (Bq)	Curie (Ci)	1 Bq = 1/3.7 $\times$ 10^{10} Ci

principle where ALARA is an abbreviation for "As Low As Reasonably Achievable."[32] Exposure to radiation during a specific activity can be decreased by limiting its duration and by maximizing the distance between the person and the source of radiation. In fact, the radiation dose is inversely proportional to the square of the distance from the source. At times, shielding from the radiation is possible, using plastics, concrete or lead (for all types of radiation except neutrons).[33]

Emergency department staff members who initially evaluate patients contaminated with radioactive material (first receivers) should work closely with the hospital radiation safety officer or nuclear medicine technologists, who are an integral part of the team receiving patients in a dedicated area of the emergency department. The radiation safety officer or nuclear medicine technologist advises staff on the following items:

- Set up of the work area (also called a radiation emergency area)
- Necessary level of personal protective equipment, including the need for a higher level of respiratory precautions
- Use of personal dosimeters to monitor the occupational dose received
- Level of contamination detected on patients
- Extent and efficacy of decontamination procedures
- Shielding, storage, and disposal of waste, including patient contaminated belongings or waste water

Personal protective equipment protects staff from becoming externally and or internally contaminated with radioactive material during the care of patients. Unfortunately, it does not protect staff from exposure to gamma radiation emitted from the patients' body, skin surface, or clothing. Maximizing the distance from the patient and minimizing the time of exposure to the radiation source can significantly decrease the radiation dose received by the first responders or receivers.[34]

Providers use appropriate garments that cover their skin, mouth, and eyes. Respiratory protection should be in the form of a full-face piece air purifying respirator with a P-100 or high-efficiency particulate air (HEPA) filter. Based on initial assessment of the level and extent of external contamination, the radiation safety officer can advise on whether a lower level of respiratory protection using an N-95 or surgical mask are appropriate.[34] Although health care providers may be concerned about secondary hazards of caring for patients who are contaminated with radioactive material, the risk posed to them is minimal and should not delay the performance of life-saving medical evaluation and interventions.

- Mr Alexander Litvinenko came into contact with 43 health care providers during his 3-week illness who were not aware of the cause of his illness. These providers used standard precautions during their contact with the victim and were tested for internal contamination after his death. Using a 24-h urine collection bioassay, none were found to have been internally contaminated with any significant amount of polonium that would expose them to a radiation dose above the acceptable dose limit to the public.[12]
- Patients who were contaminated with cesium-137 during the Goiania incident, were treated by health care providers who were using standard precautions for several weeks. During this incident, providers used standard precautions and respiratory precautions were not deemed necessary.[35]

Radiation dose limits
Dose limits to the public and workers including emergency responders and health care providers are determined using a conservative assessment of the risk of clinical effects after exposure to a specific radiation dose. The goal of these limits is to serve

as a guideline for assessing the risk from a dose and should include consideration of the duration and nature of the activity during which the dose would be received. For example, the recommended dose limit to the public is 1 mSv. The occupational total effective dose equivalent annual limit to a worker is 50 mSv.[36,37]

In an emergency, the National Council on Radiation Protection and Measurements (NCRP) does not set a dose limit dose when performing life-saving activities. Instead, it lists a cumulative dose of 0.5 Gy as a decision point at which the team leader or incident commander needs to consider various aspects of this specific response and decide accordingly how to proceed.[31]

Decontamination

After the patient's emergent, life-threatening conditions are stabilized, the patient is surveyed for contamination with radioactive material. Contaminated clothes are removed carefully and stored away in a double (usually plastic) bag for possible later analysis and forensics if necessary. Removal of clothing eliminates any contamination deposited on the garments.

The radiation survey is then repeated to locate any facial orifice, skin, or wound contamination. If radiation is detected, decontamination of the nose/mouth, skin, and/or wound follows using soap and water. The goal of decontaminating the skin is to decrease the risk of additional intake of radioactive material into the body and to decrease the radiation exposure to the skin (eg, when the radioactive material emits beta particles or gamma rays) and internal organs (eg, when the radioactive material emits gamma rays). Decontamination also decreases the risk to health care providers of being exposed to radiation or becoming secondarily contaminated with radioactive material.

After decontaminating the skin, the radiation survey is repeated. Additional decontamination can be performed if persistent contamination is detected. However, this process can be discontinued when the level of contamination ceases to decrease or when the decontamination procedure starts to cause any e trauma to the skin (eg, erythema, abrasions). The survey detection and decontamination procedures are covered in other publications and are demonstrated in accompanying online videos.[38,39]

Health care providers should also decontaminate wounds that are contaminated with radioactive material by irrigation with saline, with care taken to ensure no additional tissue trauma. Gross foreign bodies should be removed using a forceps. Because foreign bodies can be radioactive, they should be placed in a specimen bag or, preferably, a leaded container and saved in an isolated location for later analysis and proper disposal. If a repeat radiation survey of the wound fails to show additional decrease in the amount of radiation detected, decontamination should cease and the wound should be repaired as medically indicated without significant regard for the contamination.

Diagnosis and Assessment of Internal Contamination

After the patient's external surface is decontaminated, the clinician needs to assess whether the patient is internally contaminated with radioactive material. The clinician also needs to consider whether the patient is at risk of developing ARS. The ARS component of the assessment is covered in previous publications and will not be discussed in this paper.[23,40]

The goal of assessing for internal contamination is to determine whether the patient has taken up enough of the material to deliver a significant dose of radiation to the body or to specific organs like the thyroid gland in the case of radioactive iodine.

The clinical concern is for deterministic diseases like ARS or stochastic consequences like cancer. These result from the cumulative radiation dose absorbed by the body or a specific organ over the duration of residency of the element inside the body. The duration of radiation exposure is influenced in part by the physical and biological half-lives, as discussed. Consequently, the clinician considers therapies that facilitate the removal of the radioactive material and therefore mitigate the radiation dose absorbed by the patient.

External contamination is associated with a greater risk of concomitant internal contamination. Detecting radioactive material on 2 swabs of both nasal cavities can point toward internal contamination by inhalation. Unfortunately, this method is not practical for a large number of patients after a mass casualty incident. Additionally, the natural variation is nasal cavity size, the delay before evaluation and the natural nasal mucosa clearance rates make this method less favorable than in the occupational setting where it is used traditionally.

Once the patient is no longer externally contaminated, the presence, identity, and amount of radioactive material inside the body can be measured directly by using an external radiation detector when the element emits gamma rays. There are currently several radiation detectors that can be used for this purpose by a radiation safety specialist. Examples of these detectors are whole body counters, and some hand-held instruments. Additionally, hospital nuclear medicine departments potentially have equipment that can be adapted and used for the diagnosis of internal contamination and internal dose assessment in an emergency. Examples of such equipment include thyroid scanner and gamma cameras used in positron emission tomography scanning technology and cardiology departments performing stress tests. Additional guidance on the use of hospital equipment to detect internal contamination is available at the US Centers for Disease Control and Prevention website.[41] It is important to note that radioactive chemicals that decay by emitting only beta particles or alpha particles cannot be detected in this manner.

Alternatively, the amount of internalized material can be measured indirectly by using a urinary or fecal bioassay. Ideally, a 24-hour urine or feces collection can be used to produce a measurement of the activity of the specific radioactive element per liter of urine or feces. The Centers for Disease Control and Prevention has developed relatively rapid assays that can use a spot urine sample and measure the activity of several radionuclides. The activity measured in the urine can be then compared to guidance values (eg, clinical decision guide [CDG]) that translates into a radiation dose. The Centers for Disease Control and Prevention has developed a downloadable android and iOS application that can be used by clinicians for this purpose.[42] Using this assessment, the clinician can better determine the risk from the contamination and potential management options if available.[43]

Use of the clinical decision guide

The CDG has been defined by the NCRP (2008) as the maximum once-in-a-lifetime intake (in Bq) of a radionuclide that represents a stochastic risk and avoidance of deterministic effects. The CDG is a tool intended to guide physicians during their assessment of the clinical significance of a specific radionuclide intake by a patient. The NCRP states that the objective of using a CDG is "to reduce the risk of stochastic effects, cancer, to a level consistent with current regulatory guidance for responding to emergency situations and to prevent the risks of deterministic effects."[44] When a patient intake of a specific radionuclide is greater than the corresponding CDG value, decorporation therapy can be used, if one exists for the radionuclide in question. Additionally, the patient will be monitored long term for the development of any clinical consequences like cancer. The CDG values for children and pregnant females are set at a more protective level (one fifth of the CDG adult values). The duration of exposure for a child is assumed to be 70 years as opposed to 50 years for adults.

Use of the annual limit on intake

Before the introduction of the CDG by the NCRP in its report number 161, the annual limit on intake (ALI) values were relied on to assess the significance of a potential contamination with a radioactive chemical. This value is still used by radiation experts to assess the severity of an intake although it is primarily an annual regulatory limit used for workers. The Health Physics Society defines the ALI as follows: "The derived limit for the permissible amount of radioactive material taken into the body of an adult radiation worker by inhalation or ingestion in a year. The ALI is the smaller value of intake of a given radionuclide in a year by the reference man that would result in either a committed effective dose of 50 mSv or a committed equivalent dose of 500 mSv to any individual organ or tissue."[45]

Note that the CDG relates to a total body committed effective dose of 250 mSv compared with a committed effective dose of 50 mSv for the ALI. The CDG also relates to a single intake over a lifetime, whether the ALI relates to the limit on an annual intake of a specific radionuclide. The CDG value was created to assist clinicians in determining whether a certain amount of radioactive chemical inside the body is significant clinically during an emergency. The ALI is more useful when evaluating workers who may have become contaminated with a radioactive chemical.

Management Strategies for Internal Contamination

The management of internal contamination includes, in addition to supportive care, measures to decrease the radiation dose that is delivered to body organs and tissues. This measurement can be achieved by decreasing the absorption of the radioactive element from the gastrointestinal tract, the lungs, or an open wound, enhancing excretion in urine or feces, or blocking incorporation into specific organs.

The use of gastric lavage, charcoal, and cathartics are not well-studied. They are possibly efficacious when the route is via ingestion and when the patient presents for care shortly after the incident. Additionally, bronchoalveolar lavage is recommended in specific situations in which a patient has inhaled a large amount of insoluble forms of a radioactive element like plutonium oxide that is absorbed poorly through the pulmonary epithelium and can cause local damage instead. Because of the complexity of this procedure, it is unlikely to be used except in rare circumstances.[44]

Specific Therapies

Certain radioactive elements can be amenable to specific additional therapies. Currently, the US Food and Drug Administration (FDA) has approved the use of the following drugs for the treatment of internal contamination with a specific set of radioactive elements (**Table 4**):

- Prussian blue (**Fig. 1**)
    - Prussian blue-insoluble is currently approved by the FDA for the treatment of internal contamination with radioactive cesium and thallium (radioactive and nonradioactive). More commonly, it is used for nonradioactive thallium poisoning. The drug is administered orally and binds cesium or thallium in the intestinal tract during enterohepatic circulation. The resulting complex shifts excretion from the urine to the feces reducing the effective time of residence of the radioactive element inside the body and secondary radiation dose delivered to the body. The dose in adults is 3 g every 8 hours for at least

Table 4
Therapies approved by the US Food and Drug Administration

Drug	Indication	Dose	End Point	Pediatric	Pregnancy Category	Precautions and Adverse Effects	Available Forms
Prussian Blue	Internal contamination with radioactive Cesium	3 g PO, every 8 h	30 d of therapy, guided by urinary and fecal excretion of cesium	1 g PO every 8 h	C	Constipation Hypokalemia Bluish discoloration of sweat and feces Bluish discoloration of teeth when capsule is ruptured in the mouth	Radiogardase Available through the United States Strategic National Stockpile
Calcium DTPA Pentetate Calcium Trisodium	Internal contamination with plutonium, americium, and curium	1 g IV or by nebulizer every 24 h	Duration of therapy guided by urinary excretion of the radionuclide	14 mg/kg IV per day not to exceed 1 g per day	C; zinc DTPA is preferred	Depletion of essential minerals like zinc Bronchoconstriction in asthmatic receiving the dose by nebulizer	Available through the United States Strategic National Stockpile
Zinc DTPA Pentetate Zinc Trisodium	Internal contamination with plutonium, americium, and curium	1 g IV every 24 h	Duration of therapy guided by urinary excretion of the radionuclide	14 mg/kg per day, not to exceed 1 g per day	C	Adverse effects not common Headache, lightheadedness, and pelvic reported by one patient who received Zn DTPA	Available through the United States Strategic National Stockpile
Potassium Iodide	Prevent uptake of radioactive iodine by the thyroid	Dose varies by age See FDA	Until risk of exposure to radioactive iodine has gone away	Dose varies by age See FDA	C	Hypothyroidism GI Upset Rash	Over the Counter Thyroshield Thyrosafe Iosat

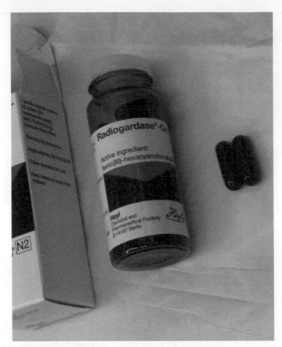

Fig. 1. Prussian blue.

30 days. The duration of therapy is guided by the amount of radioactive cesium or thallium that is being removed.[46]

- Pentetate calcium trisodium (calcium DTPA) and pentetate zinc trisodium (Zinc DTPA; **Fig. 2**)[47,48]
  - Calcium and zinc DTPA are currently approved by the FDA for the treatment of internal contamination with americium, plutonium, and curium. These drugs enhance the renal elimination of these elements when internalized. The dose is 1 g IV every 24 hours. The duration of therapy is guided by the amount of radioactive material that is being removed from the body. Calcium DTPA may also be given by nebulizer. Calcium DTPA is preferred over zinc DTPA during the initial 24 hours after contamination. Zinc DTPA is preferred over calcium DTPA in pregnant women and children owing to the concern for associated depletion of essential elements like manganese and zinc.
- Potassium iodide
  - Potassium iodide (KI) is used to saturate the thyroid gland with stable iodine and prevent additional subsequent uptake of radioactive iodine. To be efficacious, KI should be taken shortly before or shortly after the internalization of radioactive iodine. It can also be given before a potential exposure or internal contamination. The dose of KI depends on the age of the patient. Children younger than 18 years of age and pregnant women (because of the fetus they are carrying) are more vulnerable to the effects of radioactive iodine and should be prioritized to receiving this therapy when indicated.[49,50]
  - The recent nuclear power plant accident in Fukushima highlighted the common misconception that KI is an antiradiation pill. Many people took KI without any proper indication. These actions can cause harm to patients and need to be mitigated by proactive public health messaging.[51]

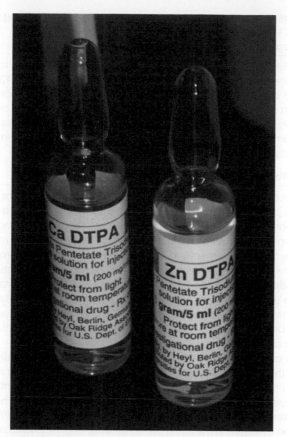

Fig. 2. Calcium and zinc diethylenetriamine pentaacetic acid (DTPA).

There are other drugs available that are FDA approved for other indications that are not related to internal contamination. The use of these drugs would be off-label in these situations (**Table 5**). Last, increasing urinary output increases the elimination of internalized tritium, which behaves inside the body primarily like water does.[52] On the other hand, alkalinizing the urine can be used to prevent the renal toxicity from internalized uranium. As mentioned, toxicity from internal contamination with isotopes of uranium is generally chemical and not related to emitted radiation.[53,54]

Table 5
Some of the therapies recommended by the National Council for Radiation Protection and Measurements report number 161 and the Radiation Emergency Assistance Center and Training Site

Drug	Indication
Alginates	Internal contamination with radioactive strontium
British anti-Lewisite (BAL)	Internal contamination with polonium
N-Acetylcysteine	Internal contamination with radioactive cobalt

These therapies are not approved by the US Food and Drug Administration.

SPECIAL CONSIDERATIONS REGARDING CHILDREN, PREGNANT WOMEN, AND BREASTFEEDING WOMEN
Children and Pregnant Women

A child and the fetus carried by pregnant woman are more sensitive to the stochastic effects of radiation. For example, internal contamination with iodine-131 is more likely to cause thyroid cancer in children compared with adults.[55] Therefore, children and pregnant women should be prioritized during the implementation of protective action measures like evacuation and KI administration. Additionally, when assessing the level of internal contamination, the CDG used is 20% of the value used in an adult. Last, dose adjustments need to be followed for available drug therapies.

Breastfeeding Women

Breastfeeding is extremely beneficial to nursing infants and mothers and is encouraged by several professional organizations and societies.[56,57] After a radiologic incident that involves the dispersal of radioactive material in the environment, breastfeeding women can become internally contaminated with 1 or more radioactive elements. Some of these elements, depending on their biokinetic properties, can be transferred to the child in the breast milk. This can lead to the internal contamination of the child. Additionally, the child can be secondarily exposed to radiation emitted from the mother's body during breastfeeding if she is internally contaminated with a radioactive element that emits gamma rays. These conditions may lead to the recommendation that breastfeeding be temporarily discontinued if alternative noncontaminated foods are available.[58]

However, the child is usually at a similar risk of becoming internally contaminated like the mother through other routes. For this reason, breastfeeding may be acceptable especially if no other source of food is available including noncontaminated water to prepare formula. Ideally, the level of internal contamination in the mother should be assessed to determine the expected amount in breast milk. Unfortunately, this information will not be available in the initial period of an emergency. Breastfeeding recommendations and guidance will need to be made by public health officials using the best evidence available to them.

Long-Term Monitoring

Victims involved in a radiologic emergency need to be monitored for a number of health effects, some of which may be tracked for several decades. For example, the Radiation Effects Research Foundation is tracking the health of the Hiroshima and Nagasaki atomic bomb survivors.[59] Additionally, victims who were exposed to radiation during the recent nuclear power plant accident in Fukushima, Japan, will be monitored for health effects for several years to come. This process is complex and requires a national plan that includes participation from a large number of stakeholders.

Risk Communication

Patients involved in a radiologic emergency have been subjected to a variety of stressors and likely display signs and symptoms that are at times out of proportion to the degree and severity of their injuries. Many of these patients are at risk for mental illness, as seen after previous incidents such as the nuclear power plant in Chernobyl in 1986.[60] Additionally, a disproportionate number of concerned uninjured survivors will present to emergency departments for evaluation and reassurance. For example, after the criticality accident in Tokai Mura, Japan (1999), that led to 2 fatalities (out of 3 workers who were involved in the accident), approximately 75,000 people were monitored for contamination with radioactive material and 1844 were provided with a medical evaluation.[61]

The emergency physician who is caring for these patients will need to be skilled at risk communication. The article by McCormick discusses psychological aspects of radiologic disasters. Additionally, the physician can seek assistance from experts in the area of radiation exposure that are available in his hospital or state. The Radiation Emergency Assistance and Training Site is also available to offer medical advice and should be contacted when necessary.

SUMMARY

Internal contamination with radioactive material can expose patients to radiation leading to short- and long-term clinical consequences. After the patient's emergency conditions are addressed and the skin is decontaminated, the treating physicians assess the amount of radioactive material that has been internalized. This evaluation allows the estimation of the radiation dose that is delivered the specific radionuclide inside the body and supports the need for additional therapies and monitoring. These complex assessments warrant the reliance on a multidisciplinary approach that incorporates local, regional, and national experts in radiation medicine and emergencies.

ACKNOWLEDGMENTS

The authors acknowledge the following individuals for their contributions to this paper: Dr Adam Pomerleau and Mr Paul Charp, from the Centers for Disease Control and Prevention.

REFERENCES

1. National Planning Guidelines. The United States Federal Emergency Management Agency. Accessed July 28, 2014. Available at: http://www.fema.gov/pdf/emergency/nrf/National_Preparedness_Guidelines.pdf. Published in 2007.
2. Balicer RD, Catlett CL, Barnett DJ, et al. Characterizing hospital workers' willingness to respond to a radiological event. PLoS One 2011;6(10):e25327. http://dx.doi.org/10.1371/journal.pone.0025327.
3. Watson CM, Barnett DJ, Thompson CB, et al. Characterizing public health emergency perceptions and influential modifiers of willingness to respond among pediatric healthcare staff. Am J Disaster Med 2011;6(5):299–308.
4. Errett NA, Barnett DJ, Thompson CB, et al. Assessment of medical reserve corps volunteers' emergency response willingness using a threat- and efficacy-based model. Biosecur Bioterror 2013;11(1):29–40. http://dx.doi.org/10.1089/bsp.2012.0047.
5. Sheikh S, McCormick LC, Pevear J, et al. Radiological preparedness-awareness and attitudes: a cross-sectional survey of emergency medicine residents and physicians at three academic institutions in the United States. Clin Toxicol (Phila) 2012;50(1):34–8. http://dx.doi.org/10.3109/15563650.2011.637047.
6. Sadigh G, Khan R, Kassin MT, et al. Radiation safety knowledge and perceptions among residents: a potential improvement opportunity for graduate medical education in the United States. Acad Radiol 2014;21(7):869–78. http://dx.doi.org/10.1016/j.acra.2014.01.016.
7. Natural Sources of Radiation. The United States Centers for Disease Control and Prevention. Available at: http://www.cdc.gov/nceh/radiation/natural.htm. Accessed July 28, 2014. Page last updated: March 10, 2014.

8. Press Release. The International Atomic Energy Agency. Available at: http://www.iaea.org/newscenter/pressreleases/2002/prn0209.shtml. Accessed February 5, 2014. Published September 2002.

9. Video: Radiological Contamination and Exposure. The United States Centers for Disease Control and Prevention. Available at: http://www.bt.cdc.gov/radiation/resourcelibrary/all.asp. Accessed June 17, 2014.

10. The Radiological Incident in Goiania, Brazil (1987). The International Atomic Energy Agency. Available at: http://www-pub.iaea.org/MTCD/publications/PDF/Pub815_web.pdf. Accessed April 21, 2014. Published in 1988.

11. Fuini SC, Souto R, Amaral GF, et al. Quality of life in individuals exposed to cesium-137 in Goiânia, Goiás State, Brazil. Cad Saude Publica 2013;29(7): 1301–10.

12. Fraser G, Giraudon I, Cohuet S, et al. Epidemiology of internal contamination with polonium-210 in the London incident, 2006. J Epidemiol Community Health 2012; 66(2):114–20.

13. Miller CW, Whitcomb RC, Ansari A, et al. Murder by radiation poisoning: implications for public health. J Environ Health 2012;74(10):8–13.

14. Trivedi A. Percutaneous absorption of tritium-gas-contaminated pump oil. Health Phys 1995;69(2):202–9.

15. The National Council on Radiation Protection and Measurements Report Number 161 Volume I, page 29.

16. Biological Half life of Iodine in Normal and Athyroidic persons. The Los Alamos National Laboratory. Available at: http://www.lanl.gov/BAER-Conference/BAERCon-46p027.htm. Accessed May 16, 2014.

17. Farina R, Brandão-Mello CE, Oliveira AR. Medical aspects of 137Cs decorporation: the Goiânia radiological accident. Health Phys 1991;60(1):63–6.

18. Toxicological Profile for Strontium. The Agency for Toxic Substances and Disease Registry. Available at: http://www.atsdr.cdc.gov/ToxProfiles/tp159.pdf. Appendix D page 4. Accessed June 16, 2014.

19. Iodine. The United States Environmental Protection Agency. Available at: http://www.epa.gov/radiation/radionuclides/iodine.html. Accessed June 17, 2014. Last updated on 3/6/2012.

20. Cesium. The United States Environmental Protection Agency. Available at: http://www.epa.gov/rpdweb00/radionuclides/cesium.html. Accessed June 17, 2014. Last updated on 3/6/2012.

21. Effective Half Life. The Health Physics Society. Available at: http://hps.org/publicinformation/radterms/radfact64.html. Accessed June 17, 2014. Last updated 27 August 2011.

22. Hall EJ, Giaccia AJ. Radiobiology for the radiologist. 7th edition. Philadelphia: Lippincott Williams & Wilkins; 2012.

23. Christensen DM, Iddins CJ, Sugarman SL. Ionizing radiation injuries and illnesses. Emerg Med Clin North Am 2014;32(1):245–65. http://dx.doi.org/10.1016/j.emc.2013.10.002.

24. The International Atomic Energy Agency. Available at: http://www.iaea.org/Publications/Factsheets/English/polonium210.html. Accessed June 17, 2014.

25. Radiation Terms and Definitions. The Health Physics Society. Available at: http://www.hps.org/publicinformation/radterms. Accessed May 16, 2014. Last updated 27 August 2011.

26. Quality Factor. The Health Physics Society. Available at: http://hps.org/publicinformation/radterms/radfact116.html. Accessed May 16, 2014. Last updated 27 August 2011.

27. International Commission on Radiological Protection (ICRP). 1990 recommenda-tions of the international commission on radiological Protection. ICRP Publication 60. Pergamon Press; 1991. Ann. ICRP 21 (1-3).
28. Exclusive Use of the S.I. Units to Express Radiological Quantities. Position State-ment of the Health Physics Society. The United States Health Physics Society. Available at: http://hps.org/documents/SIunits_ps025-0.pdf. Accessed June 17, 2014. Adapted February 2012.
29. The National Council on Radiation Protection and Measurements Report Number 161, 2011 Volume I, Page 14.
30. Pavlakis N, Pollock CA, McLean G, et al. Deliberate overdose of uranium: toxicity and treatment. Nephron 1996;72(2):313–7.
31. The National Council on Radiation Protection and Measurements Report Number 165. Section 3.2.2, Pages 20, 21.
32. As Low As Reasonably Achievable (ALARA). The Health Physics Society. Avail-able at: http://www.hps.org/publicinformation/radterms/radfact1.html. Last up-dated August 27, 2011. Accessed June 20, 2014.
33. The Medical Aspects of Radiation Incidents. The Radiation Emergency Assistance Center/Training Site. Available at: http://orise.orau.gov/files/reacts/medical-aspects-of-radiation-incidents.pdf. Accessed June 20, 2014. Revised 9/25/2013.
34. Personal Protective Equipment (PPE) in a Radiation Emergency. Radiation Emer-gency Medical Management. Available at: http://www.remm.nlm.gov/radiation_ppe.htm#firstresponder. Accessed May 27, 2014. Last updated May 4, 2014.
35. Oliveira AR, Hunt JG, Valverde NJ, et al. Medical and related aspects of the Goiâ-nia accident: an overview. Health Phys 1991;60(1):17–24.
36. Regulatory Dose Limits. The Health Physics Society. Available at: http://www.hps.org/publicinformation/ate/faqs/regdoselimits.html. Accessed June 20, 2014. Last updated December 7, 2013.
37. NRC Regulations 10 Code of Federal Regulations. The Nuclear Regulatory Com-mission. Available at: http://www.nrc.gov/reading-rm/doc-collections/cfr/part020/part020-1201.html. Accessed June 20, 2014. Last updated July 21, 2014.
38. Procedure Demonstrations. The Radiation Emergency Assistance/Training Site. Available at: http://orise.orau.gov/reacts/guide/procedures.htm. Accessed June 20, 2014.
39. Radiation Basics Made Simple. The Centers for Disease Control and Prevention. Available at: http://orau.gov/rsb/radbasics. Accessed June 20, 2014.
40. Donnelly EH, Nemhauser JB, Smith JM, et al. Acute radiation syndrome: assess-ment and management. Southampt Med J 2010;103(6):541–6. http://dx.doi.org/10.1097/SMJ.0b013e3181ddd571.
41. Use of Radiation Detection, Measuring, and Imaging Instruments to Assess Inter-nal Contamination from Intakes of Radionuclides. The Centers for Disease Control and Prevention. Available at: http://emergency.cdc.gov/radiation/clinicians/evaluation. Accessed June 20, 2014.
42. Internal Contamination Clinical Reference Application. The Centers for Disease Control and Prevention. Available at: http://emergency.cdc.gov/radiation/iccr.asp. Accessed June 20, 2014.
43. Pillai SK, Chang A, Murphy MW, et al. 2011 investigation of internal contamination with radioactive strontium following rubidium Rb 82 cardiac PET scan. Biosecur Bioterror 2014;12(1):42–8. http://dx.doi.org/10.1089/bsp.2013.0072.
44. Management of Persons Contaminated with Radionuclides: Handbook. The Na-tional Council on Radiation Protection and Measurements Report Number 161 Volume I (2008) pages 6, 179.

45. Annual Limit on Intake. The Health Physics Society. Available at: http://hps.org/publicinformation/radterms/radfact30.html. Accessed May 27, 2014. Last updated August 27, 2011.

46. Prussian Blue. The United States Centers for Disease Control and Prevention. Available at: http://www.bt.cdc.gov/radiation/prussianblue.asp. Accessed June 26, 2014. Last update February 2014.

47. DTPA (Diethylenetriamine pentaacetate). The United States Centers for Disease Control and Prevention. Available at: http://www.bt.cdc.gov/radiation/dtpa.asp. Accessed June 26, 2014. Last updated August 22, 2013.

48. Kazzi ZN, Heyl A, Ruprecht J. Calcium and zinc DTPA administration for internal contamination with plutonium-238 and americium-241. Curr Pharm Biotechnol 2012;13(10):1957–63.

49. Potassium Iodide. The United States Centers for Disease Control and Prevention. Available at: http://emergency.cdc.gov/radiation/ki.asp. Accessed June 26, 2014. Last updated February 4, 2014.

50. Guidance Potassium Iodide as a Thyroid Blocking Agent in Radiation Emergencies. The United State Food and Drug Administration. Available at: http://www.fda.gov/downloads/Drugs/GuidanceComplianceRegulatoryInformation/Guidances/UCM080542.pdf. Accessed July 28, 2014

51. Law RK, Schier JG, Martin CA, et al. National surveillance for radiological exposures and intentional potassium iodide and iodine product ingestions in the United States associated with the 2011 Japan radiological incident. Clin Toxicol (Phila) 2013;51(1):41–6. http://dx.doi.org/10.3109/15563650.2012.732701.

52. Tritium. The Health Physics Society. Available at: http://hps.org/documents/tritium_fact_sheet.pdf. Accessed June 26, 2014. Published March 2011.

53. Fatome M. Management of accidental internal exposure. J Radiol 1994;75(11):571–5.

54. Agency for Toxic Substances Disease Registry (ATSDR). Case studies in Environmental medicine (CSEM). Uranium toxicity. Atlanta (GA): US Department of Health and Human Services, Public Health Service; 2009. Available at: http://www.atsdr.cdc.gov/csem/uranium/docs/uranium.pdf.

55. The Chernobyl Accident. The United Nations Scientific Committee on the Effects of Atomic Radiation. Available at: http://www.unscear.org/unscear/en/chernobyl.html. Accessed June 11, 2014.

56. Breastfeeding. The American Congress of Obstetricians and Gynecologists. Available at: http://www.acog.org/About_ACOG/ACOG_Departments/Breastfeeding. Accessed June 26, 2014.

57. Breastfeeding. The American Academy of Pediatrics. Available at: http://www2.aap.org/breastfeeding. Accessed June 26, 2014.

58. Gartner LM, Morton J, Lawrence RA, et al. American Academy of Pediatrics Section on Breastfeeding. Breastfeeding and the use of human milk. Pediatrics 2005;115(2):496–506.

59. The Radiation Effects Research Foundation. Available at: http://www.rerf.jp/index_e.html. Accessed June 13, 2014.

60. Bromet EJ. Mental health consequences of the Chernobyl disaster. J Radiol Prot 2012;32(1):N71–5. http://dx.doi.org/10.1088/0952-4746/32/1/N71.

61. Lessons Learned from the JCO Nuclear Criticality Accident in Japan in 1999. The International Atomic Energy Agency. Available at: http://www-ns.iaea.org/downloads/iec/tokaimura-report.pdf. Accessed June 16, 2014.

Mental Health Consequences of Chemical and Radiologic Emergencies

A Systematic Review

Lisa C. MCCormick, DrPH[a],*, Gabriel S. Tajeu, MPH[a],
Joshua Klapow, PhD[a,b]

KEYWORDS

- Mental health • Disasters • Psychological impacts • Somatic symptoms
- Psychosocial interventions

KEY POINTS

- Mental health assessments should focus on identifying the spectrum of problems ranging from moderate distress to acute psychiatric illness in disaster-affected groups.
- Clinical mental health assessment following technological disasters is resource intensive; therefore, it is necessary to keep screening methods uncomplicated and broad based.
- Minimally, assessments should cover the individual's disaster experience, a brief mental status examination, and history of preexisting disorders, and other trauma exposures/stressors.
- Triage should identify those who need immediate linkage to formal mental health intervention, treatment, or care.
- Informal psychosocial community interactions should not be used in place of formal treatment of those who are at risk of developing more serious psychological illnesses.

INTRODUCTION

A disaster can be defined as any event that causes substantial loss of life, physical damage, or widespread change in the environment and leads to economic, political, and social consequences.[1–3] The United Nations expands the definition to include the inability of the affected community to cope with the aftermath.[1] Researchers differentiate disasters into two distinct categories: natural versus technological or manmade. Natural disasters are caused by naturally occurring events, such as hurricanes,

Disclosure Statement: The authors have nothing to disclose.
[a] Department of Health Care Organization and Policy, University of Alabama at Birmingham School of Public Health, RPHB 330, 1720 Second Avenue South, Birmingham, AL 35294–0022, USA; [b] Chip Rewards, Inc, 2901 2nd Avenue South, Suite 210, Birmingham, AL 35233, USA
* Corresponding author.
E-mail address: lmccormick@uab.edu

Emerg Med Clin N Am 33 (2015) 197–211
http://dx.doi.org/10.1016/j.emc.2014.09.012
0733-8627/15/$ – see front matter © 2015 Elsevier Inc. All rights reserved.

earthquakes, or tsunamis. Technological disasters, however, are the result of man-made processes, triggered by human error or accidents. Examples include oil spills, releases of radioactive isotopes, and chemical spills.

Although disasters can have considerable impact on physical wellness, property, and economics, they also can have significant and far-reaching psychosocial impacts. The primary focus of most disaster responses generally concentrates on physical damage, whereas emotional and psychological effects in the affected population are often overlooked.[4] An increase in symptoms of psychological distress and psychiatric illness, including substance abuse and domestic violence, tends to follow most major natural and technological disasters. Examples of specific disasters where increased symptoms were documented include Hurricane Katrina, the 2004 Indian Ocean tsunami, the Deepwater Horizon oil spill in the Gulf of Mexico, and the September 11, 2001 terrorist attacks.[4-6] Even though the increase in psychological distress and psychiatric symptomatology in the aftermath of disasters has been well documented, the consequences of these increases have not received extensive emergency planning consideration in the United States. This is despite a consensus among most experts that disasters result in a substantial psychological burden for those affected[1,7-9] and that early behavioral health interventions should be routinely incorporated into the response to disasters.[4,10] For instance, the 2006 Chernobyl Forum Report evaluating the effects of the Chernobyl nuclear disaster concluded that mental health was the most common public health problem unleashed by the accident, with issues including depression, anxiety, posttraumatic stress disorder, medically unexplained somatic symptoms, and stigma.[1,11,12]

Although attention has been given to the mental health effects of natural disasters,[13] there is a more limited, albeit growing, literature on the mental health effects of technological disasters, specifically those resulting from chemical and radiologic releases. This article provides a comprehensive review of the literature on the immediate psychological and mental health consequences that emergency department physicians and first responders may encounter in the aftermath of a technological disaster. A disaster does not need to be as severe as those of Bhopal or Fukushima to result in a significantly large, affected population. First responders and first receivers can see a wide spectrum of psychological distress, including acute onset of psychiatric disorders, the exacerbation of existing psychological and psychiatric conditions, and widespread symptomatology even in the absence of a diagnosable disorder. Furthermore, the informal community support systems that may exist after a natural disaster may not be available to communities affected by a technological disaster, leading to a need for more formal mental health supportive services.[2,14]

Estimates suggest that much of the population of the United States will be exposed to a natural or technological disaster in their lifetime. The immediate and lasting trauma from these disasters has underlined the need for not only an effective community response to immediate physical effects, but also mental health effects.[10,15] The importance of integrating mental health into disaster preparedness response plans has become more recognized since the September 11, 2001 terrorist attacks and the Fukushima Daiichi nuclear power plant accident.[16-18] Recent advances in the recognition and understanding of the mental health consequences of disasters have led to advancements in individual treatment options, population-based approaches, and public health intervention strategies for disaster-affected communities.[19] However, most of the literature has historically focused on the mental health consequences after natural disasters as opposed to technological disasters, such as chemical or radiologic releases, resulting in general guidelines developed to help prepare for and respond to most disasters in a homogenized all-hazard fashion. This is despite that reasons exist to look at the mental health effects of technological disasters differently.[1,20,21]

AGENTS OF TOXICITY AND CLINICAL MANIFESTATIONS
Psychological Effects of Natural and Technological Disasters

Natural and technological disasters differ substantially in their psychological effects (**Table 1**). Most regard natural disasters as "acts of God" that cannot be prevented, but can only be mitigated and endured.[2] In areas that are particularly prone to natural disasters, formal and informal frameworks exist that allow community members to assist each other in preparation and recovery. For instance, in areas where hurricanes and wildfires are common, community members may assist each other in preparing homes for evacuation. A subculture forms where community volunteers and laymen assist in preventative and recovery-based efforts. This presence of a disaster subculture can then culminate into the development of a therapeutic community that represents mass social and physical support.[13] Communities tend to bond for the good of all-social connectedness, which in turn fosters a return to predisaster conditions.[22]

Technological disasters, however, are the result of man-made processes. Technological disasters are triggered by human error or accidents or by natural disasters. For instance, in 1984 more than 40 tons of methyl isocyanate gas leaked from a Union Carbide Corporation plant in Bhopal, India, immediately killing thousands of people. This accident was attributed to the lack of maintenance in the plant including faulty valves, lack of an operational scrubber, lack of a working refrigeration system, and an offline gas flare safety system.[23] It is estimated that more than 200,000 people were exposed to the methyl isocyanate gas with 50,000 suffering from long-term health effects.[24] Literature at the time identified an immediate need for mental health treatment of the affected population and the lack of formal and informal networks to aid victims. This disaster resulted in significant psychological distress including confusion, anxiety, depression reactions, and grief reactions, and in some cases reactive psychoses. These symptoms, when not addressed, increased the risk of more chronic conditions including posttraumatic stress disorders.[25]

Chemical and Radiologic Disasters

Although technological and natural disasters can result in widespread symptomatology, chemical and radiologic disasters may have a unique psychological footprint not seen after natural disasters. Chemical and radiologic disasters often occur without warning, produce unfamiliar or unknown health effects, and can pose more long-term threats to the community at large. Furthermore, chemical and radiologic events, compared with natural disasters, result in higher levels of fear and uncertainty about exposure and its health effects.[26] Increased feelings of blame, loss of control, and questions of self-esteem have been associated with technological disasters because these disasters are usually caused by malicious intent or human error.[27] Chemical and radiologic disasters can also uniquely pose specific dangers to children and prolonged effects to future generations. Because of this, the resulting psychiatric and psychosocial effects can be extensive and prolonged.[28] The Centers for Disease Control and Prevention has developed an online training module that focuses on the unique psychological effects of radiation disasters (http://www.orau.gov/RSB/RMH/).

Technological Disaster: A Spectrum of Response

Mild and moderate symptoms of distress (eg, fear, worry, anger, sleep difficulties, nightmares, emotional numbness, depressed mood, fatigue, increased use of tobacco

Table 1
Differences between natural and technological disasters

Natural Disasters	Technological Disasters
Naturally occurring events, such as hurricanes, earthquakes, or tsunamis; "acts of God"	Oil spills, chemical spills, radiologic disasters; result of man-made processes
Predisaster Considerations	
Individuals and communities may have ability to preplan for the disaster and its aftermath.	Usually no or minimal preplanning occurs and usually not at the individual level.
Community Effects	
Community offers immediate help to one another and resources are often pooled.	Outreach from others may be slow, waiting for an entity involved in the disaster to take responsibility; have to rely on community resources, which may be scarce or inadequate to meet the demands of the event.
Therapeutic community: community and individuals pull together for the good of all. High levels of community coordination and social connectedness.	Corrosive community: community and individual recovery is not the focus of the response; response and recovery efforts may be led by outsiders with little or no connection to the community; individuals develop fears of the ongoing consequences of the disaster leading to high levels of stress, anxiety, and conflict. Community members believe they have to seek out help; may be involved in long-term litigation; no social support systems and a lack of social connectedness; some individuals directly impacted may be eligible for recompense, whereas others may not, creating community conflicts.
Closure: closure is attainable and individuals and the community can rebuild toward a predisaster state.	Lack of closure: impacts of the disaster are long-term and often unknown, possible ongoing physical and mental health issues, economic and ecologic problems/damage.
Psychological Symptoms	
Continued stress following the disaster related to indirect effects of disaster including supply and housing shortages, job loss, and disruptions in daily life.	Continued stress following the disaster related to indirect effects of disaster including supply and housing shortages, job loss, and disruptions in daily life. This stress may be compounded because of lack of social support following technological disasters. High levels of fear and anxiety resulting from uncertainty about exposure and long-term health effects including birth defects. Increased feelings of blame, loss of control, and low self-esteem as a result of these disasters usually being caused by malicious intent or human error.

Adapted from Center L. Gulf oil spill: get the facts. 2014. Lakeview Center Baptist Healthcare, Pensacola, FL. Gulf oil spill: get the facts. Available at: https://www.santarosa.fl.gov/coad/documents/FactSheetNaturalDisasters.pdf.

or alcohol) following a disaster are common in most people.[19] **Table 2** presents selected conditions that may be relevant to disaster exposures and specific interventions that should be considered. Responses to traumatic events vary from person to person. Genetic differences, past experiences, and the social context of the event all interact with the specifics of the disaster including cause, intensity, duration of exposure, and the availability of medical and psychosocial support to determine psychological and behavioral responses in each individual.[13,29] Although distress symptoms may cause temporary decrements in psychosocial functioning, most people manage their distress following a disaster without treatment or intervention.

A subsection of the population with symptoms of distress may have more significant difficulties functioning in work, school, or home. Increased frequency and intensity of distress symptoms coupled with decrements in daily functioning are important criteria for the need of more formal psychological intervention. An even smaller portion of the population may see symptoms persist over time with continued and significant decrements in functioning. These individuals may go on to develop well-defined psychiatric illnesses including posttraumatic stress disorder or major depression requiring specialized treatment and follow-up.[30-34] Proximity, duration, and intensity of exposure to the disaster, and possibly the media coverage surrounding the disaster, may be significant predictors of mental health outcome severity.[19]

Fig. 1 presents a comparison of the psychological phases of natural and technological disasters. After the impact of a natural disaster, public confidence levels actually rise during what is considered the "heroic" phase, when community members form a therapeutic community and tend to assist and support each other, and peaks at what is considered the "honeymoon" phase, when volunteers from outside the community may be plentiful. At the conclusion of the honeymoon phase, public confidence tends to drop as those living in the affected area start to really understand and take inventory of the impact that they and their community have sustained. After any natural disaster, as fewer and fewer responders and volunteers from outside the community are

Table 2		
Mental health conditions associated with disaster exposure and corresponding mental health intervention recommendations		
	Disaster Response	
Condition	General Intervention Type	Specific Intervention[a]
Posttraumatic stress disorder	Psychotherapy	Cognitive-behavioral Exposure-based
	Pharmacotherapy	Antidepressants Adjunctive medications
Major depression	Psychotherapy	Cognitive-behavioral
	Pharmacotherapy	Antidepressants
Traumatic grief	Psychotherapy	—
	Pharmacotherapy	—
Psychological distress	Psychosocial interventions	Debriefing Psychoeducation Psychological first aid Crisis counseling
	Pharmacotherapy	—

[a] Please refer to the article for more information about literature sources for intervention recommendations.

Adapted from North CS, Pfefferbaum B. Mental health response to community disasters: a systematic review. JAMA 2013;310(5):507–18.

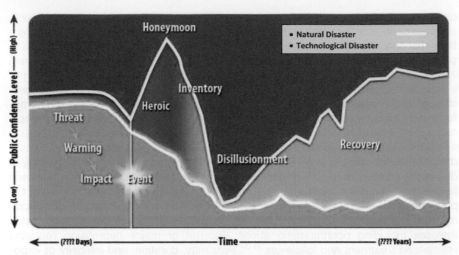

Fig. 1. Psychological phases of a disaster: differences between natural and technological disasters. (*Courtesy of* Centers for Disease Control and Prevention.)

available and as the realization that the community may not be able to immediately get back to a predisaster state, public confidence remains low in what is considered the "disillusionment" phase. But over time, public confidence begins to rise during recovery. This is not necessarily the case during technological disasters.

Because of the sudden onset of most technological disasters, there is usually little or no warning or preparation at the individual level. Additionally, after impact, no heroic or honeymoon phase is experienced because of a decreased willingness to respond to affected areas out of fear from environmental contamination and hazards. Public confidence tends to decrease straight into an extended "disillusionment" phase. Technological disasters can persist for extended periods of time with primary and secondary effects not observable for months or years.[5,11,12,23] Formal, organized outreach from others may be slow in coming to the affected communities as assessments of the situation continue and officials wait for the responsible party to take action. This delay can result in excess strain on public services. Past studies have shown emergency medicine residents and physicians do not feel adequately prepared to respond to some types of technological disaster[35,36] and that Medical Reserve Corps volunteers may not be willing to respond particularly to disasters involving radiologic materials.[37] Because of this, communities and individuals then may have to rely on limited community resources for an extended period of time, which may not be adequate to meet demands. During the assessment and triage stages, it is common to see collective community frustration and the rise of a lack of trust. As more agencies become involved, and to the extent that information is not disseminated, feelings of disruption and loss of control arise. Disrupted daily activities, changes to daily commerce, and an inability to meet routine needs lead to feelings of helplessness, isolation, and future uncertainty, all of which persist as the assessment of the disaster plays out.[22]

Technological Disasters and Sociogenic Illness

In addition to direct physical and mental health consequences for individuals, chemical and radiologic disasters can come with the added effect of somatic symptoms in unexposed or uninvolved populations, which may result in an added strain on the medical system.[1] Events occurring in or near schools and health care facilities seem to be particularly vulnerable to this phenomenon.[38] The presence of somatic symptoms en masse is sometimes called epidemic hysteria, or mass sociogenic illness, which describes the rapid spread of illness symptoms affecting members of a cohesive group despite no exposure.[39] However, there is no widely agreed on definition of mass sociogenic illness because previous studies are limited to mostly case reports.[38,40,41] Mass sociogenic illness has been seen in past events including the 1987 Goiânia, Brazil, cesium-137 accident; the 1990 missile attack on Israel by Iraq, which was feared to contain chemical agents but did not; and during the 1995 sarin attacks in a subway in Tokyo, Japan. All of these events resulted in an added strain on local medical systems from thousands of unexposed people, many of whom displayed somatic systems.[3,39,42,43]

Table 3 presents common characteristics, predominate symptoms, and recommended approaches to mass sociogenic illness. Page and colleagues[38] reported that mass sociogenic illness can be best managed by "reassurance, separating symptomatic from non-symptomatic persons, minimizing unnecessary medical procedures, and providing a credible explanation for symptoms."

MANAGEMENT
Preparing for Intervention: The Process of Triage

Immediately after a disaster, it is necessary to include considerations of community and individual concerns in an assessment to help identify those within disaster-affected groups who need intervention. Assessments should focus on identifying the mental health problems of the disaster-affected groups and any related needs.[44,45] Accurate prevalence measurements of mental health conditions should be obtained through population surveillance as part of a community assessment.[45] This community assessment could then aid the local public health and mental health system in allocating necessary and usually limited resources.[44] Those coordinating the response should have baseline knowledge of "the community's mental health, vulnerabilities, and resources and capacities before the disaster."[10]

North and Pfefferbaum[10] state that "psychological wounds are often not apparent and therefore require concerted efforts and different procedures for identification and assessment" and that the "type of assessment varies in different post disaster time frames because new disorders arising after disasters develop over weeks." Posttraumatic stress disorder and major depression are the most likely psychiatric disorders to occur after a disaster and can take weeks to develop and be diagnosed. Therefore, initial assessments completed during the first 2 to 4 weeks postdisaster "can meaningfully address distress and psychosocial issues arising in the early post disaster phases, as well as preexisting psychiatric disorders such as alcohol addiction and bipolar disorder, but are too early to fully capture new psychiatric disorders."[10]

Individual assessment entails personal clinical evaluation and a brief mental health diagnostic assessment, such as the Mental Health Triage Scale. Clinical evaluation is achieved through a personal interview by a clinician to determine the most appropriate intervention. Suggested interventions are presented in Table 2 and discussed in the next section. In disasters where many may require assessment, such as after a technological disaster, resources may be spread thin even when mental health responders from outside the local area are available. In these situations, it is necessary to keep screening methods uncomplicated and tailored to the specific context and disaster phase, such as the Mental Health Triage Scale (http://www.health.vic.gov.au/mentalhealth/triage/scale0510.pdf). These evaluations should at a minimum help physicians identify those at risk of rapid decompensation and/or those needing immediate treatment.

Table 3
Common characteristics of psychogenic illness, predominant symptoms, and recommended approach to patients with psychogenic illness

Common Characteristics	Predominant Symptoms	Management Recommendations
• Often occurs after exposure to an environmental trigger (e.g., odor, emergency response, rumor, reported toxin, etc.)	• Headache	• Attempt to separate persons with illness associated with the outbreak
• Women affected disproportionately more often than men	• Dizziness or light-headedness	• Promptly perform physical examination and basic laboratory testing sufficient to exclude serious acute illness
• Adolescents and children affected	• Nausea	• Monitor and provide oxygen as necessary for hyperventilation
• Patients with psychological or physical stress affected	• Abdominal cramps or pain	• Minimize unnecessary exposure to medical procedures, emergency personnel, media or other potential anxiety-stimulating situations
• Symptoms spread and resolve rapidly	• Cough	• Notify public health authorities of apparent outbreak
• Symptoms inconsistent with a single biologic etiology	• Fatigue, drowsiness or weakness	• Openly communicate with physicians caring for other patients
• Symptoms may include hyperventilation or syncope	• Sore or burning throat	• Promptly communicate results of laboratory and environmental testing to patients
• Symptoms associated with minimal physical or laboratory findings	• Hyperventilation or difficulty breathing	• While maintaining confidentiality, explain that other people are experiencing similar symptoms and improving without complications
• Symptoms spread by "line-of-sight" transmission (i.e., seeing or hearing of another ill person causes symptoms)	• Watery or irritated eyes	• Remind patients that rumors and reports of "suspected causes" are not equivalent to confirmed results
• Illness may recur with return to environment of initial outbreak	• Chest tightness/chest pain	• Acknowledge that symptoms experienced by the patient are real
• Illness may escalate with vigorous or prolonged emergency or media response	• Inability to concentrate/ trouble thinking	• Explain potential contribution of anxiety to the patient's symptoms
	• Vomiting	• Reassure patient that long-term sequelae from current illness are not expected

(continued on next page)

Table 3 (continued)		
Common Characteristics	Predominant Symptoms	Management Recommendations
	• Anxiety or nervousness	• As appropriate, reassure patient that thorough clinical, epidemiologic and environmental investigations have identified no toxic cause for the outbreak or reason for further concern

Adapted from Jones TF. Mass psychogenic illness: role of the individual physician. Am Fam Physician 2000;62(12):2649–53.

Specific groups of people may be more prone to immediate psychosocial problems after technical disaster than after natural disasters.[46–51] These groups included pregnant women, mothers of young children, children, and evacuees from contaminated areas. It may be helpful for first receivers to identify members of these groups for mental health assessment and intervention.

Mental Health Interventions

Early disaster mental health interventions can reduce distress and provide emotional support to affected individuals before any new psychiatric disorders have time to develop. Most people who have been affected by a disaster do not develop psychiatric disorders; however, "almost everyone with exposure to severe disaster trauma will experience distress for at least a brief period."[10] Disaster mental health interventions may include formal psychiatric treatment or informal psychosocial community interactions such as psychological first aid (PFA), psychological debriefing, and crisis counseling. These informal psychosocial community interactions are not considered formal treatment of psychiatric disorders, although they may be appropriate before or in addition to treatment.[10]

Psychological First Aid

PFA is a set of empirically derived standards that provide first responders and receivers with a framework to support afflicted children and adults after disasters with practical and social support with linkages to mental health care.[52] The aim of PFA is "to reduce initial distress, meet current needs, promote flexible coping and encourage adjustment."[53] There is a general shortage of first responders and receivers trained in PFA, no standard PFA curricula, and no widely accepted model for training health care and public health workers in PFA competencies.[54] This lack of mental health–related provisions in postdisaster situations has been associated with mental health morbidity and increased rates of suicide.[55,56] However, trained and competent PFA responders, receivers, and Medical Reserve Corps volunteers who are able to provide immediate mental health triage during the response phase of a disaster can reduce the acute and long-term mental health effects of disasters and other emergency situations.[54–56] A literature review conducted in by Fox and colleagues[54] concluded that evidence for PFA "is widely supported by available objective observations."

According to the National Association of County and City Health Officials the core components of PFA include the following:

• Providing comfort care
• Recognizing basic needs and helping to solve problems and complete practical tasks

- Validating survivors' feelings and thoughts
- Providing accurate and timely information
- Connecting people with their support systems
- Providing education about anticipated stress reactions
- Reinforcing strengths and positive coping strategies

Online training on PFA is found in the *Psychological First Aid: Helping People Cope During Disasters and Public Health Emergencies* module on the National Association of County and City Health Officials Web site (http://pfa.naccho.org/pfa/pfa_start.html). The American Psychiatric Association on its Web site also provides a PFA Field Operations Guide and other important resources (http://www.psychiatry.org/practice/professional-interests/disaster-psychiatry). The Centers for Disease Control and Prevention also has a training module entitled *Psychological First Aid in Radiation Disasters* that deals specifically with applying PFA during a radiation emergency (http://www.orau.gov/RSB/RMH/).

Psychological Debriefing

Psychological debriefing is an intervention provided hours or days after a traumatic event that can consist of one or more individual or group sessions. These sessions provide survivors with psychoeducation and assist survivors or affected individuals in sharing their experiences or venting their emotional reaction, with further intervention encouraged if appropriate.[57,58] Although this type of intervention is popular, the literature suggests that psychological debriefing may actually worsen the risk of posttraumatic stress disorder for those most at-risk individuals.[59] Therefore, high-risk individuals should be identified and referred for psychiatric services instead.[10,57]

Crisis Counseling

Crisis counseling is a brief intervention delivered by trained crisis workers (which may or may not be mental health professionals) and other paraprofessionals. It is delivered in an individual or group setting, such as a shelter or church, and seeks to support survivors by enhancing coping and connecting them to other needed mental health services.[60–62] Crisis counseling is not a sufficient treatment of those who may require formal mental health treatment, although it can be broadly helpful to large groups.[62]

SPECIAL CONSIDERATIONS AND RECOMMENDATIONS

Having evaluated the literature on posttechnological disaster psychosocial issues, the authors have identified the most common recommendations for first responders and emergency department physicians in the event of such an incident.

- Assessments should focus on identifying the spectrum of mental health problems in disaster-affected groups and any related needs, taking into consideration community and individual assessments.[44,45] It is advisable for first receivers to identify the most vulnerable populations, such as individuals with comorbid psychiatric illnesses, pregnant women, mothers of young children, children, and evacuees.
- Initial assessments can be completed during the first 2 to 4 weeks postdisaster. The phase of the disaster matters because different symptoms are expected, so assessments should be tailored appropriately. Clinical assessment is resource intensive; therefore, it is necessary to keep screening methods uncomplicated and broad based.

- Assessments at a minimum should cover details of the individual's disaster experience, full diagnostic assessment for the most prevalent of disorders (ie, acute stress disorder, depression), a mental status examination, and history of preexisting disorders and other trauma exposures and stressors.[10]
- Following assessment, triage should identify those who need immediate linkage to formal mental health intervention, treatment, or care. The intensity of the interventions ranging from basic PFA to formal psychiatric interventions is contingent on the presenting symptom profile. However, the literature has shown that appropriate interventions can reduce the acute and long-term mental health effects of disasters and other emergency situations.[54–56]
- Informal psychosocial community interactions should not be used in place of formal treatment of those who are at risk of developing more serious psychological illnesses.

SUMMARY

Increases in psychological distress and psychiatric symptomatology in the aftermath of disasters have been documented and found to be the most common public health issue following a disaster. Although there is a growing literature on the mental health effects of technological disasters, most of the literature has historically focused on the mental health consequences after natural disasters. There are reasons to examine the differential impact of these two categories of disaster. For instance, although informal mental health support systems may exist following natural disasters, this is generally not the case following technological disasters. In fact, often victims of technological disasters are met with societal opposition and stigma, leading to a greater need for mental health support services. In addition to limited research on the mental health consequences after technological disasters, little attention has been given to mental health issues that emergency department physicians and first responders might potentially encounter.

Mild and moderate symptoms of distress following a disaster are common. Responses vary from person to person depending on personal characteristics and the specific circumstances surrounding the disaster. More severe symptoms include persistent insomnia and anxiety with an even smaller portion of the population developing severe psychiatric illness, such as posttraumatic stress disorder or major depression. The duration of technological disasters is generally more prolonged compared with natural disasters, and long-term health impacts of the disaster are often unknown. This prolonged impact can translate into longer periods of psychological distress, compounding traumatic experiences, and increased probability of negative psychiatric sequelae. In turn the strain on the care delivery system, including the mental health system, can be greater.

Although there is still a limited amount of literature pertaining to the psychological and mental health consequences in the aftermath of a technological disaster, it is growing, particularly in the wake of such events as the Fukushima Daiichi nuclear disaster in 2011.[63] As future generations are affected by technological disaster and as populations grow more aware of the risks, further research will be conducted on the effects in the hopes of mitigating symptoms of psychological distress and psychiatric illness that could manifest following such an event. The authors believe there is enough known about the potential psychosocial effects to develop guidelines and formal frameworks, and there is a gap in the first responder and first receiver community. Because these professionals are the first point of contact for affected individuals in the public health and health care systems, they are most important in identifying those suffering from psychosocial effects.

ACKNOWLEDGMENTS

The authors thank Rongbing Xie for her assistance with the literature search and Corey A. Craft for his assistance with article editing.

REFERENCES

1. Gouweloos J, Duckers M, Te Brake H, et al. Psychosocial care to affected citizens and communities in case of CBRN incidents: a systematic review. Environ Int 2014;72:46–65.
2. Kasperson RE, Pijawka KD. Societal response to hazards and major hazard events: comparing natural and technological hazards. Public Adm Rev 1985;7–18.
3. Petterson JS. Perception vs. reality of radiological impact: the Goiania model. Nuclear News 1988;31(14):84–90.
4. Yun K, Lurie N, Hyde PS. Moving mental health into the disaster-preparedness spotlight. N Engl J Med 2010;363(13):1193–5.
5. Grattan LM, Roberts S, Mahan WT Jr, et al. The early psychological impacts of the Deepwater Horizon oil spill on Florida and Alabama communities. Environ Health Perspect 2011;119(6):838–43.
6. Osofsky HJ, Osofsky JD, Hansel TC. Deepwater horizon oil spill: mental health effects on residents in heavily affected areas. Disaster Med Public Health Prep 2011;5(4):280–6.
7. Bonanno GA, Brewin CR, Kaniasty K, et al. Weighing the costs of disaster consequences, risks, and resilience in individuals, families, and communities. Psychol Sci Public Interest 2010;11(1):1–49.
8. Grievink L, van der Velden PG, Stellato RK, et al. A longitudinal comparative study of the physical and mental health problems of affected residents of the firework disaster Enschede, The Netherlands. Public Health 2007;121(5):367–74.
9. Norris FH, Friedman MJ, Watson PJ, et al. 60,000 disaster victims speak: part I. An empirical review of the empirical literature, 1981-2001. Psychiatry 2002;65(3):207–39.
10. North CS, Pfefferbaum B. Mental health response to community disasters: a systematic review. JAMA 2013;310(5):507–18.
11. Bromet EJ. Mental health consequences of the Chernobyl disaster. J Radiol Prot 2012;32(1):N71–5.
12. Bromet EJ, Havenaar JM, Guey LT. A 25 year retrospective review of the psychological consequences of the Chernobyl accident. Clin Oncol 2011;23(4):297–305.
13. Perry RW, Lindell MK. The psychological consequences of natural disaster: a review of research on American communities. Mass Emergencies 1978;3(3):105–15.
14. Picou JS, Marshall BK, Gill DA. Disaster, litigation, and the corrosive community. Soc Forces 2004;82(4):1493–522.
15. Breslau N, Kessler RC, Chilcoat HD, et al. Trauma and posttraumatic stress disorder in the community: the 1996 Detroit Area Survey of Trauma. Arch Gen Psychiatry 1998;55(7):626–32.
16. Inglesby TV. Progress in disaster planning and preparedness since 2001. JAMA 2011;306(12):1372–3.
17. Lowrey W, Evans W, Gower KK, et al. Effective media communication of disasters: pressing problems and recommendations. BMC Public Health 2007;7:97.
18. Yamashita J, Shigemura J. The Great East Japan Earthquake, tsunami, and Fukushima Daiichi nuclear power plant accident: a triple disaster affecting the mental health of the country. Psychiatr Clin North Am 2013;36(3):351–70.

19. Benedek DM, Fullerton C, Ursano RJ. First responders: mental health consequences of natural and human-made disasters for public health and public safety workers. Annu Rev Public Health 2007;28:55–68.

20. Duckers ML. Five essential principles of post-disaster psychosocial care: looking back and forward with Stevan Hobfoll. Eur J Psychotraumatol 2013;4:21914.

21. Hobfoll SE, Watson P, Bell CC, et al. Five essential elements of immediate and mid-term mass trauma intervention: empirical evidence. Psychiatry 2007;70(4): 283–315 [discussion: 316–69].

22. Committee PWSRCsA. Coping with technological disasters: a user friendly guidebook. 2004. Available at: http://www.pwsrcac.org/wp-content/uploads/filebase/ programs/oil_spill_prevention_planning/coping_with_technological_disasters.pdf. Accessed June 12, 2014.

23. Broughton E. The Bhopal disaster and its aftermath: a review. Environ Health 2005;4(1):6.

24. Dhara VR, Dhara R, Acquilla SD, et al. Personal exposure and long-term health effects in survivors of the union carbide disaster at Bhopal. Environ Health Perspect 2002;110(5):487–500.

25. Murthy RS, Isaac MK. Mental health needs of Bhopal disaster victims & training of medical officers in mental health aspects. Indian J Med Res 1987;86(Suppl):51–8.

26. Havenaar JM, van den Brink W. Psychological factors affecting health after toxicological disasters. Clin Psychol Rev 1997;17(4):359–74.

27. Weisaeth L, Tonnessen A. Responses of individuals and groups to consequences of technological disasters and radiation exposure. In: Ursano RJ, Fullerton CS, Norwood AE, editors. Terrorism and disaster: individual and community mental health interventions. Cambridge: Cambridge University Press; 2003. p. 209–35.

28. Hyams KC, Murphy FM, Wessely S. Responding to chemical, biological, or nuclear terrorism: the indirect and long-term health effects may present the greatest challenge. J Health Polit Policy Law 2002;27(2):273–91.

29. Panzer AM, Butler AS, Goldfrank LR. Preparing for the psychological consequences of terrorism: a public health strategy. Washington (DC): National Academies Press; 2003.

30. Galea S, Nandi A, Vlahov D. The epidemiology of post-traumatic stress disorder after disasters. Epidemiol Rev 2005;27:78–91.

31. Green BL. Psychological responses to disasters: conceptualization and identification of high-risk survivors. Psychiatry Clin Neurosci 1998;52(S1):S25–31.

32. Norris FH, Friedman MJ, Watson PJ. 60,000 disaster victims speak: part II. Summary and implications of the disaster mental health research. Psychiatry 2002; 65(3):240–60.

33. North CS. Addressing the psychiatric sequelae of catastrophic trauma. US Psychiatry 2007;35–7.

34. North CS, Oliver J, Pandya A. Examining a comprehensive model of disaster-related posttraumatic stress disorder in systematically studied survivors of 10 disasters. Am J Public Health 2012;102(10):e40–8.

35. Kaiser HE, Barnett DJ, Hsu EB, et al. Perspectives of future physicians on disaster medicine and public health preparedness: challenges of building a capable and sustainable auxiliary medical workforce. Disaster Med Public Health Prep 2009;3(4):210–6.

36. Sheikh S, McCormick LC, Pevear J, et al. Radiological preparedness-awareness and attitudes: a cross-sectional survey of emergency medicine residents and physicians at three academic institutions in the United States. Clin Toxicol 2012;50(1):34–8.

37. Errett NA, Barnett DJ, Thompson CB, et al. Assessment of medical reserve corps volunteers' emergency response willingness using a threat- and efficacy-based model. Biosecur Bioterror 2013;11(1):29–40.
38. Page LA, Keshishian C, Leonardi G, et al. Frequency and predictors of mass psychogenic illness. Epidemiology 2010;21(5):744–7.
39. Bartholomew RE, Wessely S. Protean nature of mass sociogenic illness: from possessed nuns to chemical and biological terrorism fears. Br J Psychiatry 2002;180:300–6.
40. Boss LP. Epidemic hysteria: a review of the published literature. Epidemiol Rev 1997;19(2):233–43.
41. Wessely S. Mass hysteria: two syndromes? Psychol Med 1987;17(1):109–20.
42. Ohbu S, Yamashina A, Takasu N, et al. Sarin poisoning on Tokyo subway. South Med J 1997;90(6):587–93.
43. Smithson AE, Levy LA, Center HL. Ataxia: the chemical and biological terrorism threat and the US response. Washington, DC: Henry L. Stimson Center; 2000.
44. Nucifora FC Jr, Hall RC, Everly GS Jr. Reexamining the role of the traumatic stressor and the trajectory of posttraumatic distress in the wake of disaster. Disaster Med Public Health Prep 2011;5(Suppl 2):S172–5.
45. Ruzek JI, Young BH, Cordova MJ, et al. Integration of disaster mental health services with emergency medicine. Prehospital Disaster Med 2004;19(1):46–53.
46. Auvinen A, Vahteristo M, Arvela H, et al. Chernobyl fallout and outcome of pregnancy in Finland. Environ Health Perspect 2001;109(2):179–85.
47. Bertollini R, Di Lallo D, Mastroiacovo P, et al. Reduction of births in Italy after the Chernobyl accident. Scand J Work Environ Health 1990;16(2):96–101.
48. Bromet EJ, Havenaar J. The long-term mental health impacts of the Chernobyl accident. In: Neria Y, Galea S, Norris F, editors. Mental health and disasters. Cambridge: Cambridge University Press; 2009. p. 441–53.
49. Havenaar JM, Van den Brink W, Van den Bout J, et al. Mental health problems in the Gomel region (Belarus): an analysis of risk factors in an area affected by the Chernobyl disaster. Psychol Med 1996;26(4):845–55.
50. Knudsen LB. Legally induced abortions in Denmark after Chernobyl. Biomed Pharmacother 1991;45(6):229–31.
51. Lemyre L, Corneil W, Johnson C, et al. Psychosocial considerations about children and radiological events. Radiat Prot Dosimetry 2010;142(1):70–6.
52. Reyes G, Elhai JD. Psychosocial interventions in the early phases of disasters. Psychotherapy 2004;41(4):399.
53. Taylor M, Wells G, Howell G, et al. The role of social media as psychological first aid as a support to community resilience building. AJEM 2012;27(1):20.
54. Fox JH, Burkle FM Jr, Bass J, et al. The effectiveness of psychological first aid as a disaster intervention tool: research analysis of peer-reviewed literature from 1990-2010. Disaster Med Public Health Prep 2012;6(3):247–52.
55. Chandra A, Kim J, Pieters HC, et al. Implementing psychological first-aid training for medical reserve corps volunteers. Disaster Med Public Health Prep 2014;8(1): 95–100.
56. McCabe OL, Everly GS Jr, Brown LM, et al. Psychological first aid: a consensus-derived, empirically supported, competency-based training model. Am J Public Health 2014;104(4):621–8.
57. Bisson JI, McFarlane AC, Rose S, et al. Psychological debriefing for adults. In: Foa EB, Keane TM, Terence M, et al, editors. Effective treatments for PTSD: practice guidelines from the International Society for Traumatic Stress Studies. 2nd edition. New York (NY): Guilford Press; 2009; 2:83–105.

58. Regel S. Post-trauma support in the workplace: the current status and practice of critical incident stress management (CISM) and psychological debriefing (PD) within organizations in the UK. Occup Med 2007;57(6):411–6.
59. Rose S, Bisson J, Churchill R, et al. Psychological debriefing for preventing post traumatic stress disorder (PTSD). Cochrane Database Syst Rev 2002;(2): CD000560.
60. Center SAaMHSADTA. Crisis Counseling Assistance and Training Program (CCP). 2009. Available at: http://store.samhsa.gov/shin/content/SMA09-4373/ SMA09-4373.pdf. Accessed June 13, 2014.
61. Norris FH, Hamblen JL, Rosen CS. Service characteristics and counseling outcomes: lessons from a cross-site evaluation of crisis counseling after Hurricanes Katrina, Rita and Wilma. Adm Policy Ment Health 2009;36(3):176–85.
62. Norris FH, Rosen CS. Innovations in disaster mental health services and evaluation: national, state, and local responses to Hurricane Katrina (introduction to the special issue). Adm Policy Ment Health 2009;36(3):159–64.
63. Tsubokura M, Hara K, Matsumura T, et al. The immediate physical and mental health crisis in residents proximal to the evacuation zone after Japan's nuclear disaster: an observational pilot study. Disaster Med Public Health Prep 2014; 8(1):30–6.

Checklists for Hazardous Materials Emergency Preparedness

Stephen W. Borron, MD, MS

KEYWORDS

- Checklist • Emergency management plan • Hazard vulnerability analysis
- Human resources • Antidote stocking • Personal protective equipment

CHECKLIST 1: GENERAL AND HAZARDOUS MATERIALS DISASTER PREPAREDNESS

Adapted from article 3, "Hospital Preparedness for Chemical and Radiological Disasters," with thanks to Drs Robert Geller and Brooks Moore, and Ms Charlotte Clark.

The following is a checklist for development of hospital preparedness for chemical and radiological hazardous materials and other disaster preparedness. It is not intended to be comprehensive, but should help to guide preparation. Selected Web resources are provided without implied endorsement.

- Mitigation
  - Review Joint Commission requirements for emergency management
    - http://www.jointcommission.org/emergency_management.aspx
  - Designate hospital emergency manager and emergency management team
    - https://cdp.dhs.gov/training/courses/frame
    - https://cdp.dhs.gov/training/courses/ic
    - https://cdp.dhs.gov/training/courses/hert
    - http://www.calhospitalprepare.org/hics
  - Conduct hazards vulnerability analysis (HVA)
    - http://www.calhospitalprepare.org/post/hazard-vulnerability-analysis-tool
  - Draft hospital all-hazards response plan
    - http://www.cdc.gov/phpr/healthcare/documents/HAH_508_Compliant_Final.pdf
    - http://www.calhospitalprepare.org/emergency-operations-plan
    - http://www.fema.gov/pdf/plan/slg101.pdf
    - http://www.acep.org/clinical–practice-management/hospital-disaster-preparedness-self-assessment-tool
  - Detail specific chemical and radiological emergency annexes to plan
    - https://www.osha.gov/Publications/osha3249.pdf
    - http://www.acep.org/ems/

Department of Emergency Medicine, Paul L. Foster School of Medicine, Texas Tech University Health Sciences Center, 4801 Alberta Avenue, Suite B3200, El Paso, TX 79905, USA
E-mail address: stephen.borron@ttuhsc.edu

Emerg Med Clin N Am 33 (2015) 213–232
http://dx.doi.org/10.1016/j.emc.2014.09.013
0733-8627/15/$ – see front matter © 2015 Elsevier Inc. All rights reserved.
emed.theclinics.com

- o Appoint subject matter expert for chemical and radiological events
  - http://acmt.net/cgi/page.cgi/findtoxicologist.html
  - http://www.aapcc.org/centers/
  - http://clintox.org/contact.cfm
- o Establish communications plan
  - http://www.calhospitalprepare.org/communications
- o Conduct bed and surge capacity survey
  - http://archive.ahrq.gov/news/ulp/btbriefs/btbrief3.pdf
  - http://www.nyc.gov/html/doh/downloads/pdf/bhpp/bhpp-hospital-cbcbpp-plan.pdf
  - http://www.calhospitalprepare.org/healthcare-surge
  - http://www.calhospitalprepare.org/mass-fatality-planning
- o Establish regional partners for specialty care
  - http://www.ameriburn.org/verification_verifiedcenters.php
  - http://orise.orau.gov/reacts/
  - http://www.facs.org/trauma/verified.html
  - http://www.aapcc.org/centers/
  - http://www.ritn.net/About
- o Develop memoranda of understanding with regional partners, transfer criteria, and patient tracking system
  - http://www.aha.org/content/00-10/ModelHospitalMou.pdf
  - http://www.calhospitalprepare.org/memoranda-understanding
  - http://www.emsystems.com/info/emtrack.html
- Preparation
  - o Educate frontline staff on toxidromes of common chemical and radiological exposures and injuries
    - http://www.ahls.org/ahls/ecs/courses/courses.html
    - http://training.fema.gov/EMIWeb/IS/courseOverview.aspx?code=is-346
    - https://www.osha.gov/dts/osta/bestpractices/html/hospital_firstreceivers.html
  - o Purchase, train, and maintain personal protective equipment (PPE)
    - See checklists 2 to 5
    - http://www.remm.nlm.gov/radiation_ppe.htm#emergencies
    - https://www.osha.gov/dts/osta/bestpractices/firstreceivers_hospital.pdf
    - See checklist 8
  - o Purchase and maintain antidote stockpile
    - http://cjem-online.ca/v4/n1/p23
    - http://cjem-online.ca/sites/cjem-online.ca/files/v4n1-AppendixA.pdf
  - o Designate procedures to access Strategic National Stockpile
    - http://chemm.nlm.nih.gov/sns.htm
    - http://chemm.nlm.nih.gov/chempack.htm
- Response
  - o Develop security protocols for hospital lockdown
    - http://www.acep.org/search.aspx?searchtext=lockdown
    - http://www.ahcancal.org/searchcenter/Pages/Results.aspx?k=lockdown
  - o Specify decontamination area, with temporary or fixed decontamination facility
    - http://www.hsph.harvard.edu/wp-content/uploads/sites/1435/2013/01/Hospital-Decontamination-Self-Assessment-Tool-2013.pdf
    - https://www.osha.gov/dts/osta/bestpractices/html/hospital_firstreceivers.html

- ○ Conduct drill using decontamination teams and equipment, refine procedure
  - ■ http://ems2.dhs.lacounty.gov/manualsprotocols/Drills/ConductingDrills_Exercise30806.pdf
  - ■ http://www.hsph.harvard.edu/wp-content/uploads/sites/1435/2013/01/Strategies-for-First-Receiver-Decontamination-2013.pdf
- Recovery
  - ○ Conduct poststress mental health screening and assessment in responders
    - ■ http://www.info-trauma.org/flash/media-e/mitchellCriticalIncidentStressDebriefing.pdf
    - ■ http://store.samhsa.gov/product/Disaster-Behavioral-Health-Preparedness-and-Response-Resources/DTAC11-CATALOG
    - ■ http://learn.nctsn.org/course/index.php?categoryid=11
    - ■ http://whqlibdoc.who.int/publications/2011/9789241548205_eng.pdf
  - ○ Restock used supplies from local vendors or national stockpile
    - ■ http://archive.ahrq.gov/prep/hosprecovery/hosprecovery.pdf
  - ○ Develop an after-action report
    - ■ http://archive.ahrq.gov/research/hospdrills/
    - ■ http://www.au.af.mil/au/awc/awcgate/doj/sample_aar.pdf

CHECKLIST 2: OCCUPATIONAL SAFETY AND HEALTH ADMINISTRATION MINIMUM PERSONAL PROTECTIVE EQUIPMENT SELECTIONS FOR THE HOSPITAL DECONTAMINATION ZONE AND SPECIFIC CONDITIONS NECESSARY FOR HOSPITALS TO RELY ON THEM (OCCUPATIONAL SAFETY AND HEALTH ADMINISTRATION, 2005 #1)

Adapted from article 4, "Personnel Protection and Decontamination of Adults and Children," with thanks to Drs Michael G. Holland and David Cawthon. Selected Web resources are provided without endorsement.

Hospital Decontamination Zone

- Powered air-purifying respirator that provides a protection factor of 1000. The respirator must be National Institute for Occupational Safety and Health (NIOSH) approved.
- Combination 99.97% high-efficiency particulate air/organic vapor/acid gas respirator cartridges (also NIOSH approved).
- Double-layer protective gloves.
- Chemical-resistant suit.
- Head covering and eye/face protection (if not part of the respirator).
- Chemical-protective boots.
- Suit openings sealed with tape.

Conditions

1. Thorough and complete HVA and emergency management plan (EMP) that consider community input and have been conducted/developed and updated within the past year.
   - http://www.calhospitalprepare.org/post/hazard-vulnerability-analysis-tool
   - https://www.osha.gov/dts/osta/bestpractices/html/hospital_firstreceivers.html#appf

2. The EMP includes plans to assist the numbers of patients that the community anticipates might seek treatment at this hospital, keeping in mind that most patients may self-refer to the nearest hospital.
   • http://www.calhospitalprepare.org/emergency-operations-plan
3. Preparations specified in the EMP have been implemented (eg, employee training, equipment selection, maintenance, and a respiratory protection program).
4. The EMP includes methods for handling the numbers of ambulatory and nonambulatory patients anticipated by the community.
5. The hazardous substance was not released in close proximity to the hospital, and the elapsed time between the patients' exposure and patients' arrival at the hospital exceeds approximately 10 minutes, thereby permitting substantial levels of gases and vapors from volatile substances time to dissipate.
6. Patients' contaminated clothing and possessions are promptly removed and contained (eg, in an approved hazardous waste container that is isolated outdoors), and decontamination is initiated promptly on arrival at the hospital. Hospital EMP includes shelter, tepid water, soap, privacy, and coverings to promote patient compliance with decontamination procedures.
7. EMP procedures are in place to ensure that contaminated medical waste and waste water do not become secondary sources of employee exposure.
8. The decontamination system and predecontamination patient waiting areas are designed and used in a manner that promotes constant fresh air circulation through the system to limit hazardous substance accumulation. Air exchange from a clean source has been considered in the design of fully enclosed systems (ie, through consultation with a professional engineer or certified industrial hygienist) and air is not recirculated.

CHECKLIST 3: OCCUPATIONAL SAFETY AND HEALTH ADMINISTRATION MINIMUM PERSONAL PROTECTIVE EQUIPMENT SELECTIONS IN THE HOSPITAL POSTDECONTAMINATION ZONE AND SPECIFIC CONDITIONS NECESSARY FOR HOSPITALS TO RELY ON THEM. (OCCUPATIONAL SAFETY AND HEALTH ADMINISTRATION, 2005 #1)

Adapted from article 4, "Personnel Protection and Decontamination of Adults and Children," with thanks to Drs Michael G. Holland and David Cawthon. Selected Web resources are provided without endorsement.

Hospital Postdecontamination Zone

• Normal work clothes and PPE, as necessary, for infection control purposes (eg, gloves, gown, and appropriate respirator).

Conditions

The hospital postdecontamination zone is defined as an area considered to be uncontaminated, and equipment and personnel are not expected to become contaminated in this area (Occupational Safety and Health Administration [OSHA], 2005). This zone requires 6 conditions that the hospital must meet to comply with the OSHA minimum PPE selections:

1. EMP is developed and followed in a way that minimizes the emergency department (ED) personnel's reasonably anticipated contact with contaminated patients (eg, with drills that test communication between the hospital and

emergency responders at the incident site to reduce the likelihood of unanticipated casualties).

2. Decontamination system (in the hospital decontamination zone) and hospital security can be activated promptly to minimize the chance that patients will enter the ED and contact unprotected staff before decontamination.

3. EMP procedures specify that unannounced patients (once identified as possibly contaminated) disrobe in the appropriate decontamination area (not the ED) and follow hospital decontamination procedures before admission (or readmission) to the ED.

4. Patients in this area were previously decontaminated by a shower with soap and water, including a minimum of 5 minutes under running water. Shower instructions are clearly presented and enforced. Shower facility encourages patient compliance (eg, shelter, tepid water, reasonable degree of privacy).

5. EMP procedures clearly specify actions for ED clerks or staff to take if they suspect a patient is contaminated. For example: (1) do not physically contact the patient, (2) immediately notify supervisor and safety officer of possible hospital contamination, and (3) allow qualified personnel to isolate and decontaminate the patient.

6. The EMP requires that, if the ED becomes contaminated, that space is no longer eligible to be considered a hospital postdecontamination zone. Instead, it should be considered contaminated and all employees working in this area should use PPE as described for the hospital decontamination zone.

CHECKLIST 4: SELECTION OF PERSONAL PROTECTIVE EQUIPMENT

Adapted from article 4, "Personnel Protection and Decontamination of Adults and Children," with thanks to Drs Michael G. Holland and David Cawthon. Selected Web resources are provided without implied endorsement.

Various government agencies and manufacturers' databases are available to aid in the selection of specific PPE:

General

- US Centers for Disease Control and Prevention (CDC): http://www.cdc.gov/niosh/ncpc/
- US Department of Health and Human Services (HHS): http://chemm.nlm.nih.gov/ppe.htm
- OSHA: https://www.osha.gov/dts/osta/otm/otm_viii/otm_viii_1.html
- Grainger: http://www.grainger.com/content/qt-190-chemical-protective-clothing

Respirators

- NIOSH: http://www.cdc.gov/niosh/npptl/respusers.html
- OSHA: https://www.osha.gov/SLTC/etools/respiratory/respirator_selection.html
- 3M: http://multimedia.3m.com/mws/mediawebserver?mwsId=SSSSSufSevTs ZxtUOxmG4x_SevUqevTSevTSevTSeSSSSSS–
- Mine Safety Appliances: http://webapps.msanet.com/responseguide/
- Scott: http://www.scottsurelife.com

Boots

- Bata: http://bataindustrials.com/

- Honeywell: http://www.honeywellsafety.com/USA/Products-by-Hazard/Chemical.aspx?tid=977&bid=0&hid=114&iid=209
- Tingley: http://www.tingleyrubber.com/images/4049%HazProof.pdf

Gloves

- Ansell: http://www.ansellpro.com/download/Ansell_7thEditionChemicalResistanceGuide.pdf
- Best: http://www.chemrest.com/
- Kimberly-Clark: http://www.kcproductselector.com/Gloves
- http://ezguide.northsafety.com/indglovesmain.aspx
- Shield: http://www.shieldscientific.com/public/chemical-resistance-guide/

Suits

- 3M: http://solutions.3m.com/wps/portal/3M/en_US/3M-PPE-Safety-Solutions/Personal-Protective-Equipment/
- Ansell: http://protective.ansell.com/en/Products/Trellchem
- Blauer: http://blauer.com/chembio
- DuPont: http://www.SafeSPEC.DuPont.com
- Kappler: http://www.kappler.com/index.php/hazmatch
- Kimberly-Clark: http://www.kcprofessional.com/products/ppe/disposable
- Lakeland: http://www.lakeland.com/chemmax_search.aspx
- Lion: http://lionconnects.com
- St Gobain: http://www.protectivesystems.saint-gobain.com

CHECKLIST 5: PREPARING A WRITTEN RESPIRATORY PROTECTION PROGRAM

Adapted from article 4, "Personnel Protection and Decontamination of Adults and Children," with thanks to Drs Michael G. Holland and David Cawthon. Selected Web resources are provided without endorsement.

A formal written respiratory protection program is required by 29 CFR 1910.134 (https://www.osha.gov/dte/library/respirators/major_requirements.pdf) and shall include the following elements:

- Procedures for selecting respirators for use in the workplace
- Medical evaluations of employees required to use respirators
- Fit testing procedures for tight-fitting respirators
- Procedures for proper use of respirators in routine and reasonably foreseeable emergency situations
- Procedures and schedules for cleaning, disinfecting, storing, inspecting, repairing, discarding, and otherwise maintaining respirators
- Procedures to ensure adequate air quality and flow of breathing air for atmosphere-supplying respirators
- Training of employees in the respiratory hazards to which they are potentially exposed during routine and emergency situations
- Training of employees in the proper use of respirators, including putting on and removing them (donning and doffing), any limitations on their use, and their maintenance
  - https://www.osha.gov/dts/osta/bestpractices/html/hospital_firstreceivers.html#appk

- Procedures for regularly evaluating the effectiveness of the program

The California Department of Public Health has developed a tool kit and template for respiratory protection for health care workers and an evaluation checklist.

- http://www.cdph.ca.gov/programs/ohb/Pages/RespToolkit.aspx
- http://www.cdph.ca.gov/programs/ohb/Documents/HCResp-RPP-Template. docx
- http://www.cdph.ca.gov/programs/ohb/Documents/HCResp-EvalChecklist.pdf

First responders, including firefighters, law enforcement, and emergency medical personnel, and many first receivers at public hospitals, are usually employees of local, municipal, or state governments. Although Federal OSHA's standards and enforcement authority do not extend to such state and local governments, these employers and employees are covered by the 26 states that operate OSHA-approved state plans and, in states without state plans, by the Environmental Protection Agency (EPA) with regard to HAZWOPER (Hazardous Waste Operations and Emergency Response: 29 CFR 1910.120). State plan states set and enforce standards, such as the HAZWOPER and respiratory protection standards, which are identical to, or at least as effective as, federal OSHA standards, and therefore may have more stringent or supplemental requirements. EPA's HAZWOPER parallel standard was adopted to cover emergency responders who would not be covered by the OSHA standard, including volunteers who work for a governmental agency engaged in emergency response, such as firefighters. For consistency, OSHA interprets the HAZWOPER standard for the EPA. Federal OSHA administers the safety and health program for the private sector in the remaining states and territories, and also retains authority with regard to safety and health conditions for federal employees throughout the nation.

CHECKLIST 6: RESOURCES FOR CHEMICAL EMERGENCIES AND PLANNING

Adapted from article 5, "Resources for toxicologic information and assistance," with thanks to Drs Mark A. Kirk and Carol J. Iddins. The opinions expressed herein are those of the authors and are not necessarily those of the US Government (USG) or its agencies. Neither the USG nor its agencies, nor any of their employees, makes any warranty, expressed or implied, or assumes any legal liability or responsibility for the accuracy, completeness, or usefulness of the information contained herein or represents that its use would not infringe on privately owned rights. Selected Web and/or telephonic resources are provided without implied endorsement.

Chemical Emergency Speed Dial: 24/7 On-call Resources

- Regional Poison Center: 1-800-222-1222 (any chemical emergency)
- Chemtrec: 1-800-424-9300 (hazardous material spills)
- National Response Center: 1-800-424-8802 (major oil or chemical release)
- Local and state health departments: (report unusual illness, suspected epidemics, obtain epidemiologic and laboratory support):
  - Local health departments: _____. For a map with directory for your locality go to: http://www.naccho.org/about/lhd/
  - State Health Departments: _____. For a map with directory for your state go to: http://www.cdc.gov/mmwr/international/relres.html

Chemical Assets (Alphabetical)

Resource	URL	Best Use
Advanced HAZMAT Life Support Course	http://www.ahls.org/ahls/ecs/main/ahls_home.html	Education and training
American College of Medical Toxicology: Chemical Agents of Opportunity Course	http://acmt.net/Chemical_Agents_of_Opportunity.html	Education and training
American College of Medical Toxicology Consultation Services	Directory of Inpatient Medical Toxicology Services: http://acmt.net/Directory_of_Inpatient_Medical_Toxicology_Services.html Agency for Toxic Substance and Disease Registry Consultation Network: http://acmt.net/ATSDR_Consultation_Network.html	Toxicant management Consultation
ATSDR Medical Management Guidelines	http://www.atsdr.cdc.gov/MMG/index.asp	Toxicant management
ATSDR's Toxicology FAQs for Chemical Agents	http://www.atsdr.cdc.gov/toxfaqs/index.asp	Crisis communication
CBRNE-enhanced Response Force Packages teams	http://www.army.mil/aps/08/information_papers/transform/ARNG_CERFP.html	Specialized response teams
CDC Chempack	http://chemm.nlm.nih.gov/chempack.htm	Incident preplanning: Toxicant management Antidotes
CDC Clinical Laboratory Response Network	http://emergency.cdc.gov/chemical/lab.asp	Toxicant management Diagnostics
CDC's Crisis and Emergency Risk Communication Quick Guide	http://www.bt.cdc.gov/cerc/	Crisis communication
Center for Domestic Preparedness	https://cdp.dhs.gov/	Education and training
Chemical Hazards Emergency Medical Management	http://chemm.nlm.nih.gov/	Toxicant management
Chemical Hazards Emergency Medical Management Intelligent Syndrome Tool	http://chemm.nlm.nih.gov/chemmist.htm	Toxicant management
Department of Homeland Security and HHS. Patient Decontamination in a Mass Chemical Exposure Incident: National Planning Guidance for Communities; draft, 2014	Web release pending (Draft document available at: http://www.regulations.gov/#!documentDetail;D=DHS-2014-0012-0002. Accessed October 22, 2014.)	Incident preplanning: Decontamination
DOT Emergency Response Guidebook: A Guidebook for First Responders During the Initial Phase of a Dangerous Goods/Hazardous Materials Transportation Incident. 2012	http://phmsa.dot.gov/pv_obj_cache/pv_obj_id_7410989F4294AE44A2EBF6A80ADB640BCA8E4200/filename/ERG2012.pdf	Toxicant management
Edgewood Chemical Biological Center. Guidelines for Mass Casualty Decontamination During a HAZMAT/Weapon of Mass Destruction Incident, Volumes I & II	http://www.nfpa.org/~/media/Files/Research/Resource links/First responders/Decontamination/ecbc_Guide_MassCasualtyDecontam_0813.pdf	Incident preplanning: Decontamination

Resource	URL	Function
EPA National Decontamination Team	http://www.epa.gov/OEM/index.htm	Specialized response teams
Federal Bureau of Investigation Hazardous Materials Response Unit/Hazardous Evidence Response Team Unit	http://www.fbi.gov/about-us/investigate/terrorism/terrorism	Specialized response teams
Local and city health departments; directory	http://www.naccho.org/topics/emergency/	Toxicant management; Consultation
Local emergency planning committees	http://www2.epa.gov/epcra/local-emergency-planning-committees	Incident preplanning: HVA/situational awareness
National Disaster Life Support Course	http://www.ndlsf.org/index.php/courses/adls	Education and training
National Guard Bureau Civil Support Team-V/MD	http://www.army.mil/aps/08/information_papers/transform/ARNG_Civil_Support_Teams.html	Specialized response teams
National Library of Medicine's Special Information Services: Disaster Course Digital Go Bag	http://disaster.nlm.nih.gov/dimrc/disastercourse_digitalgobag.html	Education and training
National Library of Medicine's Special Information Services: Environmental Health and Toxicology	http://sis.nlm.nih.gov/enviro.html	Toxicant management
NIOSH Pocket Guide to Chemical Hazards. HHS, CDC, NIOSH, 2010	http://www.cdc.gov/niosh/npg/	Toxicant management
OSHA Best Practices for Hospital-based First Receivers of Victims from Mass Casualty Incidents Involving the Release of Hazardous Substances	https://www.osha.gov/dts/osta/bestpractices/html/hospital_firstreceivers.html	Incident preplanning: Decontamination
Regional poison centers	http://www.aapcc.org/centers/	Toxicant management; Consultation
Technical Support Working Group, Best Practices and Guidelines for CBR Mass Personnel Decontamination. US Department of Defense, 2004	http://www.cttso.gov/?q=node/247	Incident preplanning: Decontamination
US Army Medical Research Institute of Chemical Defense's Chemical Casualty Care Division	http://ccc.apgea.army.mil/default.htm	Education and training
US Army Medical Research Institute of Chemical Defense Consultation Services	http://chemdef.apgea.army.mil/Default.aspx	Toxicant management; Consultation
US Marine Corps Chemical Biological Incident Response Force team	http://www.cbirf.marines.mil/	Specialized response teams
Wireless Information System for Emergency Responders	http://wiser.nlm.nih.gov/	Toxicant management

Abbreviations: ATSDR, Agency for Toxic Substances and Disease Registry; CBR, chemical, biological, radiological; CBRNE, chemical, biological, radiological, nuclear, and high-yield-explosive; DOT, US Department of Transportation; FAQ, frequently asked questions.

CHECKLIST 7: CHEMPACK CONTENTS

Pharmaceuticals under this program may be used by the hosting hospital or released to another hospital or emergency response agency in the same city in the event of an accidental or intentional release of nerve agent (also applies to exposure to agricultural organophosphorous and carbamate pesticides).

1. Threatens the medical security of the community.
2. Puts multiple lives at risk.
3. Hospital or local pharmaceutical resources are insufficient to meet the demand.

Readers should contact their local emergency management authorities in advance of a disaster to obtain contact information for the Chempack coordinator and availability of these assets in the region.

Hospital Chempack Container for 1000 Casualties			
	Quantity	Unit Pack	Cases
Mark 1 autoinjector	480	240	2
Atropine sulfate 0.4 mg/mL 20 mL	900	100	9
Pralidoxime 1-g for injection 20 mL	2760	276	10
AtroPen 0.5 mg	144	144	1
AtroPen 1.0 mg	144	144	1
Diazepam 5 mg/mL autoinjector[a]	150	150	1
Diazepam 5 mg/mL vial, 10 mL[a]	650	25	26
Sterile water for injection, 20-mL vials	2800	100	28
Sensaphone 2050	1	1	1
Satco B DEA container	1	1	1

Abbreviation: DEA, US Drug Enforcement Administration.
[a] DEA schedule IV controlled substance and needs a custody transfer document.
Source: North Dakota Department of Health (http://ndhealth.gov/DoH/Publications.asp).

EMS Chempack Container for 454 Casualties			
	Quantity	Unit Pack	Cases
Mark 1 autoinjector	1200	240	5
Atropine sulfate 0.4 mg/mL 20 mL	100	100	1
Pralidoxime 1-g injector 20 mL	276	276	1
AtroPen 0.5 mg	144	144	1
AtroPen 1.0 mg	144	144	1
Diazepam 5 mg/mL autoinjector[a]	300	150	2
Diazepam 5 mg/mL vial, 10 mL[a]	50	25	2
Sterile water for injection 20-mL vials	200	100	2
Sensaphone 2050	1	1	1
Satco B DEA container	1	1	1

[a] DEA schedule IV controlled substance and needs a custody transfer document.

CHECKLIST 8: ANTIDOTE RECOMMENDATIONS FOR STOCKING OF FACILITIES THAT ACCEPT EMERGENCY PATIENTS

Antidote	Poisoning Indications	Recommendation			Class of Evidence[b]
		Should Be Stocked	Available Within 60 min	Immediately Available[a]	
Acetylcysteine	Acetaminophen	Yes	Yes	No	I (IV) II (oral)
Antivenin (Crotalidae) Polyvalent, Wyeth, or	North American crotaline snake envenomation	Yes	Yes	No	III
Crotalidae Polyvalent, Immune Fab, ovine[c]	North American crotaline snake envenomation	Yes	Yes	No	II
Antivenin (Latrodectus mactans)	Black widow spider envenomation	Yes	No	No	III
Antivenin (Micrurus fulvius)	Eastern and Texas coral snake envenomation	Yes	Yes	No	III
Atropine sulfate	Organophosphorus and N-methyl carbamate insecticides	Yes	Yes	Yes	III
Botulism antitoxin, equine (A, B)	Botulism	No	NA	NA	III
Botulism immune globulin (BabyBIG)	Infant botulism	No	NA	NA	I
Calcium chloride[d]	Fluoride, calcium channel blocking agent	Yes	Yes	Yes	III
Calcium gluconate[d]		Yes	Yes	Yes	III
Calcium disodium EDTA	Lead	Yes	No	No	II
Calcium trisodium pentetate (calcium DTPA)	Internal contamination with plutonium, americium, or curium	Yes	No	No	III
Cyanide antidote kit or	Cyanide poisoning	Yes	Yes	Yes	III
Hydroxocobalamin hydrochloride[c]	Cyanide poisoning	Yes	Yes	Yes	II
Deferoxamine mesylate	Acute iron poisoning	Yes	Yes	No	II
Digoxin Immune Fab	Cardiac glycosides/steroid toxicity	Yes	Yes	Yes	II
Dimercaprol	Heavy metal toxicity (arsenic, mercury, lead)	Yes	Yes	No	II
Ethanol[d] or	Methanol, or ethylene glycol poisoning	Yes	Yes	No	III
Fomepizole[c]	Methanol, or ethylene glycol poisoning	Yes	Yes	No	II
Flumazenil	Benzodiazepine toxicity	Yes	Yes	Yes	III

(continued on next page)

(continued)

Antidote	Poisoning Indications	Recommendation			Class of Evidence[b]
		Should Be Stocked	Available Within 60 min	Immediately Available[a]	
Glucagon hydrochloride[d]	β-Blocker, calcium channel blocker	Yes	Yes	Yes	III
Methylene blue	Methemoglobinemia	Yes	Yes	Yes	II
Naloxone hydrochloride	Opioid and opiate drugs	Yes	Yes	Yes	I
Octreotide acetate[d]	Sulfonylurea-induced hypoglycemia	Yes	Yes	No	II
Physostigmine salicylate	Anticholinergic syndrome	Yes	Yes	Yes	II
Potassium iodide	Thyroid radioiodine protection	Yes	Yes	No	III
Pralidoxime chloride	Organophosphorus insecticide poisoning	Yes	Yes	NC	II
Pyridoxine hydrochloride	Isoniazid, hydrazine and derivatives	Yes	Yes	Yes	III
Prussian blue	Thallium/radiocesium	NC	NC	NC	II
Sodium bicarbonate[d]	Sodium channel blocking drugs, urine or serum alkalization	Yes	Yes	Yes	II

Cyanide antidote kit: conventional kit composed of amyl nitrite, sodium nitrite, and sodium thiosulfate. Class of evidence: class I, good-quality randomized and blinded clinical trials and good-quality systematic reviews of good-quality randomized trials; class II, prospective, nonrandomized, or nonblinded clinical trials, cohort or well-designed case-control studies, good-quality observational or volunteer studies; class III, retrospective case series, case studies, relevant expert opinions, or animal studies.

Abbreviations: DTPA, diethylene triamine pentaacetic acid; EDTA, ethylene diamine tetra-acetic acid; IV, intravenous; NA, not applicable because panel did not recommend stocking; NC, panel could not reach consensus.

[a] In most hospitals, immediate availability means that the antidote should be stocked in the ED.

[b] Class of evidence was defined as the highest level of evidence observed.

[c] Preferred agent.

[d] Indication listed in package label does not include its antidotal use.

From Dart RC, Borron SW, Caravati EM, et al. Expert consensus guidelines for stocking of antidotes in hospitals that provide emergency care. Ann Emerg Med 2009;54:386–94.e1. Table 2; with permission.

CHECKLIST 9: AMOUNT OF ANTIDOTE TYPICALLY NEEDED TO TREAT 1 PATIENT WEIGHING 100 KG

Pharmaceutical shortages have become more common since this list was published in 2009. Ready access to alternative and/or backup supplies should be considered in stocking.

Antidote	Stocking Recommendation		Notes and Considerations for HVA
	8 h[a]	24 h[a]	
Acetylcysteine	28 g	56 g	Note: this recommendation applies to stocking of either oral or intravenous products
			Note: administer intravenously for hepatic failure
Antivenin (Crotalidae) polyvalent	30 Vials	30 Vials	Note: product has been discontinued by manufacturer; some supplies remain
			HVA: geographic/endemic areas, history/experience with exotic bites, consider casualties with simultaneous bites (checklist 10)
Crotalidae Polyvalent Immune Fab, ovine	12 Vial	18 Vial	Note: less common acute and delayed antivenom reactions, faster mixing, use in equine serum hypersensitivity
			HVA: geographic/endemic areas, history/experience with exotic bites, consider casualties with simultaneous bites (see checklist 10)
Antivenin (L mactans)	1 Vial	1 Vial	HVA: geographic/endemic areas (see checklist 10)
Antivenin (M fulvius)	5 Vials	10 Vials	Note: product has been discontinued by manufacturer; some supplies remaining. Antivenoms from Mexico or Costa Rica are likely effective. Contact regional poison center to locate antivenom sources. HVA: Geographic/endemic areas (see checklist 10)
Atropine sulfate	45 mg	165 mg	—
Botulism antitoxin, equine (A, B)[b]	NA	NA	Note: contact your state health department to assist with procurement from the CDC
Botulism Immune globulin (BabyBIG)	NA	NA	Information from the Infant Botulism Treatment and Prevention Program, telephone: 510-231-7600, http://www.infantbotulism.org/physician/obtain.php
Calcium chloride	10 g	10 g	Note: do not administer SQ. Should be administered by central venous IV route, if possible
Calcium gluconate	30 g	30 g	Note: may be given by IV, SQ routes. Both calcium gluconate and calcium chloride should be available

(continued on next page)

(continued)

Antidote	Stocking Recommendation		Notes and Considerations for HVA
	8 h[a]	24 h[a]	
Calcium disodium EDTA	0.75 g	2.25 g	—
Calcium DTPA	1 g	1 g	HVA: receiving hospital for research laboratory (see checklist 10)
Cyanide antidote kit	1 Kit	1 Kit	HVA: industry, history, local conditions. Community planning, facility service area (see checklist 10) Note: nitrites cause methemoglobinemia and can impair oxygen delivery, should not be used in patients with smoke inhalation with carbon monoxide poisoning; sodium thiosulfate may be used but evidence is limited, and may cause hypotension
Hydroxocobalamin hydrochloride	10 g	10 g	Note: can be used safely in patients with smoke inhalation. Red color of drug causes laboratory test interference, red discoloration of skin and urine HVA: industry, history, local conditions. community planning, facility service area (see checklist 10)
Deferoxamine mesylate	12 g	36 g	—
Digoxin Immune Fab	15 Vials	15 Vials	—
Dimercaprol	500 mg	1.5 g	—
Ethanol	180 g	360 g	Note: ethanol is an effective antidote. It is only available as 95% concentration and required compounding at use. Loading dose, maintenance infusion, and frequent dose adjustments required. Medication errors are common
Fomepizole	1.5 g	4.5 g	Note: fomepizole preferred for simplicity of use, lack of need for compounding in pharmacy, reduction in medication errors, potential for avoiding hemodialysis in selected patients, and anticipated safety in children

	6 mg	12 mg	
Flumazenil			Note: primary use is for iatrogenic oversedation. Risks may outweigh benefits in patients with mixed/unknown overdose, chronic benzodiazepine use, seizure disorders, head injury
Glucagon hydrochloride	90 mg	250 mg	—
Methylene blue	400 mg	600 mg	—
Naloxone hydrochloride	20 mg	40 mg	—
Octreotide acetate	75 μg	225 μg	—
Physostigmine salicylate	4 mg	4 mg	—
Potassium iodide	130 mg	130 mg	—
Pralidoxime chloride	7 g	18 g	—
Pyridoxine hydrochloride	8 g	24 g	HVA: industry, history, endemic conditions, community planning facility service area (see checklist 10)
Prussian blue	NA	NA	—
Sodium bicarbonate	63 g	84 g	—

Cyanide antidote kit: conventional kit composed of amyl nitrite, sodium nitrite, and sodium thiosulfate. These minimum stocking recommendations are made to apply to all hospitals; any facilities with an HVA indicating greater or lesser need should stock appropriately.

Abbreviations: PO, by mouth; SQ, subcutaneous.

[a] Facilities should plan for a minimum of 8 hours unless they have mechanisms for more rapid resupply or transfer already in place. Facilities should plan for 24 hours if they will maintain patients for longer periods or will provide definitive care. Caution: 24-hour amount may not be sufficient for the entire treatment course.

[b] Botulinum antitoxin, equine (A,B) has been replaced by CDC with USA Heptavalent Botulinum Antitoxin (HBAT; for types A,B,C,D,F,G), an F(ab)'2 product.

From Dart RC, Borron SW, Caravati EM, et al. Expert consensus guidelines for stocking of antidotes in hospitals that provide emergency care. Ann Emerg Med 2009;54:386–94.e1. Table 3; with permission.

CHECKLIST 10: HAZARD VULNERABILITY ASSESSMENT FOR EMERGENCY ANTIDOTES

Factor	Principle	Example
Pharmaceutical products used as therapeutic agents	Agents that are widely available should generally have the antidote stocked because important geographic differences are not anticipated	Acetaminophen Anticholinergic agents Benzodiazepines Dapsone Digoxin Iron Isoniazid Lidocaine Opioid analgesics Sulfonylurea hypoglycemic agents
Characteristics of hospital catchment area	Industries, practices, activities, and indigenous fauna indicate potential need for antidote	Industries generating or using cyanide, heavy metals, hydrogen fluoride, organophosphorus chemicals, radionuclides, thallium Chemical transportation routes Indigenous fauna and flora (snakes, spiders, plants) Agricultural practices (organophosphate insecticides, cyanide baits, mining)
Referral patterns	Many hospitals accept referrals from remote areas, which should be included in risk assessment	Transfers to urban hospital from agricultural areas Referral from mining region
History or experience of use	Some modes of suicide or abuse become locally prevalent without a specific industry being present	Popularity of cyanide or other specific agents as a suicide agent Amateur snake keepers in area Residential or commercial fires (eg, older buildings, lack of fire alarms)
Anticipated volume of use	Depending on characteristics of area, more than 1 patient of a poisoning may be anticipated	Multiple-casualty incidents (eg, smoke inhalation involving treatment with cyanide antidotes) Indigenous crotaline snakebite in areas with frequent occurrences, such as the southeastern or southwestern United States
Anticipated time to restocking or resupply of antidote	Time to restocking varies greatly among hospitals	Hospitals that stabilize and refer patients to other institutions should stock for the anticipated period Hospitals that provide tertiary or definitive treatment should stock for anticipated duration of illness or until restocking from another hospital or distributor can occur Time to restocking varies by antidote. Some may have prolonged periods before restocking can occur

From Dart RC, Borron SW, Caravati EM, et al. Expert consensus guidelines for stocking of antidotes in hospitals that provide emergency care. Ann Emerg Med 2009;54:386–94.e1. Table 4; with permission.

CHECKLIST 11: IDENTIFICATION OF A POTENTIAL FOOD, WATER, OR MEDICATION CONTAMINATION EVENT

Adapted from article 9, "Intentional and Unintentional Food, Drug, and Water Contamination," with thanks to Drs Charles McKay and Elizabeth J. Scharman. Selected Web resources are provided without implied endorsement.

- Obtain a history of onset of symptoms and any association with new medication refills or purchases, or eating/drinking
- Identify any concerns regarding food, water, or medication appearance or taste
- Query as to others who shared these items and their condition
- Identify any prominent organ effects or laboratory findings of concern
- If possible, obtain sample of potentially contaminated material
- If assessment raises concern regarding contamination, contact the regional poison control center (PCC) at 1-800-222-1222 and report concerns
- If a toxidrome with a specific antidote is being considered, the PCC can assist in identifying and/or locating these medical countermeasures. The PCC can also identify additional resources, such as medical toxicologists, if the hospital does not have a medical toxicologist on staff
- If other reports from regional caregivers, or consistent with notices on American Association of Poison Control Centers (AAPCC) listserv, Epi-X (http://www.cdc.gov/epix/), or other reporting sources, the PCC directors may draft a press release for dissemination to hospitals in conjunction with state department of public health notification to assist in defining clinical picture, possible diagnostic studies, and treatment
- Additional public health, laboratory, and investigative resources can be brought in as appropriate:
  - National Association of County and City Health Officials Directory of Local Health Departments: http://www.naccho.org/about/lhd/
  - CDC Directory of State and Territorial Health Departments: http://www.cdc.gov/mmwr/international/relres.html

CHECKLIST 12: PREPAREDNESS FOR RADIOLOGICAL/NUCLEAR EMERGENCIES

Adapted from article 10, "Emergency Department Management of Patients Internally Contaminated with Radioactive Material," with thanks to Drs Ziad Kazzi, Jennifer Buzzell, Luiz Bertelli, and Doran Christenson. The opinions expressed herein are those of the authors and are not necessarily those of the USG or its agencies. Neither the USG nor its agencies, nor any of their employees, makes any warranty, expressed or implied, or assumes any legal liability or responsibility for the accuracy, completeness, or usefulness of the information contained herein or represents that its use would not infringe on privately owned rights. Selected Web and/or telephonic resources are provided without implied endorsement.

- Perform a radiation HVA (local and regional radiological hazards).
- Prepare and exercise plan to receive patients of a radiological/nuclear emergency.
- Predesignate shelter-in-place areas that can be used in an emergency to protect staff and patients from hazardous radioactive plume.
- Predesignate a radiation emergency area to receive contaminated patients.
- Maintain availability of appropriate PPE (level C and D).
- Train staff on radiological decontamination.

- Maintain a list of available and calibrated radiation detectors. Regularly train staff on their proper use. Maintain several personal dosimeters and the corresponding dosimetry program that is to be used in an emergency.
- Prepare for managing waste contaminated with radioactive material.
- Maintain roster of hospital radiation experts (radiation safety officer, nuclear medicine technologist, radiation oncologist, radiology technicians, radiologist, clinical toxicologist, hematology-oncology specialist).
- Maintain roster of state resources (state radiation control officer, regional poison center, public health agency).
- Maintain roster of federal resources (the Radiation Emergency Assistance Center/Training Site: http://orise.orau.gov/reacts/default.aspx and the CDC: http://emergency.cdc.gov/radiation/professionals.asp) and include mechanism to request specific radiation medical countermeasures from the Strategic National Stockpile through the state health official.
- Train medical staff on the diagnosis and management of radiation exposure, internal contamination and the acute radiation syndrome. Identify the regional Radiation Injury Treatment Network Centers for possible assistance (http://www.ritn.net/).
- Prepare to provide mental health support to survivors and staff after a radiological/nuclear incident.
- Prepare initial messages that can be used in a radiological/nuclear incident.

CHECKLIST 13: RESOURCES FOR RADIOLOGICAL/NUCLEAR EMERGENCIES AND PLANNING

Adapted from article 5, "Resources for toxicologic information and assistance," with thanks to Drs Mark A. Kirk and Carol J. Iddins. Selected Web resources are provided without implied endorsement. The opinions expressed herein are those of the authors and are not necessarily those of the USG or its agencies. Neither the USG nor its agencies, nor any of their employees, makes any warranty, expressed or implied, or assumes any legal liability or responsibility for the accuracy, completeness, or usefulness of the information contained herein or represents that its use would not infringe on privately owned rights. Selected Web and/or telephonic resources are provided without implied endorsement.

Radiological/Nuclear Emergency Speed Dial: 24/7 On-call Resources

- Radiation Emergency Assistance Center/Training Site (REAC/TS): 865-576-1005 ask for REAC/TS
- Regional Poison Center: 1-800-222-1222
- Armed Forces Radiobiology Research Institute (AFRRI) Emergency Operations Center (for military and civilian command and control centers): 301-295-0530
- CDC Emergency Operations Center: 770-488-7100
- State Radiological Health: _____. For a map with directory for your state go to: http://www.crcpd.org/Map/default.aspx.

Organization	Radiological/Nuclear Assets (Alphabetical) Contact Information	Best Use
Advanced HAZMAT Life Support for Radiological Incidents and Terrorism	http://www.ahls.org/ahls/ecs/courses/description.html?ctid=225	Education
American Red Cross	http://www.redcross.org/find-help	Response
AFRRI Medical Radiobiology Advisory Team	http://www.usuhs.edu/afrri/outreach/emergency_response.html	Response
Medical Effects of Ionizing Radiation	http://www.usuhs.edu/afrri/outreach/meir/meir.htm	Education
Biodosimetry Assessment Tool/First-responder Radiological Assessment Tool	http://www.usuhs.edu/afrri/outreach/biodostools.htm http://www.usuhs.edu/afrri/register/index.html	Dose calculators
Conference of Radiation Control Program Directors	http://www.crcpd.org/Map/default.aspx	Response
Medical Reserve Corps	https://www.medicalreservecorps.gov/HomePage	Response
National Alliance for Radiation Readiness	http://www.radiationready.org/	Information
National Disaster Life Support Foundation	http://register.ndlsf.org/	Training
National Disaster Medical System:	http://ndms.fhpr.osd.mil/	Response
Disaster Medical Assistance Teams, Disaster Mortuary Response Teams or National Veterinary Response Teams		
National Guard Weapons of Mass Destruction Civil Support Teams	http://www.army.mil/aps/08/information_papers/transform/ARNG_Civil_Support_Teams.html	Response
Oak Ridge Institute for Science and Education Radiation Emergency Assistance Center/Training Site (REAC/TS)	http://orise.orau.gov/files/reacts/medical-aspects-of-radiation-incidents.pdf http://orise.orau.gov/files/reacts/triage.pdf http://orise.orau.gov/reacts/capabilities/continuing-medical-education/	Triage Education
Radiation Emergency Medical Management:	www.remm.nlm.gov	Response Information
RADAR dose calculator	http://www.doseinfo-radar.com/RADARHome.html	Dose calculator
RadPro	http://www.radprocalculator.com/	Dose calculator
Radiation Injury Treatment Network	http://www.ritn.net/	Response Education

(continued on next page)

(continued)

Radiological/Nuclear Assets (Alphabetical)

Organization	Contact Information	Best Use
State of California	http://www.emsa.ca.gov/disaster_medical_services_division_hospital_incident_command_system_resources	ICS
US Department of Agriculture	http://www.usda.gov/wps/portal/usda/usdahome?contentidonly=true&contentid=Emergency_Preparedness_and_Response.html	Response
US Department of Energy/National Nuclear Security Administration	http://nnsa.energy.gov/	Response
HHS Assistant Secretary for Preparedness and Response	http://www.phe.gov/Preparedness/planning/hpp/Documents/hpp-healthcare-coalitions.pdf	Response
HHS	http://emergency.cdc.gov/radiation/?s_cid=cdc_homepage_topmenu_004,	Response Education
US Department of Homeland Security Federal Emergency Management Agency Center for Domestic Preparedness	http://www.fema.gov/ http://training.fema.gov/IS/crslist.aspx https://cdp.dhs.gov/	Response ICS Education
EPA	http://www.epa.gov/radiation/docs/er/planning-guidance-for-response-to-nuclear-detonation-2-edition-final.pdf	Response Triage
US Food and Drug Administration	http://www.fda.gov/Radiation-EmittingProducts/default.htm http://www.fda.gov/Drugs/EmergencyPreparedness/default.htm	Response
US Nuclear Regulatory Commission	http://www.nrc.gov/	Response
US Public Health Service Rapid Deployment Force	http://ccrf.hhs.gov/ccrf/FactSheets/RDF_Fact_Sheet_FINAL.pdf	Response

Abbreviation: ICS, incident command system; RADAR, RAdiation Dose Assessment Resource.

Index

Note: Page numbers of article titles are in **boldface** type.

Emerg Med Clin N Am 33 (2015) 233–239
http://dx.doi.org/10.1016/S0733-8627(14)00113-8
0733-8627/15/$ – see front matter © 2015 Elsevier Inc. All rights reserved.

emed.theclinics.com

Moving?

Make sure your subscription moves with you!

To notify us of your new address, find your **Clinics Account Number** (located on your mailing label above your name), and contact customer service at:

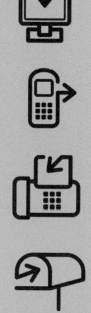

Email: journalscustomerservice-usa@elsevier.com

800-654-2452 (subscribers in the U.S. & Canada)
314-447-8871 (subscribers outside of the U.S. & Canada)

Fax number: 314-447-8029

Elsevier Health Sciences Division
Subscription Customer Service
3251 Riverport Lane
Maryland Heights, MO 63043

*To ensure uninterrupted delivery of your subscription, please notify us at least 4 weeks in advance of move.

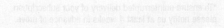